COGNITIVE THERAPY TECHNIQUES

Cognitive Therapy Techniques

A PRACTITIONER'S GUIDE

Robert L. Leahy

THE GUILFORD PRESS
New York   London

Published by The Guilford Press
A Division of Guilford Publications, Inc.
72 Spring Street, New York, NY 10012
www.guilford.com

Printed in the United States of America

This book is printed on acid-free paper.

Last digit is print number: 9 8 7 6 5 4 3 2 1

Library of Congress Cataloging-in-Publication Data

Leahy, Robert L.
    Cognitive therapy techniques : a practitioner's guide / Robert L. Leahy.
        p. cm.
    Includes bibliographical references and index.
    ISBN 1-57230-905-9 (paper)
    1. Cognitive therapy.   I. Title.
RC489.C63L382 2003
616.89′ 142—dc21

                                                    2003006945

For David Burns

About the Author

Robert L. Leahy, PhD, is President of the International Association for Cognitive Psychotherapy, Founder and Director of the American Institute for Cognitive Therapy in New York City (*www. CognitiveTherapyNYC.com*), Clinical Associate Professor of Psychology in Psychiatry at Cornell University Medical School, and former Editor of the *Journal of Cognitive Psychotherapy*. Dr. Leahy's recent books include *Cognitive Therapy: Basic Principles and Applications, Practicing Cognitive Therapy, Treatment Plans and Interventions for Depression and Anxiety Disorders* (with Stephen J. Holland), *Overcoming Resistance in Cognitive Therapy, Bipolar Disorder: A Cognitive Therapy Approach* (with Cory F. Newman, Aaron T. Beck, Noreen A. Reilly-Harrington, and Laslo Gyulai), *Clinical Applications of Cognitive Psychotherapy* (edited with E. Thomas Dowd), *Psychology and the Economic Mind*, and the forthcoming *Roadblocks in Cognitive-Behavioral Therapy: Transforming Challenges into Opportunities for Change* and *Psychological Treatment of Bipolar Disorder* (edited with Sheri L. Johnson).

Acknowledgments

I would like to thank Seymour Weingarten, Editor in Chief of The Guilford Press, for being a supportive publisher. My experience with Guilford has been uniformly positive. My editor at Guilford, Jim Nageotte, helped me organize the presentation of the concepts in this book. I look forward to further collaborations with Jim, Seymour, and Guilford.

The idea of this book grew over discussions at an excellent restaurant in Soho in New York City—over a Vietnamese meal at "Can." An advantage of being a New York author is the treat of an occasional free meal accompanied by excellent discussion. We were discussing the project *Treatment Plans and Interventions for Depression and Anxiety Disorders*, which I coauthored with Stephen J. Holland. Seymour and his staff thought there might be a need for a separate book on techniques, especially given that I had listed almost 100 techniques with examples in *Treatment Plans*. The present book is a result of that discussion.

I would like to thank my colleagues at the American Institute for Cognitive Therapy in New York City—especially my long-time colleague Laura Oliff. At weekly case conferences over the last 10 years, I have discussed almost everything that I later published. Professionals interested in advanced training in cognitive therapy can contact us through our website at *www.CognitiveTherapyNYC.com*. My editorial and research assistants—Randye Semple and David Fazzari (both from Columbia University)—were immensely helpful in putting together the completed manuscript.

Perhaps the most influential person in the development of my thinking about techniques is my earlier mentor and now good friend David Burns. Many of the readers of this book will recognize David's enormously important contribution to the development of, and training in, many of the techniques in this book. Having David as a supervisor was one of the single most important experiences in my professional life.

I also had a the good fortune to receive training from Aaron "Tim" Beck at the Center for Cognitive Therapy at the University of Pennsylvania. Tim served as a wise role model for the practice of digging deeper to understand the underlying logic of patients' beliefs. My work today is still influenced by this inquisitive, theory-building style of thinking. The entire field of cognitive therapy began with Tim's early work in the 1960s. Even today he continues to make contributions to our understanding of schizophrenia, personality disorders, and depression.

Preface

Do you find yourself using the same cognitive techniques with most—if not all—of your patients? Do you feel stuck using the same tried and true bag of "tricks" with few alternatives? I think these are feelings all of us have had. Many of us get stuck in familiar patterns, using clinical tactics that have worked most of the time or some of the time. In so doing, we overlook the range of approaches that can give us great flexibility and make a world of difference for our patients.

I have asked many cognitive therapists, "What techniques do you generally use?" The same few techniques come up over and over: identify the thought, look at the costs and benefits of the thought, examine the evidence. These are valid techniques, and I am not suggesting you discard them. But if you have a narrow repertoire of interventions to draw on, therapy can get a bit stuck, and even remain superficial. What could be worse, your own enthusiasm for the process could be undermined by the routine you establish.

I wrote this book both for new clinicians who do not want to be limited to a simple list of a few techniques and for experienced clinicians who can derive from it ideas of how to expand cognitive therapy by employing techniques that will appear new to them.

An exciting reality about cognitive therapy is that there are new techniques, new strategies and new conceptualizations being developed all of the time. As work in this field has grown, researchers and clinicians have refined and tested dozens of therapeutic interventions that can be applied to work with our clients. I have organized this book around certain categories of interventions or techniques, beginning with many of the traditional techniques for identifying and evaluating thoughts and assumptions. I have drawn on the recent work on cognitive models of worry and rumination, as well as some techniques from a schema-focused model, to examine how novel cognitive therapy techniques can help with a range of client problems.

Given the philosophical bent of much of cognitive therapy, it should come as no surprise that I devote a separate chapter to identifying and modifying logical errors and faulty information processing, as well as putting things into a historical and philosophical perspective. I believe emotional processing is as key to psychopathology as "cognitive distortions." With that in mind, I have written the chapter on emotional and experiential techniques with the intention of broadening the "feeling" component and the ecological validity of cognitive therapy. The chapter on examining and challenging cognitive distortions will serve as a useful tool for therapists looking for a quick guide. If the patient is "fortune telling," what are the techniques you can use?

Finally, I have provided two chapters with in-session dialogues to give the reader a sense of what the techniques I describe actually sound like in action. I have chosen need for approval and self-criticism as the target problems, since these common issues underlie depression and much of anxiety.

The first eight chapters share a common organizing framework—identifying and defining the technique, providing examples of questions to pose, illustrating the application of the technique through a clinical dialogue, assigning homework to the patient, possible problems that can arise and how to address them, cross-reference to other techniques, and self-help forms for patients

Finally, a brief caveat. I do not believe in "technique therapy." I view each technique as the beginning of an investigation into the patient's thinking and feeling. Each technique allows us to collect new data, create and expand our conceptualization, and broaden and deepen our relationship with the patient. Techniques can be used to open a window, to look more closely, and to see things in a different way. Cognitive therapy is not reducible to techniques: rather, techniques allow us to *begin* cognitive therapy. With this new range of techniques you should be able to work collaboratively with your patients at different "entry points" to test and modify thoughts and assumptions and to provide them with more effective self-help skills. When your patient tries a technique that does not quite work at the time, it will be reassuring if he or she can utilize another 10 techniques.

Contents

List of Forms

Introduction

The cognitive therapy model is based on the view that stressful states such as depression, anxiety, and anger are often maintained or exacerbated by exaggerated or biased ways of thinking. The therapist's role is to help the patient recognize his or her idiosyncratic style of thinking and modify it through the application of evidence and logic. Thus cognitive therapy follows from a long and esteemed line of reason-based models, such as the Socratic logic-based dialogues and Aristotle's method of collecting and categorizing information about the real world. The cognitive model—which stresses the central role of (1) cognition in emotion and (2) schematic processing as a determining factor in information processing—reflects the cognitive revolution that occurred in the field of psychology in the 1970s (Leahy, 1996).

Cognitive therapists engage patients in scientific and rational thinking by asking them to examine the presuppositions that lead to depressive or anxious states. In addition, these therapists assist patients in examining the validity of statements by collecting evidence that contradicts the statements. Moreover, cognitive therapists examine the meaning, or the lack of meaning, in the salient concepts with which depressed or anxious individuals berate themselves. These might include concepts that have no empirical referent, such as "worthless person" or "loser."

Cognitive therapy owes a conceptual debt to earlier philosophical work on phenomenology by Husserl (1960); indeed, cognitive therapy *is* phenomenology in that it describes and analyzes the categories of experience. The difference between cognitive therapy pioneer Beck and philosopher Husserl is that Beck provides a method for testing out the phenomenological experience by testing one's thoughts against reality.

This "reality" is an *open system*. Thus the cognitive model is constructivist to the extent that the "knower"—here, the therapist and the patient—will never have all of the facts. There is no exhaustive test of information. *Knowing* in the empirical world is a statement more of probabilities than of certainties. Predictions are based on incomplete information—always. This recognition that inferential thinking is always incomplete, indeterminative, and probabilistic is an essential component of the cognitive therapist's perspective. Thus, when the patient demands certainty—"Yes, but I could be the one whose plane crashes!"—the cognitive therapist should recognize that existential probabilities do exist and cannot be eliminated. The real question, for the patient demanding certainty, is why is it difficult to accept uncertainty? This leads to a new approach to the patient's "knowledge needs"—the need to predict with certainty. Often examining this need reveals that the patient views "certainty" as part of a desire for absolute control—without which disasters will occur.

The therapist asks the patient to look at the preponderance of the evidence to reach tentative conclusions and to remain skeptical about all ways of knowing. I emphasize this attitude to underscore my view that the cognitive therapist should not become a "cheer-leader" for positive thinking. We should avoid the impression caricatured by Stuart Smalley of NBC's *Saturday Night Live*, who wants his guests to think, "You are good enough, smart enough, and people like you!" Cognitive therapy is not a process of bolstering defenses or proselytizing about "the power of positive thinking." Rather, it demonstrates the power of realistic thinking—that is, to the extent that we can know reality.

The system of knowledge upon which cognitive therapy is based is an open one. New facts, new experiences, even new needs and preferences may arise at any point. Thus, the cognitive therapist introduces the patient to a *pragmatic* view of knowing—in essence, presenting the central question "How will this thought affect you?" For example, the cognitive therapist may ask: "What consequences (i.e., the tradeoffs or costs and benefits) will you experience by believing that you should get everyone's approval?" Similarly, the therapist might invite the patient to test the belief that the consequences of not getting approval will be disastrous. This testing would involve behavioral experiments such as assertiveness exercises, through which the patient learns that experiencing disapproval (or giving disapproval) often results in no change in real life. Such experiments put the dread evoked by the belief to a pragmatic test.

A pragmatic test for the kind of repetitive intrusive thoughts that occur in obsessive–compulsive disorder includes thought flooding. That is, the fear of thoughts—or the thought–action fusion (Rachman, 1993)—can be tested by having the patient repeat those feared thoughts. Thus the obsession (e.g., "If I tell the Devil to go to Hell, I will be struck down") can be reversed by abandoning suppression of the thought and doing the opposite: inviting the thought into full awareness and repeating it 500 times. Similarly, just as intrusive thoughts can be "tested" by exposure, so also can feared sensations, such as those that induce panic (Wells, 1997a).

The cognitive therapist recognizes that rational analysis and descriptions of thought processes may not be sufficient to medicate change. Evocation of emotion, development of motivation, and experiential techniques that activate new phenomenological experiences and feelings also may be essential. The patient may need to confront reality with new thoughts and behaviors in order to experience, on an emotional level, the existential importance of a "rational" response or simply a new way of thinking. Cognitive therapists help clients put thoughts into action by engaging in behavioral experiments that translate insight into practice.

Some critics of cognitive therapy argue that it is too rational and too simplistic, more an exercise of words than an exercise of emotion. I have included a chapter on the experiential techniques of emotion-focused therapy as well as some of my work on emotional processing. It is essential to balance the techniques of cognitive therapy with empathy, validation, and motivational interviewing—styles of conducting therapy that will assist the patient in viewing cognitive interventions as emotionally relevant. I often wonder, though, how such critics can account for the dramatic changes in emotion which cognitive therapy facilitates in individuals who are depressed and anxious. After all, if cognitive therapy helps people become less depressed and anxious, it *is* addressing emotion in the most important way—by changing negative feelings.

Therapists who practice cognitive therapy often seem to have their "favorite techniques." Some rely heavily on activity scheduling, examining the evidence and daily records of dysfunctional thoughts, whereas others may rely more on the techniques of rational role play, double standard, and testing predictions. The problem with this circumscribed repertoire is that different techniques work for different clients and problems. When I become obsessive and ruminative (my favorite hobbies), I create a dysfunctional thought record and set up problem-solving strategies. It works for me, but it might not work for others with the same pattern. The current book is an attempt to provide the clinician with a range of cognitive therapy techniques that might be useful for various problems that are confronted in therapy.

A number of years ago I recall a trainee commenting, "But how do you know which question to ask?" I assumed that he was referring to "which technique" to use. Initially I thought it was not a very good question—probably because I did not have a ready answer—but I realized it was an excellent question (and I regretted not asking it myself). Years later, I still do not have the answer, but I do have a lot of techniques. Interested readers may find numerous techniques they have never used (or even heard of). But most likely, readers will find this compendium of techniques a valuable "refresher"— that is, something that will jog their memory and help them recognize that the, say, five techniques they are using on their current patient can be augmented by 50 other techniques that they have not used in recent months (or years).

The first three chapters—"Eliciting Thoughts and Assumptions," "Evaluating and Challenging Thoughts," and "Evaluating Assumptions and Rules"—provide an overview of the basic techniques used in cognitive therapy. These chapters should be read in sequence. The next chapter, "Evaluating Worries," may seem focused on the problems associated with anxiety disorders—especially generalized anxiety disorders—but the techniques covered therein are applicable to any problems in which negative predictions are activated. The fifth and sixth chapters, "Information Processing and Logical Errors" and "Putting Things in Perspective," will help clinicians assist those patients who jump to conclusions that are not justified by facts, logic, or context. The seventh chapter, "Schema-Focused Therapy," reviews some of the techniques that are helpful in evaluating personal schemas. Chapter 8, "Emotional Processing Techniques" reviews the different emotional or experiential techniques that can be used to activate and modify emotionally salient material. Chapters 9 through 11 review specific applications to specific problem areas. In Chapter 9, "Examining and Challenging Cognitive Distortions," I present various questions and interventions to challenge the different cognitive distortions. Chapter 10, "Modifying Need for Approval," and Chapter 11, "Challenging Self-Criticism," provide case examples of how to modify these negative patterns. Many of the techniques mentioned in the earlier chapters are utilized here. Specific intervention strategies for Axis I disorders—such as panic, social phobia, and obsessive–compulsive disorder—are not covered here but may be referenced in Leahy and Holland (2000), *Treatment Plans and Interventions for Depression and Anxiety Disorders.* Detailed description of a specific case, utilizing many cognitive therapy techniques, is available in Judith Beck's (1995) excellent *Cognitive Therapy: Basics and Beyond.* A general introduction to cognitive therapy can be found in Leahy's (1996), *Cognitive Therapy: Basic Principles and Applications.*

Critics may be eager to point out that cognitive therapy is already too technique-oriented and too formulaic. I agree that cognitive therapy can become mechanical, invalidating, nonconceptual, shallow, and just plain boring. That is why I wrote a book on resistance in cognitive therapy, emphasizing validation concerns, risk aversion, victim roles, schematic processing, self-limitation, and self-consistency (Leahy, 2001b). Countertransference issues can be conceptualized and addressed within a cognitive therapy framework and may assist the therapist in utilizing his or her countertransference response to understand the patient's interpersonal world and interpersonal strategies. But we should keep in mind that there is something essential in the utilization of techniques that elicit, examine, test, challenge, and modify thoughts and behaviors. Cognitive therapy is based on these established—and proven—approaches.

I say this to remind readers—and myself, as I often get led astray by my own imagination—that deep philosophical discussions with patients about the origins of problems and the bold insights for which so many of us strive can be pursued by abandoning the active, Socratic style of cognitive therapy. The first judgment call I ponder, when I reach a therapeutic impasse, is whether I need to go back to basics: activity scheduling, pleasure predicting, categorizing automatic thoughts, examining the costs and benefits, looking at the evidence, and so many other basic techniques (Beck, 1976; Beck, Rush, Shaw, & Emery, 1979; Beck, 1995; Burns, 1989; Leahy, 1997). After I have tried the basics, I can shift to other techniques and interventions—such as case conceptualization, schema-focused therapy, and emotion-focused techniques—which may provide a richness and depth.

Many therapists prefer to practice their own style of therapy and their own integration of models. Independence and innovation are laudable, but they should take second place to starting the patient with empirically supported treatments. For example, it might make sense to postpone the schema work until the treatment modules for depression and anxiety disorders—interventions that have proven effective—have been given a vigorous trial. Don't we owe it to our patients to employ, as our first line of treatment, those techniques we know actually work (based on outcome literature)? I recall how one of our trainees, who was quite intelligent but thought she could do cognitive therapy "her way," had a significantly high premature termination rate with her patients. To her credit, she modified her eclectic style (which did not include homework assignments) to utilize a more basic cognitive therapy model, focused on techniques, structure, and homework assignments. Her effectiveness and premature termination rate improved dramatically.

Essentially, I recommend that therapists first master the techniques and treatment approaches that have been shown to be effective. Before developing a grand theoretical scheme about how cognitive therapy needs to be modified for a particular patient, it would be valuable to utilize the interventions that have already been shown to be empirically valid.

In conducting cognitive therapy, I often utilize several techniques with a patient—even after the patient has seemed to change a negative thought. I believe in *overpractice* or *overlearning*—especially when it comes to modifying habits of thinking that have persisted for years. An advantage of utilizing a variety of techniques to test or challenge a single negative thought is that the patient has alternative techniques for future use, should his or her initial challenge not work. This approach was impressed on me years ago when I was learning cognitive therapy in individual supervision with the master of technique, David Burns. I would present a problem with a patient, let's say, a hard-wired negative thought, and David would say, "Tell me 10 techniques that you could use." In actual practice, I found this reliance on a multiplicity of techniques to serve as a very powerful way of structuring sessions that had an enormous impact on patients. They were getting a lot of ideas about how to cope with their negative thoughts!

I have found that it is essential to elicit ongoing feedback from patients. In addition, it is useful for the patient and therapist to intermittently summarize the techniques they have used, write them down, and examine which were useful and which were not, and why. For example, it is always helpful to examine why weighing the evidence for an automatic thought does *not* work. Perhaps there is a more fundamental belief, conditional rule, or demand for absolute certainty that needs to be explored. When techniques fail, the failure allows us to discover something even more fundamental, such as schemas or absolute rules. In fact, the ambitious and curious clinician should look forward to the failure of techniques, because failure (and resistance) in therapy can be windows into more fundamental problems that provide excellent opportunities to develop case conceptualizations, and then bring to bear more techniques to examine patients' core beliefs.

I think behavioral techniques are essential, and I have included a list of these in Appendix A of *Treatment Plans and Interventions for Depression and Anxiety Disorders* (Leahy & Holland, 2000). Because my focus is primarily on the cognitive aspects of therapy, I suggest that readers interested in the behavioral components consult the excellent book on behavioral therapy edited by Hersen (2002) as well as Leahy and Holland (2000).

As a cognitive therapist (or cognitive-behavioral therapist), I view the behavioral techniques as serving the purpose of testing out negative thoughts. For example, activity scheduling, graded task assignments, and pleasure predicting are behavioral interventions that allow the patient to test out negative beliefs, such as "I don't enjoy anything" or "I am always depressed." Assertiveness training is used to test out the thoughts "No one likes me" and "I'm just shy." Attentional distraction is used to test out the idea that "I have no control over my thoughts" or "I just worry all the time." Exposure hierarchies can modify the belief that a specific stimulus is dangerous and cannot be tolerated. Imaginal exposure challenges the idea that even thinking about something is unbearable. Relaxation training can accomplish several goals: (1) it can test the thought that (for example) "I am always nervous"; (2) it can help the patient induce more calming thoughts or moods that can be used to challenge the negative thoughts; (3) it can reduce overall level of arousal, thereby reducing the likelihood of emotional priming for negative thoughts. Finally, self-reward and self-contingency management can be helpful in modifying negative beliefs about competence. In each case when using behavioral techniques, it is helpful to have the patient identify the automatic negative thoughts and to use behavioral tests as a challenge to these thoughts.

The text includes examples of therapist–patient dialogues for each technique. I always find it helpful to see how a therapist actually talks with a patient—for me, it provides a good role model of what to do. Although I hope this volume will prove to be helpful, it cannot substitute for direct training and supervision. I have been impressed that clinicians I have trained for postdoctoral fellowships at the American Institute for Cognitive Therapy in New York City have been wise enough to continue their individual supervision with more experienced clinicians. Getting a license to practice should never be considered the completion of one's training. I hope this volume will prove to be a useful reference tool, as well, allowing the reader to reexamine alternatives that may have been overlooked.

CHAPTER 1

—

Eliciting Thoughts and Assumptions

Beck's cognitive model of psychopathology stresses the central role of thinking in the elicitation and maintenance of depression, anxiety, and anger (Beck, 1970, 1976; Beck, Emery, & Greenberg, 1985; Beck et al., 1979). Cognitive biases impute vulnerability to negative life events, such that a loss or impediment will more likely be interpreted in an exaggerated, personalized, and negative fashion. Beck's cognitive model suggests that there are several levels of cognitive assessment. At the most immediate level are the automatic thoughts that come spontaneously, appear valid, and are associated with problematic behavior or disturbing emotions. These automatic thoughts can be classified according to their specific biases or distortions—for example, mind reading, personalizing, labeling, fortune telling, catastrophizing, or dichotomous (all-or-nothing) thinking (see Beck, 1976; Beck et al., 1985; Beck, 1995; Leahy & Holland, 2000). Automatic thoughts can be true or false—that is, the automatic thought "She doesn't like me" may be based on mind reading (i.e., I lack sufficient evidence to derive this belief), but nonetheless it may prove to be true.

The emotional vulnerability to this thought will result from the underlying assumptions or rules (e.g., "I must get the approval of everyone to be worthwhile") and the underlying personal schemas (e.g., "I am unlovable" or "I am worthless") held by the individual. Underlying maladaptive assumptions or rules are typically rigid, overinclusive, impossible to attain, and impute vulnerability to future depressive episodes or to anxiety states (see Ingram, Miranda, & Segal, 1997; Persons & Miranda, 1992). Thus individuals who believe that they must gain the approval of everyone are more vulnerable to depression and anxiety because they inevitably will fail to live up to these standards. Their mind reading and personalizing will make them more likely to perceive rejection when it is not there.

Incoming information is channeled through these automatic thoughts (e.g., "Did she reject me?") and then evaluated according to the underlying assumptions (e.g., "If I don't get approval, then I am worthless"). The underlying assumptions are linked to the personal schema (e.g., "I am unlovable"), further reinforcing the negative personal belief and adding confirmation to the distrust and fear of others. These negative personal schemas ("I am unlovable," "worthless," "defective") create selective attention and memory—that is, these individuals will be more likely to detect or interpret and recall information consistent with the schema thereby further strengthening the schema. Thus depressive and anxious styles of thinking are "theory-driven" and "research-based," in that they are continually looking for information to confirm the schema. This model is consistent with the considerable literature on the schematic processes underlying attention and memory (Hastie, 1980; Segal, Williams, & Teasdale, 2002). Like personal schemes, scientific theories are often guided by paradigms that direct the misinterpretation of information and that conserve themselves even in the face of contradictory data (Hanson, 1958; Kuhn, 1970). The cognitive model of therapy is based on George Kelly's (1955) model of "man (or woman) as scientist"—that is, that humans can identify their personal "constructs" or beliefs and test them. The current cognitive model, advanced by Beck and his colleagues, stresses the aspect of scientific thinking that seeks "disconfirmation" or "falsification" of a belief—that is, examining how a belief could be proven wrong or inadequate, rather than simply seeking out confirmatory evidence (see Popper, 1959). The depressed individual may focus selectively on information consistent with the negative state of feeling depressed, ignoring the relevance of disconfirming evidence. The cognitive model seeks to examine both kinds of evidence.

Although I emphasize the Beckian model of cognitive therapy in this book, I also recognize the substantial contribution made by Albert Ellis and his colleagues (see Dryden & DiGiuseppe, 1990; Ellis, 1994; Kassinove & Tafrate, 2002). Ellis's system, developed contemporaneously with Beck's model, provides a more general approach to psychopathology by emphasizing a set of common cognitive vulnerabilities. These include low frustration tolerance, "shoulds," and other demanding and irrational cognitive distortions. The current approach does not conflict with the rational–emotive behavioral model advocated by Ellis and may be usefully integrated with it.

Throughout this chapter (and the book) we examine how therapists can assist patients in identifying and evaluating thoughts of various kinds. (Appendix A contains cognitive therapy conceptualizations for the major depressive and anxiety disorders; also see Leahy & Holland, 2000.) The cognitive model of psychopathology recognizes commonalities in thinking distortions and biases across diagnostic categories (e.g., automatic thought distortions), but also recognizes that there are specific conceptualizations for each diagnostic grouping. The goal here is to help patients adapt a cognitive approach to their problem by stressing the importance of identifying patterns of thinking, rather than focusing on the expression of emotion. However, experienced cognitive therapists also recognize that emotions often contain valuable information—indeed, Leslie Greenberg and Jeremy Safran have indicated how emotional expression and the therapeutic alliance can help patients utilize their emotions as a source of information about unmet needs (Greenberg & Safran, 1987). These emotional schemas about unmet needs—often evoked by activating emotional intensity and helping patients to differentiate various emotions—can be a rich source of information about cognitions and an important part of modifying these thoughts and feelings. I describe these "experiential techniques" in a later chapter; here we focus on more traditional cognitive techniques.

TECHNIQUE: EXPLAINING HOW THOUGHTS CREATE FEELINGS

Description

The fundamental assumption guiding cognitive therapy is that the individual's interpretation of an event determines how he or she feels and behaves. Many people, in fact, are surprised to learn that their feelings are the result of how they think about an event and that by modifying their interpretation, they can have very different feelings. In this chapter, I review a variety of techniques that are useful in helping patients learn how to recognize the ways in which their thoughts and feelings interact. After all, people seek therapy not because they think they are irrational but because their feelings, behavior, and relationships are problematic. Two foundational points are worth considering:

1. *Thoughts* and *feelings* are distinct phenomena.
2. Thoughts create feelings (and behavior).

Thoughts are not the same thing as feelings. Feelings are internal experiences of emotions—for example, I may feel anxious, depressed, angry, afraid, hopeless, happy, exhilarated, indifferent, curious, helpless, regretful, or self-critical. To say I have a particular feeling or emotion is similar to saying, "This hot iron hurts" or "This scone tastes good to me." We do not challenge feelings—it would not make sense to say to a patient, "You're not really anxious." To do so would be equivalent to saying, in essence, that the hot iron did not really hurt the patient when he or she said, *Ouch.* "Ouch" is a report of a sensation—just as the words "I am happy" or "I am sad" are reports of feelings. We do not dispute feelings. We challenge and dispute the thoughts that give rise to those feelings.

Therapists can explain to patients how their thoughts may create their feelings or may increase or decrease a feeling. Consider, for example, the different feelings these two statements engender: "I think I'm unlovable and, therefore, I feel hopeless"; or "I think I'm better off without him and, therefore, I feel hopeful and relieved." Figure 1.1 provides additional explanatory examples.

Question to Pose/Intervention

Therapists can use the following wording as a model for explaining these ideas to patients in straightforward, jargon-free language: "Before you can challenge and change thoughts, you have to understand how thoughts affect your feelings. When you are feeling down or anxious, you may have certain thoughts. For example, imagine you are walking down the street in a strange part of town very late at night and you hear someone walking behind you. Glancing over your shoulder, you see that it's two very large men. Your thought might be, 'They're going to rob me.' How would you feel? Afraid? But

Thought: I think . . .	**Feeling:** Therefore, I feel . . .
I'll never be happy again.	Hopeless
Life is not worth living.	Suicidal
She left me because I was unattractive.	Hopeless
I'm going crazy.	Frightened, panicky
He's taking advantage of me.	Angry, vengeful, defensive
No one cares about me.	Lonely, rejected
I won't be able to take care of myself.	Anxious, helpless, dependent
I've solved problems before, I can solve them again.	Hopeful, energized
I don't need to be perfect.	Relieved, less pressured
I should give myself credit for trying.	Proud, happy

FIGURE 1.1. How Thoughts Create Feelings.

what if you thought, 'They're my friends from work'? How would you feel? Relieved? When you are feeling down or anxious in your day-to-day life, you have different thoughts. So, let me ask you, when you were sitting in your apartment thinking, and you noticed that you felt anxious, what were you thinking?"

Example

As indicated in Figure 1.1, thoughts can create both positive and negative feelings. Sometimes the patient may get so focused on what he or she is feeling that he or she does not recognize that it is a particular thought that creates the feeling. Consider the following dialogue:

THERAPIST: What seems to be bothering you?

PATIENT: I just feel sad.

THERAPIST: Can you tell me why you feel sad?

PATIENT: I just feel awful, like a sense of doom. I cry a lot.

THERAPIST: OK. Maybe you can help me understand what you are saying to yourself that's making you feel sad. Complete this sentence: "I feel say because I think . . . "

PATIENT: I'm unhappy.

THERAPIST: *Unhappy* is a feeling. But what are you saying to yourself that makes you feel sad? For example, are you saying anything about yourself as a person, about the future, or about this experience?

PATIENT: I guess I'm saying that I think that I'll never be happy.

In this example, the therapist was able to elicit the hopeless prediction, "I'll never be happy." This prediction can be evaluated by using the following techniques: cost–benefit analysis, examining the evidence for and against the validity of the prediction, examining logical errors (e.g., "I feel sad now, therefore, I'll always feel sad.") All of these techniques are discussed in the pages to follow.

Homework

Patients are asked to keep track of their feelings and how these feelings are related to their thoughts. The therapist can say: "I want you to keep a record of your negative feelings over the next week, using this form [Form 1.1 at the end of the chapter]. When you notice that you are having a feeling or an emotion, write down what that feeling is in the left-hand column. Examples of feelings are *sad, anxious, afraid, hopeless, angry,* and *confused.* Now, in the right-hand column, write down the thought that goes with that feeling. For example, the feeling might be 'anxious' and the thought might be 'I am afraid I'll do badly at work.' So the entire thought is, 'I feel anxious because I am afraid I'll do badly at work.' "

Possible Problems

Patients commonly confuse thoughts with feelings. It is useful to anticipate this problem by offering an example: "Sometimes people confuse a thought with a feeling. For example, someone might say, 'I feel anxious because I am nervous.' This is really a report of two feelings or emotions—that is, *anxious* and *nervous.* 'I feel anxious' is a feeling, and 'I am nervous' is another feeling. The thought might be 'I think I won't do well' or 'I think I'll always be anxious.' "

Another common problem initially is that patients are unable to identify the thoughts associated with their feelings. In these cases, the therapist might use some of the other techniques described in this chapter or in Chapter 8, which contains a section on imagery techniques.

Cross-Reference to Other Techniques

As indicated, we can utilize other techniques in this chapter—such as "guessing the thought"—or we can use the imagery induction techniques described in Chapter 8. Many patients receive assistance in identifying automatic thoughts from reading books on cognitive therapy, such as David Burns's *Feeling Good Handbook* (1989) or Dennis Greenberger and Christine Padesky's *Mind over Mood* (1995). In addition, providing patients with a list of common cognitive distortions (Figure 1.6) and a form for them to fill in (see below) is quite helpful.

Form

Form 1.1 (Self-Help Form: How Thoughts Create Feelings, p. 27).

TECHNIQUE: DISTINGUISHING THOUGHTS FROM FACTS

Description

Often, when we are angry or depressed, we treat our thoughts as if they are facts. I might say, "He thinks that he can take advantage of me," and I might think that I am absolutely right—but I could also be wrong. When I am anxious, I might think "I know I'll do poorly in this presentation"—but I could be either right or wrong. I can believe or think that I am a giraffe, but it does not mean that I am a giraffe. Just because I believe something is true does not mean that it *is* true. Thoughts are hypotheses, descriptions, perspectives, and even guesses. They can prove to be either true or false. Patients need to learn how to identify their thoughts and then examine the facts. In order to distinguish thoughts, feelings, and facts, therapists can use the A-B-C technique in which patients have an opportunity to recognize how the same *a*ctivating event can lead to different *b*eliefs (thoughts) and *c*onsequences (feelings and behavior). If I believe I can never do well on the exam (my thought), I might feel hopeless and behave accordingly—for example, by not bothering to study. On the other hand, if I believe that I have a good chance of doing well on the exam, I might feel hopeful and therefore study for it.

What is interesting about this example is that my initial thought—"I won't do well on the exam"—leads to the maladaptive behavior of not preparing for the exam, which then leads to the self-fulfilling prophecy of doing poorly on the exam.

Many people who are depressed, anxious, or angry treat their thoughts as if they were facts—that is, "It's *true* that I won't do well on the exam" or "I *know* she'll reject me." Figure 1.2 contains a number of examples of the same activating event leading to different thoughts, feelings, and behaviors.

The importance of distinguishing a negative thought from possible facts is illustrated by Figure 1.3. Here the patient is asked to imagine that he or she is having a negative thought, such as, "I am not prepared for my exam." The right-hand column prompts the patient to consider any facts that might be relevant to a valid evaluation of his or her preparedness? The initial thought is a belief; the possible facts can *become* beliefs, once they are considered. The patient can be asked, "Is it possible that your thoughts are not the only things to consider? Wouldn't you want to look at other possible facts?" Thoughts and facts are not equivalent.

A = Activating Event	B = Belief (Thought)	C = Consequence: Feelings	C = Consequence: Behaviors
I hear the window rattling.	Someone is breaking into my house.	Anxious	Lock the door, call police.
I hear the window rattling.	It's windy outside and the window is old and loose.	Slightly irritated	Try to tighten the window, go back to sleep.
A man is approaching me on a dark, empty street.	I'm going to get mugged.	Terrified	Run.
A man is approaching me on a dark, empty street.	I wonder if that's my old friend Steve.	Curious, pleased	Call out Steve's name.
My husband is sitting reading the newspaper.	He doesn't care about my feelings.	Angry, resentful	Tell him he's self-centered.
My husband is sitting reading the newspaper.	He's withdrawing from me because he's angry with me.	Upset, guilty	Avoid interacting with him.
I feel my heart beating rapidly.	I'm having a heart attack.	Anxiety, panic	Go to emergency room.
I feel my heart beating rapidly.	I've had too much coffee.	A little regretful	Try to cut back on caffeine.

FIGURE 1.2. The A-B-C Technique. The same event gives rise to different thoughts that lead to different feelings and behaviors. You determine if your thought is true by examining the facts.

Negative Thought	Other Possible Facts
It's raining outside and I'll never get home on time.	Maybe it stopped raining since I came in an hour ago. I can go outside to check out the facts.
I am not prepared for my exam.	I have read the material, gone to class, and done some work.
I'll always be alone.	I don't have all of the facts, since I don't know what is in the future. I have friends. I have a lot of qualities that people like.

FIGURE 1.3. Thoughts versus Possible Facts.

Question to Pose/Intervention

"Thoughts and facts are not the same. Just because you think something is true does not necessarily mean that it is true. I can think that I am a zebra—but my thought does not mean I am a zebra. We have to check out the thought against the facts."

Example

THERAPIST: Can you tell me what you're thinking about that's making you so anxious?

PATIENT: I think I'm going to get fired.

THERAPIST: How do you know that you will get fired?

PATIENT: I just know it. I can see it coming.

THERAPIST: You may believe or think that you'll get fired, but isn't it possible that you could be wrong about this?

PATIENT: I feel pretty strongly about this. I just know it's going to happen.

THERAPIST: Although it could be true—it could happen that you might be fired—it may also be possible that it won't happen. There's a difference between a *belief* and a *fact*. Believing it's true doesn't make it true. Would you consider the possibility of examining the reasons why you might get fired and the reasons why you might *not* get fired?

In this example, the therapist acknowledges the patient's strong belief and explains that *belief* does not equal *truth*. The therapist then invites the patient to examine the evidence and the reasoning that leads to the belief about getting fired. The recognition that thoughts are not facts is the starting point of helping the patient construct alternative interpretations of events.

Homework

The therapist can ask the patient to keep track of activating or preceding events that lead to specific beliefs and feelings by using Form 1.2 at the end of the chapter. In addition, the patient can use the Thought versus Possible Facts form (1.3) to examine how a particular thought does not always take into account all of the possible facts. For example, the thought "I am not prepared for the exam" does not include the possible facts that I am intelligent, I have attended class, and I have read the assignments.

Possible Problems

Some people believe that their thoughts are the last word on the truth. Indeed, sometimes the negative thoughts *are* true. We do not want patients to get the impression that we believe that everything they believe is false. This distinction can be made in the following way: "Sometimes your thoughts will accurately describe the facts, and sometimes your thoughts will not accurately reflect all of the facts. Wouldn't it be a good idea to use a general rule of checking out your negative thoughts against all of the relevant facts?"

Some patients respond that examining the facts seems invalidating and critical of the patient's position. I have described this problem in *Overcoming Resistance in Cognitive Therapy* (Leahy, 2001b). The feeling of invalidation can be explored directly by asking the patient if these questions about the facts seem like "put-downs" or "rejections." Again, the important point to make is that examining the facts does not necessarily mean that the patient is incorrect.

Cross-Reference to Other Techniques

Other relevant techniques include looking at the evidence for and against the validity of a thought, distinguishing thoughts from feelings, categorizing cognitive distortions, and looking at variations in believing a thought. For example, the patient who has variation in a thought such as "I am a failure" can be asked if his or her belief in the thought depends on the facts to which he or she is attending.

Forms

Forms 1.2 (Self-Help Form: The A-B-C Technique, p. 28); Form 1.3 (Thoughts versus Possible Facts, p. 29).

TECHNIQUE: RATING THE DEGREE OF EMOTION AND DEGREE OF BELIEF IN THE THOUGHT

Description

We may have many different emotions and beliefs about a single event. What is really important is how strongly we *feel* something and how strongly we hold a *belief*.

Emotions obviously vary in degree. I can feel slightly sad, somewhat sad, very sad, extremely sad, or overwhelmingly sad. Since many people who are sad, anxious, or angry are often undifferentiated in their thinking or in their observations of their own emotions, it is useful to teach them how to distinguish the various degrees of their emotions. Furthermore, given that change in therapy is often gradual, it is important that patients be able to detect various degrees of change in their feelings or emotions. For example, a patients whose feelings change from overwhelmingly sad to somewhat sad might realistically conclude that good progress has been achieved.

Question to Pose/Intervention

"How much do you feel upset, and how strongly do you hold your belief? Rate your feeling (emotion) from 0% to 100%, where 0% corresponds to having none of that feeling and 100% corresponds to the most intense experience of that feeling. The same with your beliefs: 0% corresponds to not holding that belief at all, and 100% corresponds to believing your thought 100%. To what degree do your feelings and thoughts change? What could be some reasons why you feel better at certain times than other times? Are you doing different things when you are feeling down? Or up? Are you thinking differently when you are down? Or up?"

Example

THERAPIST: You said that you are feeling sad since you and John broke up. Can you describe this sadness for me?

PATIENT: Oh, I feel very sad. Sometimes I cry when I think of how he left me.

THERAPIST: Your feelings are important, so I want to be able to really understand how you feel when you're thinking about the breakup. If you were to rate your sadness from 0% to 100%, where 0% represents absolutely no sad feelings and 100% represents the greatest sadness imaginable, how would you rate your sadness?

PATIENT: I guess I've never thought about how I rate my feelings. I'd say about 95% sadness.

Similarly, the patient may hold an absolute belief—for example, "I can never be happy without John"—but the patient's degree of belief (i.e., the credibility or strength of the belief) might be less than 100%. This recognition that beliefs vary in strength is a very important beginning in gaining distance from distressing beliefs. If I can hold a belief in which I invest less than 100% veracity, then it means that I already have some doubt about that belief. It also means that my belief can vary—it could be less than its current strength. Consequently, I can imagine changing this belief even more vividly.

THERAPIST: You said you feel very sad when you think about John leaving you. Can you complete this sentence with the first thoughts that come to your mind? "I feel very sad when I think of John leaving me because I think . . . "

PATIENT: I can never be happy without him.

THERAPIST: OK. The automatic thought is "I can never be happy without him." Why don't you write that down. [The therapist has given the patient a clipboard with paper and pen to take notes during the session.] Now let's see how much you believe that thought: "I can never be happy without him." If you were to rate that thought from 0% to 100%, where 0% represents the complete absence of that belief and 100% represents your absolute certainty that this belief is true, how would you rate it?

PATIENT: I guess I'd have to say it's a pretty high rating. I really believe this—most if the time. I'd give it about 90%.

Some people have a hard time using this kind of scale. The idea of rating emotions and beliefs is foreign to their thinking. The therapist may need to provide visual aids.

THERAPIST: You said you felt sad, but it's hard for you to use the scale. Let's define what this scale is. (*Draws the scale shown in Figure 1.4.*) Let's say that 0% represents absolutely no sadness, and that 100% represents the most sadness that anyone could imagine—you are absolutely overwhelmed with sadness, so that you can't think of anything else. Fifty percent represents a moderate amount of sadness, whereas 90% represents an extreme amount of sadness—a very disturbing amount—but you are still able to function, to a large degree. Now, when you think about John leaving you, where would you place your sadness on this scale?

PATIENT: I'd say at about 95%. I'm extremely sad, but I'm still able to function, to some degree.

Homework

The therapist can ask patients to keep track of how their degree of belief in their thoughts changes during the course of the next week. Patients are asked to use the self-help form (1.4) for rating emotions and beliefs (at the end of the chapter), on which they note what events preceded the thoughts and feel-

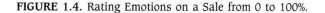

0	10	20	30	40	50	60	70	80	90	100
No sadness		Slight			Moderate		Very		Extreme overwhelming sadness	

FIGURE 1.4. Rating Emotions on a Sale from 0 to 100%.

ings and rate the degree of belief and the degree of emotion associated with each event. After this exercise has been completed, it can be suggested that patients reflect on what could account for the variation in the negative thoughts and feelings they experience.

Possible Problems

Problems that typically occur with this exercise include a lack of motivation to write down the same belief more than once during the week. Patients may think, "I've already done this." However, the purpose of the exercise is to examine carefully the variation in the belief and the feeling and what accounts for this change. This differentiation also helps us identify possible "trouble times" for patients—that is, times when they are more likely to feel depressed or anxious. This knowledge can assist the therapist in focusing treatment around these problematic times.

Cross-Reference to Other Techniques

Other relevant techniques include examining how thoughts lead to feelings, distinguishing thoughts from facts, the vertical descent technique, categorizing negative thoughts, and looking for variations in a particular thought.

Forms

Form 1.4 (Self-Help Form: Rating Emotions and Beliefs, p. 30).

TECHNIQUE: LOOKING FOR VARIATIONS IN A SPECIFIC BELIEF

Description

In order to gain distance from a belief, it is often useful to recognize that even in the present circumstances, our beliefs may change in strength or credibility. The cognitive therapist is always interested in the flexibility of beliefs; extremely depressed or anxious persons, in contrast, may think that their beliefs are fixed in concrete and never change. Consequently, the therapist directly assesses variability of belief. This technique is closely related to the technique of rating degree of emotion and degree of belief in the thought described above. The emphasis here is on a specific belief and its variation across time and situations.

Question to Pose/Intervention

"Are there times that you believe this thought with less conviction? What is going on when you believe this negative thought less? If your thought were entirely true, then how could you believe it to be less true at certain times?"

Example

THERAPIST: You said that you believe that you can never be happy without John and that you give this belief a 90% rating.

PATIENT: That's right. I really believe this. That's why I'm so unhappy.

THERAPIST: Now during the course of the day, I imagine that your moods change—sometimes you're more unhappy than at other times?

PATIENT: Yes. I'm not always crying or even thinking about John.

THERAPIST: What are you thinking about when you're not thinking of John?

PATIENT: I'm thinking about changing the apartment—maybe getting some new furniture. Or I'm thinking of having lunch with my friends.

THERAPIST: Obviously, when you're not thinking about John, the strength of the belief is 0%—since at that very moment, you're not feeling unhappy, even though John is not with you.

PATIENT: Well, that's a novel way of thinking about it. But I guess you're right.

THERAPIST: Are there times during the day when you think of John but you are not 90% unhappy?

PATIENT: Yes. Sometimes I think, "Maybe I'm better off without him."

THERAPIST: So, if I were to jump into your head at that moment and ask you, "Tell me—right now—how much do you believe 'I can never be happy without John?' how would you answer?"

PATIENT: Oh, well, at those times, my belief would be very low, maybe even 10%.

THERAPIST: So this belief that you have right now *can* change—even in the course of a few hours. What do you make of that?

PATIENT: I guess that my thoughts about the breakup might change.

THERAPIST: When people go through breakups, they often have very strong, negative, powerful beliefs. I'm sure you have friends who have gone through this experience.

PATIENT: Yes, my friend Alice got divorced 5 years ago.

THERAPIST: Perhaps she had the exact same belief that you have right now. Have her beliefs changed over the years?

PATIENT: You're right, they have! Now she can't even imagine being in the same room with her ex-husband.

THERAPIST: Well, let's keep this in mind—how your beliefs change and the beliefs of other people change.

Homework

Using Form 1.5 (at the end of the chapter), the patient can be given the homework assignment of tracking the degree of belief in a specific thought for several days. Presumably, the patient's focus and concern about a belief will vary with time of day, events, and other thoughts. This variation further reinforces the idea that a strongly held belief can be changed. Furthermore, the patient's strongly held belief may vary during the session. Periodically during the session, as the patient and therapist focus on challenging beliefs and planning behavior, the therapist can ask the patient how strong the belief is at those different points. It is not uncommon for a patient to begin the session with a belief held at 90% and end the session with the belief held at 40%.

This change in belief is then linked to the change in emotion—for example, sadness has decreased as the strength in the belief has diminished—further reinforcing the assumptions of cognitive therapy and providing hope to the patient that strongly held beliefs and unpleasant emotions can be modified.

THERAPIST: Your belief has changed from 90% to 40% in 30 minutes, and your sadness has greatly decreased. What do you make of that?

PATIENT: I guess my thoughts and feelings can change in this kind of therapy.

THERAPIST: If we were able to change your thoughts and feelings in just 30 minutes, what do you think would happen if you were able to use these techniques on your own?

PATIENT: Well, I guess I'd feel better.

THERAPIST: Why don't we see what happens, then?

Possible Problems

As with the foregoing techniques in this chapter, patients may be less motivated to write down a negative belief when he is feeling better. The therapist needs to make clear that there is a lot of useful information when they are feeling better. For example, if the patient believes "I have nothing to offer because I am a loser" but notices that his or her degree of belief in this thought is 0 % when talking with friends, the patient has gained useful information that can lead to the following intervention and question: "If your belief changes, then assign yourself tasks that are associated with more positive beliefs. If your belief changes, then it may not be accurate. What information are you considering when you are feeling less negative?"

Cross-Reference to Other Techniques

As suggested above, other relevant techniques include graded task assignment, examining all of the information or facts, challenging beliefs by examining the evidence for and against the validity of the belief, distinguishing a fact from a thought, and distinguishing a thought from a feeling.

Form

Form 1.5 (Tracking Degree of Belief in a Thought, p. 31).

TECHNIQUE: CATEGORIZING THE DISTORTION IN THINKING

Description

Continually distorting thoughts in the same manner—for example, by jumping to conclusions, personalizing bad events, or labeling oneself as a failure—are common patterns in people who are depressed or anxious. The cognitive model proposes that unpleasant emotions are often associated with these biases or distortions in thinking. Automatic thoughts (i.e., thoughts that come spontaneously) are associated with negative affect or dysfunctional behavior and seem plausible to the individual. Examples of automatic thoughts are "I'll never be happy," "I'm stupid," "No one likes me," "It's all my fault," and "She thinks I'm boring." Automatic thoughts can be true, false, or have varying degrees of validity. The same thought may contain more than one distortion—for example, "When I go to the party, she'll think I'm boring." This thought reflects both fortune telling and mind reading. Beck (Beck, 1976; Beck et al., 1979) and Burns (1989) have identified various automatic thought distortions. Form 1.6 (at end of chapter) provides common thought distortions that are associated with depression, anxiety, and anger.

Question to Pose/Intervention

"Are you continually distorting your thinking in the same way? Look at the checklist of cognitive distortions. Are there certain kinds of distortions that you are using? What are they?"

Example

The therapist elicits the patient's automatic thoughts by asking, "What were you thinking when you felt sad?" or by supplying a sentence stem for the patient to complete, such as, "I felt anxious because I thought . . . " The automatic thoughts are then categorized. The therapist explains: "Write down your negative or upsetting thought in the left-hand column and categorize the distortion in the right-hand column." See Figure 1.5 for an example.

Homework

The patient can be given the assignment of monitoring any negative automatic thoughts over the following week and categorizing them, using Forms 1.6 and 1.7 at the end of the chapter. The value of this exercise is that patients see how they repeat the same categories of automatic thoughts—for example, fortune telling: "I'll never be happy," "Nothing will work out," "No one will ever want me," "I'll always be alone." If there is a clear repetition of a specific category of negative thoughts, then the therapist and patient can develop a specific set of challenges that can be used repeatedly to depotentiate the thoughts. For example, the patient who continually engages in mind reading (e.g., "He thinks I'm a loser," "They don't like me," "I must look pathetic") might be instructed to compose a list of challenges to these repetitive thoughts. These challenges could include the following: "I don't have any evidence," "I'm jumping to conclusions," "Why should they dislike me if they don't even know me?," "I'm just as good as anyone here," "I don't need their approval," "I don't need to impress everyone," or "Maybe they're thinking about whether *I* like *them*."

Possible Problems

As indicated above, some patients believe that categorizing their thoughts as distortions implies that they are stupid or crazy. It is important to clarify that some negative thoughts are true. For example, the thought might be, "She doesn't like me." We can categorize this thought as mind reading, but it could also be true. Perhaps she doesn't like me. I indicate to patients that we use the form "cognitive distortions" because it is a handy way of categorizing thoughts—but that many negative thoughts have a degree of truth to them. Once we are able to find a pattern to the thoughts—let's say, mind reading—that is associated with feeling down, then we can develop some specific interventions for that pattern. Categorizing thoughts should not be equated with refuting or negating thoughts. We have to examine the facts.

Automatic Thought	Distortion
I'm a failure.	Mislabeling
She thinks I'm unattractive.	Mind reading
Nothing I do works out.	All-or-nothing thinking
Anyone can do this job—it doesn't mean anything.	Discounting positives

FIGURE 1.5. Examples of Automatic Thought Distortions.

Cross-Reference to Other Techniques

Other relevant techniques include the thought monitoring described above, whereby the patient keeps track of thoughts, facts, feelings, and variations in the degree of belief in a thought. In addition, the checklist of cognitive distortions can assist the therapist in planning interventions or questions, such as using vertical descent, identifying underlying assumptions and schemas, evaluating feared fantasy, looking at the costs and benefits, and considering the evidence for and against the validity of certain thoughts.

Forms

Form 1.6 (Checklist of Cognitive Distortions, p. 32); Form 1.7 (Categorizing Your Thought Distortions, p. 33).

TECHNIQUE: VERTICAL DESCENT

Description

Sometimes negative thoughts turn out to be true. Let's say that a male patient predicts he will be ignored or rebuffed at a party. This is fortune telling, but it may prove accurate. Exploring the beliefs underlying the fear of that outcome helps to depotentiate the thought. With this technique, the therapist continues to ask about that thought or event: "What would then happen if that were true?" or "What would that mean to you if that happened?" We refer to this process as *vertical descent* we are attempting to burrow down to the bottom-most belief. Accordingly, the therapist writes the patient's thought on the top of a page and then draws a downward arrow to the series of thoughts or events that is implied by the thought (see Figure 1.6).

Question to Pose/Intervention

"If your thought is true, why would it bother you? What would it make you think? What would happen next?"

Example

Vertical descent is a useful way at getting at the underlying fears of which patients are unaware. I use this technique frequently, because I have found that I can never really tell what the patient's underlying beliefs and fears might be. For example, most of us have a fear of dying—but what is it that each of us really fears? Consider these two patients, each of whom had a fear of dying.

THERAPIST: You said that you sometimes fear you might have cancer. Even though the doctor has reassured you that you are OK, what would it mean to you if you did have cancer?

PATIENT: I'd be afraid that I might die.

THERAPIST: Almost everyone has a fear of that, of course, but let me ask you about your own fears of dying. Complete this sentence: "I'd be afraid of dying because . . . "

PATIENT: I'd be afraid that I wasn't really dead—that I was only in a coma—and that I would wake from the coma in my grave, buried alive.

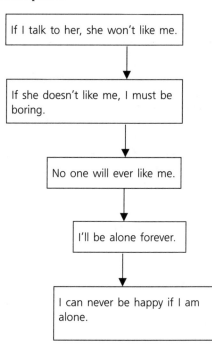

If I talk to her, she won't like me.

If she doesn't like me, I must be boring.

No one will ever like me.

I'll be alone forever.

I can never be happy if I am alone.

Event and Thought	Implication
Event: Considering going to a party. **Thought:** "I feel anxious approaching that woman at the party."	
What do you think will happen?	I'll get rejected.
If that happens, then it means . . .	I must be a loser.
If I'm a loser, then it means . . .	I'll never find anyone for a relationship.
If I never find anyone, then . . .	I'll always be alone.
If I'm always alone, then that would bother me because . . .	I can't be happy if I'm alone—I'd always be miserable.
What is my underlying assumption?	I need other people to feel happy.

FIGURE 1.6. Taking the Vertical Descent to the Implication of a Thought.

This patient's fears of being buried alive are quite symbolic (to use a noncognitive term). Many of her problems revolved around the issue of constraints on her behavior, such as food restrictions, limits set on her by her boss, and the limits of her finances. It is useful to write out on a sheet of paper or a blackboard in the office the string of thoughts showing the downward progression to the core fear. The example of the first patient, with the fear of being buried alive, is shown in Figure 1.7.

Another patient, whom I would describe as a compulsive caretaker who tries to take care of everyone's needs, also had a fear of dying. His fear revolved around the well-being of his wife and daughter, were he to die.

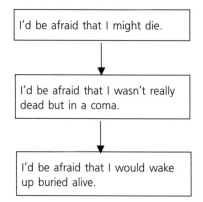

FIGURE 1.7. Taking the Vertical Descent to the Implication of a Thought.

THERAPIST: What about dying would bother you the most?

PATIENT: It's not the physical pain. I don't really worry about that. And I've already done enough for five lifetimes. It's that if I died, I would be worried that I didn't take care of everyone.

THERAPIST: Who is it that you would have to take care of?

PATIENT: My wife and my daughter. I could die if I knew they'd be alright.

THERAPIST: So you're saying that you can accept death if you know that the people you love are taken care of?

PATIENT: That's right.

THERAPIST: Are you assuming that they are helpless without you?

PATIENT: I guess I am.

The therapist can ask any number of questions about an event or thought. For example:

   Why would that be a problem for you?
   What would happen?
   Why would that bother you?
   Then what?
   What would that mean to you?

Homework

The patient is asked to draw out the implication of negative thoughts by using the vertical descent form (1.8, at the end of the chapter). This form asks the patient to identify a string of implications. The therapist might say to the patient: "Your negative thoughts are connected with other negative thoughts. We are interested in how you think and what each negative thought means to you. For example, someone might have the negative thought 'I'm not prepared for the exam,' which then leads to the thought 'I'll fail the exam,' which tumbles into the thought 'I'll have to drop out of school.' Try to identify some of your negative thoughts and then examine the string of thoughts that follows. Keep asking yourself, 'And if that were true, it would bother me because it would mean . . . ' "

Possible Problems

Some patients stop identifying their negative thoughts in the middle of the sequence. For example, the patient might stop with the thought, "I'll flunk the exam," and not go any further in the vertical descent. The patient might say "Flunking seems bad enough" or "I don't really believe I would flunk the exam." It is helpful to ask the patient to keep pushing for even "deeper" or "worse" thoughts that would follow from the first few thoughts. Often we find that the patient's thoughts about having any failure or rejection are associated with fantasies of awful or catastrophic consequences. These underlying "worst fears" fuel the anxiety about the initial thoughts.

Cross-Reference to Other Techniques

Techniques related to the vertical descent include identifying thoughts and feelings, examining the evidence for and against the thought, examining the costs and benefits of the validity of the thought, evaluating the leaps in logic underlying the thought, calculating sequential probabilities, and challenging the thought.

Form

Form 1.8 (Using the Vertical Descent, p. 34).

TECHNIQUE: ASSIGNING PROBABILITIES IN THE SEQUENCE

Description

Using the vertical descent procedure described above, the patient can now estimate the probability of each event occurring in the sequence, given that the preceding event is true. We are not only interested in the thoughts that are implied in the vertical descent but also in the subjective estimates of probabilities. These subjective estimates are usually far beyond what we would expect to be true, given our knowledge of baseline information in the general population.

Question to Pose/Intervention

"What is the probability that X would happen?" "What is the likelihood from 0% to 100%?"

Example

The therapist might introduce the idea of probability in the following way.

THERAPIST: The likelihood that something will happen is called *probability*. Probabilities can vary between 0% and 100%—there are probably very few things that have a 0% or 100% probability. For example, the probability of getting heads when I flip a coin is 50%. The question that I will ask you is, What is the probability of each of your thoughts being true? Let's take the first thought "I am not prepared for the exam." What is the probability that this thought is true?

PATIENT: I'd say about 90%.

THERAPIST: Your next thought was that you would fail the exam. What's the probability that you would fail the exam, given that you are not prepared?

PATIENT: Oh, I'd say about 30%. I actually know some of the things that will be on the test.

THERAPIST: OK. But if you *did* fail the exam, what is the probability that you would flunk out of school?

PATIENT: Probably 2%. I have already taken a lot of courses and passed them.

THERAPIST: OK, but if you *did* flunk out of school, what is the probability that you would never get a job?

PATIENT: Less than 1%.

THERAPIST: OK, now what if we got our calculator out and totaled up these probabilities. The way we do this is to take your first estimate 90%, enter .90, and multiply by each of the other probabilities. So that is .90 times .30 times .02 times .01. What do we get? The calculator says .000054.

PATIENT: That seems like an unlikely event.

THERAPIST: It's about 5 in 100,000 or about 20,000 to 1.

Possible Problems

As with the previous vertical descent exercise, the patient may stop prematurely in the sequence, claiming that he or she really doesn't believe the next thought in the sequence. Or the patient may claim that the initial thoughts would be bad enough. Again, the therapist should emphasize that even if the other thoughts don't seem credible or likely, they still should be identified because they might illustrate underlying fears that need to be examined.

Another type of problem arises when the patient claims, in essence, "Well, I know that it is unlikely, but what if *I'm* the one to whom this happens? You can't show me that it is impossible." Patients who demand "certainty" can be asked, "What are the costs and benefits of demanding certainty?" "Are there any things in your life for which you don't have certainty?" "Why do you tolerate that uncertainty?"

Cross-Reference to Other Techniques

Other relevant techniques include all of the techniques identified Chapter 4 on examining and challenging worries.

Form

Form 1.9 (Using the Vertical Descent, p. 35).

TECHNIQUE: GUESSING THE THOUGHT

Description

It is not always possible for the patient to identify the negative thought—sometimes the intensity of the emotion is so great that the patient finds it difficult to reflect on the thoughts that go with the feelings. Beck (1995) recommends having the therapist suggest some possible thoughts to the patient to determine if any of them seem consistent with how he or she is thinking and feeling. The therapist must be careful not to suggest that the patient has an "unconscious" belief that only the therapist can identify. Both therapist and patient can attempt to speculate as to the nature of the thinking underlying the thought.

Question to Pose/Intervention

"You can't say exactly what your thought is. What kinds of thoughts would go with these negative feelings? Is it possible you are saying these things to yourself? [Therapist suggests some possible thoughts.]"

Example

The patient feels overwhelmed with sadness and hopelessness after the breakup of her engagement. She focuses on her physical complaints—"I can't eat, and I feel so tired." She repeats to the therapist, "I feel so awful since we broke up. I just can't think straight." The therapist tries to elicit specific negative thoughts.

THERAPIST: You said that you felt awful since the breakup. Could you tell me what kinds of thoughts you are having?

PATIENT: I just feel terrible. I can't sleep.

THERAPIST: Yes, those are feelings that you are describing right now. But could you complete the sentence "I feel awful since the breakup because I think . . . "

PATIENT: I don't think anything. I just feel like dying.

THERAPIST: Can you identify any thoughts that go with that feeling of hopelessness?

PATIENT: No, the feeling is too intense.

THERAPIST: I wonder if we could try to guess at what those negative thoughts might be. I don't know what they are, so I'll just make some suggestions and you tell me if any of these ring a bell for you.

PATIENT: OK.

THERAPIST: Could you be saying to yourself, "I'll never be happy again"?

PATIENT: Yeah. That makes sense. That's what I'm thinking.

THERAPIST: Are you saying, then, "I can never be happy unless I have [Roger] in my life"?

PATIENT: Definitely. That's what I'm feeling.

Homework

The therapist can request that the patient list any unpleasant moods and either identify or "guess" the thought.

Possible Problems

The therapist could have tried to get the patient to review the differences between a thought and a feeling, but sometimes the patient is unable to gain enough emotional distance to identify the thought. Once the negative thoughts are identified, the therapist can continue with the vertical descent procedure: "I could never be happy without Roger because . . . Roger was unique . . . I could never love anyone like I loved him . . . I can never be happy unless I have a man in my life." Sometimes the patient insists that there are no thoughts, just feelings. The therapist can ask the patient to close her eyes and attempt to induce the negative feeling as intensely as she can. The therapist can instruct the patient to imagine the situation that has elicited this feeling—for example, "sitting at home alone thinking of [Roger]." The therapist can guide the patient toward identifying the negative thoughts while the feeling or emotion is intensely felt: "While you are feeling really sad, can you imagine what you are thinking? Could it be that you are thinking 'I can never be happy without Roger'?"

I provide a form (at the end of the chapter) for the patient and therapist to write down their "guesses" about these possible negative thoughts. These guesses need to be examined quite carefully, since many patients may believe that everything is driven by mysterious unconscious thoughts and motivations. The therapist will want to examine, with the patient, the plausibility that these are the real thoughts underlying the feeling. Furthermore, patients can verify the guesses by staying on the lookout for the problematic thoughts the next time they feel sad or hopeless.

Cross-Reference to Other Techniques

Techniques related to this one include the use of vertical descent, monitoring emotions, thoughts, and situations, reviewing the list of cognitive distortions to determine if there are any suggestions that remind the patient of the underlying thought, imagery techniques, emotional evocation, point–counterpoint, challenging the thought, and role playing negative and positive thoughts with the therapist.

Form

Form 1.10 (Guessing at the Negative Thought, p. 36).

FORM 1.1. Self-Help Form: How Thoughts Create Feelings

Thought: I think . . .	Feeling: Therefore, I feel . . .

FORM 1.2. Self-Help Form: The A-B-C Technique

"Activating event" refers to an event that precedes your thought or belief. For example, recognizing that "The exam is tomorrow" is the activating event that precedes the thought "I am not prepared," which might lead to the "Consequence: Feeling" of anxiety and worry and to the "Consequence: Behavior" of studying very hard for the exam.

A = Activating Event	B = Belief (Thought)	C = Consequence: Feelings	C = Consequence: Behaviors

FORM 1.3. Thoughts versus Possible Facts

Write out your negative thought in the left-hand column, and then write out some possible facts that you might need to consider.

Negative Thought	Other Possible Facts

FORM 1.4. Self-Help Form: Rating Emotions and Beliefs

The degree that you believe in your negative thoughts may change with different events and at different times. Write down the event or situation that you are in when you have a negative thought. For example, repeated events and situations might include "sitting alone" or "thinking of going to a party" or "trying to get some work done." Then write down your negative thoughts, how much you believe them, your emotions, and the degree of your emotions.

Event/ Situation	Negative Thought and Degree of Belief (0–100%)	Emotion and Degree of Emotion (0–100%)

FORM 1.5. Tracking Degree of Belief in a Thought

The degree to which you agree with your specific negative belief may change during the course of the day. For example, the belief "I can't do anything" may be very strong when you are lying in bed in the morning. You may believe it 95%. But when you are at work, you may believe this thought 10%. Keep track of a negative belief for a couple of days and try to note if there is any change or variation in the degree to which you agree with your belief. What are you doing when that variation occurs? Are you with anyone? Does the strength of the belief vary with the time of day?

Negative Belief:			
Time/Activity	**% Belief**	**Time/Activity**	**% Belief**
6 A.M.		4 P.M.	
7		5	
8		6	
9		7	
10		8	
11		9	
12 NOON		10	
1 P.M.		11	
2		12	
3		1 A.M.	

FORM 1.6. Checklist of Cognitive Distortions

1. **Mind reading:** You assume that you know what people think without having sufficient evidence of their thoughts. For example: "He thinks I'm a loser."

2. **Fortune telling:** You predict the future—that things will get worse or that there is danger ahead. For example: "I'll fail that exam" or "I won't get the job."

3. **Catastrophizing:** You believe that what has happened or will happen will be so awful and unbearable that you won't be able to stand it. For example: "It would be terrible if I failed."

4. **Labeling:** You assign global negative traits to yourself and others. For example: "I'm undesirable" or "He's a rotten person."

5. **Discounting positives:** You claim that the positive accomplishments you or others attain are trivial. For example: "That's what wives are supposed to do—so it doesn't count when she's nice to me" or "Those successes were easy, so they don't matter."

6. **Negative filter:** You focus almost exclusively on the negatives and seldom notice the positives. For example: "Look at all of the people who don't like me."

7. **Overgeneralizing:** You perceive a global pattern of negatives on the basis of a single incident. For example: "This generally happens to me. I seem to fail at a lot of things."

8. **Dichotomous thinking:** You view events, or people, in all-or-nothing terms. For example: "I get rejected by everyone" or "It was a waste of time."

9. **"Shoulds":** You interpret events in terms of how things should be rather than simply focusing on what is. For example: "I should do well. If I don't, then I'm a failure."

10. **Personalizing:** You attribute a disproportionate amount of the blame for negative events to yourself and fail to see that certain events are also caused by others. For example: "My marriage ended because I failed."

11. **Blaming:** You focus on the other person as the source of your negative feelings and you refuse to take responsibility for changing yourself. For example: "She's to blame for the way I feel now" or "My parents caused all my problems."

12. **Unfair comparisons:** You interpret events in terms of standards that are unrealistic by focusing primarily on others who do better than you and then judging yourself inferior in the comparison. For example: "She's more successful than I am" or "Others did better than I did on the test."

13. **Regret orientation:** You focus on the idea that you could have done better in the past, rather than on what you could do better now. For example: "I could have had a better job if I had tried" or "I shouldn't have said that."

14. **What if?:** You ask a series of questions about "what if" something happens, and you are never satisfied with any of the answers. For example: "Yeah, but what if I get anxious?" Or "What if I can't catch my breath?"

15. **Emotional reasoning:** You let your feelings guide your interpretation of reality. For example, "I feel depressed; therefore, my marriage is not working out."

16. **Inability to disconfirm:** You reject any evidence or arguments that might contradict your negative thoughts. For example, when you have the thought "I'm unlovable," you reject as irrelevant any evidence that people like you. Consequently, your thought cannot be refuted. Another example: "That's not the real issue. There are deeper problems. There are other factors."

17. **Judgment focus:** You view yourself, others, and events in terms of black/white evaluations (good–bad or superior–inferior) rather than simply describing, accepting, or understanding. You are continually measuring yourself and others according to arbitrary standards and finding that you and others fall short. You are focused on the judgments of others as well as your own judgments of yourself. For example: "I didn't perform well in college" or "If I take up tennis, I won't do well" or "Look how successful she is. I'm not successful."

From Leahy (1996). Copyright 1996 by Jason Aronson Inc. Reprinted by permission.

FORM 1.7. Categorizing Your Thought Distortions

Categories of thought distortions: Mind reading, fortune telling, catastrophizing, labeling, discounting positives, negative filter, overgeneralizing, dichotomous thinking, "shoulds," personalizing, blaming, unfair comparisons, regret orientation, what-if thinking, emotional reasoning, inability to disconfirm, judgment focus.

Automatic Thought	Distortion

FORM 1.8. Using the Vertical Descent (Why Would It Bother Me If My Thought Were True?)

Event: _____

Thought:

┌───┐
│   │
│   │
└───┘

It would bother me because it would make me think . . .

│
▼

┌───┐
│   │
│   │
└───┘

│
▼

┌───┐
│   │
│   │
└───┘

│
▼

┌───┐
│   │
│   │
└───┘

│
▼

┌───┐
│   │
│   │
└───┘

FORM 1.9. Using the Vertical Descent (Why Would It Bother Me If My Thought Were True?)—Calculating the Sequence of Probabilities

Event: _____

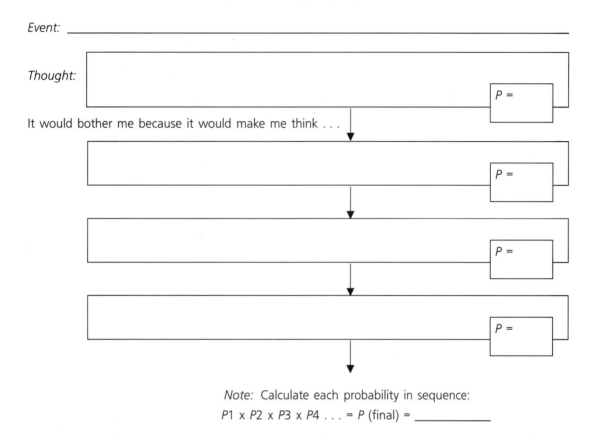

Thought:

It would bother me because it would make me think . . .

Note: Calculate each probability in sequence:

*P*1 x *P*2 x *P*3 x *P*4 . . . = *P* (final) = _____

FORM 1.10. Guessing at the Negative Thought

"Emotions" refer to feelings such as sad, anxious, angry, helpless, or hopeless. "Possible negative thoughts" refer to thoughts that you believe may go with these feelings. In the far right-hand column, rate the degree of belief that you have in each negative thought, using a scale ranging from 0% to 100%.

Emotions	Possible Negative Thoughts	Belief (0–100%)

CHAPTER 2

Evaluating and Challenging Thoughts

$\mathbf{A}$fter the patient and therapist have identified and categorized the various negative thoughts and examined how they are related to depression, anxiety, and anger, the stage is set for evaluating and challenging these thoughts. In this chapter we consider a variety of techniques that are used to test the validity of the negative thoughts, keeping in mind that negative thoughts sometimes are true. Cognitive therapy does not advocate the "power of positive thinking" but rather the power of identifying *whatever* is being thought. Some individuals underestimate the negative implications of their behaviors—for example, individuals who are abusing alcohol or drugs (Beck, Wright, Newman, & Liese, 1993) or manic individuals (Leahy, 1999, 2002). Technically, cognitive therapists evaluate or test thoughts, examining their implications, looking at the evidence, and considering alternative interpretations. The cognitive approach is constructivist in that it recognizes that the individual's construction or interpretation of reality may be based on unique information, personal categories, or biases of perception or cognition (Mahoney, 1991).

At times, however, the therapist may ask the patient to mount a more vigorous challenge, hopefully activating new and more adaptive interpretations through active disputation. In a sense, these challenges or disputations are a way of testing the validity of a negative thought. If the negative thought is valid, it should be able to withstand vigorous challenge. However, the therapist should recognize that overly disputatious debating with the patient might result in the patient feeling invalidated, dominated, humiliated, or misunderstood. With these caveats in mind, let us turn to a sampling of techniques that can help patients examine the validity of the thoughts under consideration.

TECHNIQUE: DEFINING THE TERMS

Description

The therapist might explain this next stage to patients in this way: "In order for us to examine and challenge your thoughts, we have to know what you are talking about. If you label yourself as a 'failure,' we need to know what *failure* means to you. How would you define a *failure*? Are you using terms and concepts that you have never defined for yourself or others? This technique—defining the terms—is known as the 'semantic technique' because it asks you to define the meaning of the terms you are using.

"Imagine that you are a scientist (or a psychologist) doing research. Someone says, 'Bill is a failure,' and you want to determine if this statement reflects an accurate perception of Bill. The first thing we need to do is define *failure*. For example, you might define failure as:

- Having no success
- Not able to achieve rewards
- Inferior to almost everyone on everything

"Or, if you are prone to self-criticism and depression, you might have a rather unique way of defining failure for yourself. You might define failure in a way that almost no one but you would agree constitutes a failure. For example, you might define yourself as a failure by the following criteria:

- Not doing as well as I'd like
- Giving less than 100% of myself
- Not doing as well as someone else
- Doing poorly at a single task

"So today we are going to discover your definition of failure."

Question to Pose/Intervention

"How would you define the things that are bothering you? For example, how would we know if someone is worthless, successful, a failure, and so on? How would we know if someone is not some of these things? Give a detailed definition."

Example

THERAPIST: You said that you feel like a failure since Bill left you. How would you define *failure*?
PATIENT: Well, the marriage didn't work out.
THERAPIST: So you believe that the marriage didn't work out because you, as a person, are a failure?
PATIENT: If I had been successful, then he would still be with me.
THERAPIST: So could we conclude that people whose marriages don't work out are all failures?
PATIENT: No, I guess I wouldn't go that far.
THERAPIST: Why not? Should we have one definition of failure for you and another for everyone else?

This example illustrates how simply eliciting patients' negative and extreme definitions can assist them in understanding how irrational their perspective is. Individuals who define failure as less than "extraordinarily successful" can see that their definition is a polarized one that uses all-or-nothing terms—that is, "complete success" versus "complete failure." A variation on the semantic technique is to ask patients how others would define "success" or "failure." My preference is to focus patients on the positive end of the continuum by asking them to define terms such as "success" or "worth-while."

THERAPIST: You can see that your definition of failure is quite different from the way other people might see it. Few people would say that a person who is divorced is a failure. Let's focus on the positive end right now. How would most people define success in relation to a person?

PATIENT: Well, they might say that people are successful when they accomplish some of their goals.

THERAPIST: OK. So could we say that if someone accomplishes some goals, they are successful?

PATIENT: Right.

THERAPIST: Could we also say that people have different degrees of success? Some people accomplish more goals than others?

PATIENT: That sounds right.

THERAPIST: So, if we applied these ideas to you, could we say that you have accomplished some of your goals in life?

PATIENT: Yes, I did graduate from college, and I have been working for the past 6 years. I've been busy raising Ted, and he had some medical problems a couple of years ago, but I got the right doctors for him.

THERAPIST: So could we call these successful behaviors on your part?

PATIENT: Right. I've had some successes.

THERAPIST: Is there a contradiction, then, in your thinking—calling yourself a failure but saying that you have had several successes?

PATIENT: Yes, that doesn't make sense, does it?

Homework

Using Form 2.1 (at the end of the chapter), patients can practice defining the terms of their negative thoughts. Figure 2.1 is an example of a male patient articulating his definitions in order to test out the possibility that his thinking is idiosyncratic.

Possible Problems

For some patients the feeling *is* the definition—"I feel like I'm a failure." This "emotional reasoning" is the evidence the patient summons to support his or her notion of being a failure. I suggest to patients that they examine the way that the dictionary arrives at definitions. The dictionary examines the common use of a word is—that is, how do most people go about defining *failure*? I suggest that we are trying to come up with definitions that we could use in a scientific study—that is, definitions other people could use that would allow them to look at the same facts and come up with the same conclusions. For example, if I define "cold" as "less than 30 degrees Fahrenheit," then people can determine easily

Automatic thought: "None of my relationships work out."

Terms	Definitions	Problems with my definitions
None	Not a single one	All-or-nothing thinking. I have many different kinds of relationships, with various degrees of positives and negatives.
Relationships	Romantic relationships	I have many kinds of friendships, romantic relationships, and shorter-term relationships.
Work out	End up in a permanent, blissful marriage	Working out doesn't have to mean "permanent, blissful marriage." Things can be relatively more positive than negative for various degrees of time.

FIGURE 2.1. Defining the Terms.

whether it is cold outside. If I define successful behavior as making progress toward a goal, then I can evaluate whether someone is making progress toward his or her goal and thereby determine if he or she is achieving some success as a result of that behavior.

Other problems that often occur with patients' definitions are that they are too global, vague, idiosyncratic, and inconsistent. The definitions may change with change in moods. It is helpful to point out to patients that the definition may not be clear and precise enough. One way to convey this point is to ask: "If others used your definition of 'loser,' would they be able to go out and determine the people who are losers?" It is worth stressing that patients' definitions can be so idiosyncratic that they bear little resemblance to how others define the same terms. The therapist should ask, "Is this how most people would define this term?" or "How do others use this term?"

In addition, the term may be so value-laden and subjectively determined that it is not really amenable to definition. For example, for our purposes the term "worthwhile person" is meaningless, since there is no way we can go out and determine who is a worthwhile person and who is not. We might be able to grapple with the term "worthwhile actions"—that is, actions that have value for self and others—but even here we are skating a thin ice. It is common for individuals to find that they are upset over these kinds of meaningless terms, such as "worthwhile person" or "loser" or "total failure." Helping patients focus on behaviors that are more or less desirable for them sets the stage for evaluating how these behaviors could be increased or decreased in frequency.

Cross-Reference to Other Techniques

Techniques related to this one include eliciting automatic thoughts, categorizing them into cognitive distortions, looking at the evidence for and against the validity of the thought, and examining the quality of the evidence.

Form

Form 2.1 (Defining the Terms, p. 58).

TECHNIQUE: COST–BENEFIT ANALYSIS

Description

Once the patient has identified a thought that leads to disturbing feelings, the question is, "Are you motivated to change your thought?" We are interested in directing the patient to examine the consequences—both positive and negative—of holding a particular belief. Once the consequences are clear, the patient can choose either to maintain the belief or replace it with a different one.

Question to Pose/Intervention

"What are the costs and benefits of your belief? What are the advantages and disadvantages of your thought? List them. What would change if you believed this less? If you believed this more? If you had to apportion 100% between the costs and benefits, would it be an even 50/50 split? Perhaps 60/40? 40/60? How would you apportion the 100% between those costs and benefits? Alternatively, look at a thought that is more positive or less critical. What are the costs and benefits of that thought? How does this cost–benefit analysis compare with the analysis of your original thought?"

Example

THERAPIST: Let's examine your thought "I'll get rejected if I go to that party." I'd like you to write that thought down and put a line down the middle of the page. On the left side at the top, write "advantages" and on the right, "Disadvantages." (*The patient constructs Figure 2.2.*) Now let's examine all the advantages of believing that you will be rejected at the party.

PATIENT: I can't think of any advantages.

Advantages	Disadvantages
I won't be surprised.	I'm anxious.
I avoid rejection.	My self-esteem sinks.
	I avoid people.
	I'm less assertive.
	I don't get what I want—settle for less.
	I feel inferior to others.
	I don't meet people I'd like to know.

FIGURE 2.2. Advantages and Disadvantages of the Thought: "I'll Get Rejected If I Go to That Party"

THERAPIST: There are always reasons or advantages that people have for believing something. Is there any way that this thought protects you?

PATIENT: Well, I guess if I believe that I'll get rejected, I won't be surprised—I'll be prepared for it.

THERAPIST: OK. Any other advantages?

PATIENT: I might be able to avoid rejection by avoiding the party. (*The therapist and patient then examine the disadvantages.*) If I think I'll be rejected, it makes me anxious and lowers my self-esteem. It makes me avoid people. (*The therapist and patient continue to examine if there are any other advantages or disadvantages, constructing Figure 2.2. They then divide up 100 points between the advantages and disadvantages.*) The disadvantages outweigh the advantages. If I were to divide up 100 points, I'd say it's 10% for the advantages and 90% for the disadvantages.

THERAPIST: So the disadvantages outweigh the advantages by 80 points.

The therapist is not finished with this patient. An alternative assumption or thought is examined: "I should care less about what people think of me." The therapist and patient construct a cost–benefit analysis for this new thought and weigh the tradeoffs (Figure 2.3). The patient concludes that the advantages are 95% and the disadvantages are 5%—a resultant of 90% in favor of the advantages. Clearly, the patient is better off believing she should care less about what people think of her.

What if the patient finds that the advantages outweigh the disadvantages of a maladaptive assumption? Then what? As an example, consider the following. Bill believes: "I should always meet the expectations of my boss no matter how unreasonable they may be." Bill claims that the advantages of this belief are that he will work harder, he will get himself "psyched up," and that "everyone on the job is like that," and he can't be different. The disadvantages include anxiety, self-criticalness, overwork, and subservience to his boss's irrational demands. When he weighs the advantages, he gives them 70%; the disadvantages are given 30%. Consequently, he believes that the advantages outweigh the disadvantages—that is, on balance, this thought "works" for him. Even when the therapist examines the evidence that he must believe he has to meet *all* of his boss's irrational expectations to motivate himself, he still concludes that he needs this thought to be productive on the job.

THERAPIST: You have concluded that this thought works for you?

BILL: Yes. If I didn't think this way, I couldn't work there.

Advantages	Disadvantages
I'd be less anxious at parties.	Maybe I'll meet someone who doesn't like me because I'll take too many chances.
I'd be more assertive.	
My self-esteem would fluctuate less.	
I'd meet new people.	
I'd feel less hopeless.	
I'd feel more relaxed with new people.	
It could help me at work.	

FIGURE 2.3. New Thought: "I Should Care Less about What People Think of Me."

THERAPIST: OK. Well you're entitled to believe anything that you wish. If you are committed to this thought and choose to believe it, then I assume that you are willing to absorb the costs of this thought.

BILL: What do you mean?

THERAPIST: I assume that you are willing to pay the costs of anxiety, overwork, self-criticism, and having your moods depend on the whims of your boss.

BILL: I don't *want* to feel anxious and self-critical.

THERAPIST: Yes, I know you don't like the costs of this assumption. But if that is the thought that you believe you need, there is no way of getting around the costs. *Those are the costs of that thought.*

This excerpt illustrates how patients must confront their choices—either a problematic thought must be modified or they will have to pay the costs. For this particular session, Bill decided to maintain his belief. This technique frees patients to examine the consequences of their beliefs—they can choose to hold any belief as long as they recognize the cost of the belief.

Homework

The cost–benefit analysis is useful in confronting patients' procrastination, avoidance, or underlying assumptions. Consider the example of a patient who is considering joining a health club. He is asked to list the costs and benefits of sitting at home watching television versus the costs and benefits of going to the health club. Similarly, the patient and the therapist may have identified an underlying belief that "I must be certain before I do anything." This belief can be submitted to a cost–benefit analysis and contrasted with another thought, "I can take reasonable risks." The purpose of the cost–benefit analysis is to confront patients with the issue of choosing among alternatives and to focus on the motivation to change.

Homework can consist of utilizing Form 2.2 (at the end of the chapter), shown below, in which the patient and therapist identify thoughts or choices confronting the patient and weigh their tradeoffs. The therapist can say, "We have identified several thoughts [or behaviors] that are problematic for you. I'd like you to list these and then write out the costs and benefits of each one and look at how they weigh out for you."

Possible Problems

A very common problem is denial that there is any benefit to a negative thought: "Oh, I know that it is irrational. There are no benefits. I don't know why I keep doing it." Here the therapist should insist on examining the possible "silent" benefits for the patient: "There are very few things that we do for which we see no benefit. For example, even though people may claim that cigarette smoking has very high costs and no real benefits, people who smoke actually get some short-term benefit from smoking. It helps them feel better, it staves off the craving for a smoke." The therapist can ask the patient to try *not* to be rational—"try to be neurotic when you think about the possible benefit of your negative thought." Possible benefits for negative thoughts include avoiding frustration, hopeless behavior, failure, risk, and discomfort. Possible benefits for worry include being prepared, avoiding surprises, and motivating oneself. Sometimes it is useful to ask patients to close their eyes, imagine confronting the choice (e.g., going to the health club vs. watching TV), and thinking of all the reasons and feelings that get in the way.

Another problem is that some of the benefits of a negative thought or behavior, though short-lived, confer highly reinforcing effects in their immediacy and saliency. For example, smoking, drinking, overeating, and passive behavior may confer immediate benefits of high intensity. Thus patients need to examine the longer-term negative consequences of these thoughts and behaviors. The costs of changing are "front-loaded" or up-front—using an investment analogy might be helpful—with payoffs accumulating over time (see Leahy, 2001a).

Cross-Reference to Other Techniques

Related techniques include eliciting automatic thoughts, vertical descent, role playing against the thought, and guessing at the thought. Imagery techniques can be helpful in eliciting reasons for not engaging in positive behavior or thoughts.

Form

Form 2.2 (Cost–Benefit Analysis, p. 59).

TECHNIQUE: EXAMINING THE EVIDENCE

Description

In describing this technique of examining the evidence, the therapist might say, "Now that you have defined your terms and indicated what would be a test of your thought, including what predictions you might make from your thought, you should examine the evidence both *for and against* the validity of your negative beliefs. Let's take the negative thought 'I'm a failure.' You have defined failure as 'not achieving goals' and success as 'achieving goals.' Placing a line down the center of the page, with 'I'm a failure' written at the top of the page, list all the evidence in the left-hand column that is consistent with your belief and all the evidence in the right-hand column that contradicts your belief. [Figure 2.4 provides an example.]"

Evidence for . . .	Evidence against . . .
Tom doesn't like me.	Lots of friends like me.
I did poorly on the last job report.	I'm honest and decent.
Carol is making more money than I am.	I'm doing much better than the average person.
	I graduated from college.
	I've been employed since college.
	I support myself.
For (%): 20%	Against (%): 80%
Subtract: % Against – % For = 60%	

FIGURE 2.4. Testing the Belief "I'm a Failure."

"In addition to counting the items for and against the validity of your thought, it is important to weigh them psychologically—that is, how much does this evidence convince you one way or the other? In weighing the evidence, you will notice that there is almost always some evidence to support any belief; the important point is to examine all evidence on *both* sides of the ledger.

When testing a belief, it is essential to put the belief into the form of a proposition about facts—that is, a statement about what you believe is the truth. Avoid any statements that simply refer to feelings—such as, 'I feel sad, depressed, angry, etc.'—because these are not thoughts or beliefs that we can test. It would make no sense to argue that you do not feel sad if you say that you do feel sad. Similarly, we need to avoid examining rhetorical statements, such as 'Isn't life awful?' or 'I can't believe that this is happening.' Again, these are not testable thoughts. You can rephrase them as propositions, such as 'Life is awful' or 'It's terrible that this is happening,' so that we could then collect evidence for and against the validity of these thoughts.

"Examine statements that you are testing to see if they are meaningless because they are true for almost everyone: For example, 'It is *possible* that I could have a panic attack' is meaningless because it is true for everyone. What you are really worried about—and which we *can* test against the facts—are the implied beliefs, such as 'I probably will have a panic attack' or 'It would be terrible if I had a panic attack.' Finally, we cannot collect evidence on 'what-if' statements, because these are not clear statements about reality. Consequently, you need to transpose your 'what if' statements into propositions. For example, 'What if I have a panic attack' might become 'I'm going to have a panic attack' or 'It would be terrible to have a panic attack.' "

Question to Pose/Intervention

Weigh the evidence for and against your thought. Is it 50/50? 60/40? 40/60? If you subtracted the costs from the benefits, what would the result be? In addition, you might consider an alternative, more positive thought. Conduct a similar cost–benefit analysis and compare the results."

Example

THERAPIST: You said that you are a "loser" because you and Roger got divorced. We already defined what it is to be a loser—someone who does not achieve anything.

PATIENT: Right. That sounds really extreme.

THERAPIST: OK. Let's look at the evidence for and against the validity of this thought that you have achieved something. Draw a line down the center of the page. On the top I'd like you to write "I have achieved some goals."

PATIENT: (*Draws line and writes statement.*)

THERAPIST: What is the evidence that you have achieved some goals?

PATIENT: I graduated from college, I raised my son, I worked at the office, I have some friends, and I exercise. I'm a good person—I am reliable, and I care about my friends.

THERAPIST: OK. Let's write all of that down. Now in the left-hand column let's write down evidence against the validity of the thought that you have achieved some goals.

PATIENT: Well, maybe it's irrational, but I would have to write down that I got divorced.

THERAPIST: OK. Now, in looking at the evidence for and against the validity of your thought that you have achieved some goals, how do you weigh it out? 50/50? Some other ratio?

PATIENT: I'd have to say it's 95% in favor of the positive thought.

THERAPIST: So how much do you believe now that you have achieved some goals?

PATIENT: 100%.

THERAPIST: And how much do you believe that you are a failure because you got divorced?

PATIENT: Maybe *I'm* not a failure, but the marriage failed. I'd give myself about 10%.

Homework

Using Form 2.3 (at the end of the chapter), the patient is asked to write down a negative thought each day (or to write down negative thoughts identified in the session) and to weigh the evidence for and against the validity of the negative thoughts. I tend to prefer having the patient also weigh the evidence for and against the validity of a positive thought, since this is more likely to lift his or her mood.

Possible Problems

As with other cognitive challenges to negative thoughts, the patient may say, "I know it's irrational, but I feel that it's true." As noted, this category of response is called emotional reasoning and can be addressed through a variety of techniques including double standard, cost–benefit analysis, point–counterpoint, imagery induction, imagery restructuring, feared fantasy, and role playing. Other patients may view these evaluations of negative thoughts as invalidating, dismissive, critical, or minimizing. The therapist can explain that the purpose of the exercise is simply to examine the evidence, as the patient sees it, in regard to his or her thoughts. Indeed, some negative thoughts are true, and this validity can readily lead to an examination of underlying assumptions that fuel the emotional impact of the thought, or to problem-solving endeavors that can change the external reality to which the patient responds problematically.

Cross-Reference to Other Techniques

Related techniques include eliciting and identifying automatic thoughts, cost–benefit analysis, categorizing cognitive distortions, defining the terms, double-standard technique, examining limited information searches, and examining schemas.

Form

Form 2.3 (Examining the Evidence, p. 60).

TECHNIQUE: EXAMINING THE QUALITY OF THE EVIDENCE

Description

In describing this technique of examining the quality of the evidence, the therapist might say: "You have now listed the evidence for and against the validity of your negative belief—a belief with which you may be prosecuting and punishing yourself. You may have already established that you would be better off without this belief, but as you examine the evidence that supports your belief, you find that you have many reasons for holding on to your negative thought. The question you can ask yourself then is, 'How good is this evidence?' To put it in very direct terms, would you be able to convince other people of your negative belief? Would a jury accept your evidence as valid? For example, take the negative belief 'I'm a failure.' You may have offered the following evidence in support of your belief:

- 'I feel like a failure.'
- 'Dan thinks I'm not as good as he is.'
- 'I didn't do well on the exam.'
- 'I lost the game in tennis.'

"Imagine that you are presenting these items to a jury as evidence of the case you make against yourself. You say to the jury, 'I feel like a failure—so that proves I am a failure.' Do juries accept feelings as evidence of someone's worth? No.

"Or how about saying to the jury, 'I'm a failure because Dan thinks I'm not that great.' Would the jury accept hearsay about Dan's evaluation of you as evidence? Again, no. If you pointed out that you did not do well on the exam, would the jury conclude that you are a failure as a person? Again, definitely not. Your feelings, your need for approval, or your poor exam results would not be regarded as quality evidence of your failings as a person.

"The important point to make is that you may be using, as evidence, information that is emotional, personal, debatable, and irrelevant. Just because you have come up with a lot of reasons to support your negative belief does not imply that the evidence is conclusive or even relevant. For example, you may be concluding that you are a failure because you are using emotional reasoning, personalizing an event, overgeneralizing, using perfectionistic standards, discounting your positives, filtering out your negatives, mind reading, jumping to conclusions about the future, referring to irrelevant material, or drawing illogical conclusions."

Question to Pose/Intervention

"How good is the evidence supporting and refuting your belief? Do you think that other people would consider your evidence convincing? Irrational? Extreme? Would other people think that you could convince a jury that your statement is true? Or would they think it is too extreme? Why? What are some of the errors in your thinking?"

Example

THERAPIST: You said that your evidence of being unattractive is that you feel ugly and that Roger broke up with you.

PATIENT: I just don't feel attractive.

THERAPIST: Right. You also said that the women in the magazines are more attractive than you are.

PATIENT: That's right. They look like they're perfect.

THERAPIST: What do you think about the quality of your evidence in relation to the thought "I'm ugly"? Would you be able to convince a jury that someone *is* ugly because they *felt ugly*?

PATIENT: No. I guess they would require some kind of other information.

THERAPIST: You mean, some kind of independent information—something other than the way you feel?

PATIENT: Yeah, like what other people think of that person.

THERAPIST: Are there some men who think you're attractive?

PATIENT: Well, there have been a number of men who find me attractive. But I'm not interested in them.

THERAPIST: As evidence that you are not attractive, you cite the fact that Roger broke up with you. What were the reasons for the breakup?

PATIENT: We weren't getting along. He just can't commit to anyone. And he lies.

THERAPIST: So you personalized *his* shortcomings and concluded that *you* are not attractive?

PATIENT: That's true.

THERAPIST: I wonder if we could look at the evidence that you use to support your negative beliefs and see if the evidence is relevant and convincing or if it is characterized by these kinds of distortions.

Using Form 2.4 (at the end of the chapter), the patient can list the evidence supporting the negative beliefs and evaluate its quality by ferreting out any distortions. Many patients find it helpful to recognize that their beliefs are supported by evidence that is not convincing or that is irrelevant. (See Figure 2.5 for an example.)

Homework

The patient can keep track of several thoughts during the week, identifying each negative thought and the evidence for and against the validity of that negative thought. Or the patient can review previous homework or notes from therapy sessions, wherein he or she has listed evidence for his negative thoughts. The assignment is to examine the possible problems with the evidence, focusing on whether there are cognitive distortions, biases, or illogical reasoning. The therapist might say: "After you have listed the evidence in favor of your negative thoughts, go back and use the form for examining the quality of evidence [Form 2.4 at the end of the chapter]. Now ask yourself if your evidence has any distortions in it. You can even grade each piece of evidence for its quality, as A, B, C, D, or F. You can also grade the quality of evidence against the validity of your negative thoughts."

Automatic thought: "I'm a failure."

Evidence	Possible problems with its quality or relevance
I feel like a failure.	My feelings are not proof of anything (*emotional reasoning*).
Dan thinks I'm not as good as he is.	Whatever Dan thinks is his opinion. It doesn't make sense for me to conclude that Dan's opinion makes me a failure (*personalizing an event*).
I didn't do well on the exam.	Doing well or poorly on one performance doesn't make someone a failure. I did well on several exams, but that doesn't mean I'm a genius (*overgeneralizing, using perfectionistic standards, discounting positives*).
I lost the game in tennis.	Losing a game in tennis is part of the game of tennis. It doesn't mean that I'm a failure. Everyone loses at a game of sports at some point—even world champions lose games (*discounting positives, using perfectionistic standards, drawing illogical conclusions*).

FIGURE 2.5. Examining the Quality of the Evidence.

Possible Problems

Many patients adhere to their feelings as evidence: "I feel it's true, even though I know it's not rational. I know the evidence doesn't support this view." Several questions can be raised for this kind of response. First, the therapist can utilize the point–counterpoint technique, described later in this book. Second, the therapist can point out that feelings are important, though they are not evidence, and we need to distinguish between feelings and facts. Third, the therapist can explain that *feeling* the validity or invalidity of a belief is a different level of experience from *mental* or *cognitive* knowledge. When patients really *feel* that a particular belief is truly invalid, their maladaptive belief will have changed even more. Moreover, the therapist can note that feeling an old, habitual belief is truly *not* true may come later, after examining the facts and the logic of their thinking a number of times.

Cross-Reference to Other Techniques

As indicated, it is helpful to utilize the point–counterpoint technique, the double-standard technique, role plays, vertical descent, and examining cognitive distortions and the logic or inferences drawn.

Form

Form 2.4 (Examining the Quality of the Evidence, p. 61).

TECHNIQUE: Defense Attorney

Description

In describing this technique of the defense attorney, the therapist might say: "In challenging your thoughts, you can imagine yourself brought into a trial where the prosecution (played by your automatic thoughts) has been attacking you for the last several days, labeling you as a lazy loser, an incompetent, and a generally guilty person. You are now given the task of playing the role of the defense attorney who must attack the evidence, the credibility of the witnesses against you (the defendant), and the logic of the prosecution's case. After suffering through several days of prosecution, you would not expect the defense to get up and simply say 'My client is innocent,' and then sit down and rest the case. You would expect a vigorous defense, one in which you would present your own evidence and witnesses on your own behalf. As the attorney, you do not have to believe in the innocence of your client (that is, yourself). You only have to take the job seriously." (For this analogy, see Freeman et al., 1990; Reinecke, Dattilio, & Freeman, 1996.)

Question to Pose/Intervention

"If you were trying to act as your own attorney whose job was to defend yourself, what would you say in your own defense? Try to be the best lawyer possible in defending yourself."

Example

THERAPIST: You've been criticizing yourself for much of your adult life, calling yourself a loser, a worthless person, lazy. Now I want you to imagine that you have been hired as "Tom's lawyer," and you have to defend Tom against these slanderous attacks. It's not necessary that you believe in Tom's innocence or even that you like Tom. I just want you to be a competent lawyer in your defense of Tom. I'll play the part of the prosecutor and tell you how bad Tom is. You defend Tom.

PATIENT: OK.

THERAPIST: Tom is a lazy loser who has never accomplished anything.

PATIENT: That's not true. He has graduated from college. He has a good job, he supports his family, and his boss thinks he's doing well.

THERAPIST: Well, Tom just feels like a loser to me.

PATIENT: Feelings don't count as evidence in court. The facts don't support the idea that he's a loser.

THERAPIST: Well, he's not perfect, so he's a loser.

PATIENT: If that were true, then *everyone* would be a loser.

The advantage of this defense attorney exercise is that many people find it easier to imagine being a lawyer defending someone else than defending themselves. By taking on the "professional role" of lawyer, patients can place themselves in a role of demanding proof, questioning evidence, challenging the prosecutor—that is, all the things we expect from lawyers.

Homework

The therapist can instruct the patient to imagine acting as his or her own defense attorney by posing the following questions to consider and supplying Form 2.5 (at the end of the chapter).

"You can prompt yourself in the role of defense attorney by asking the following legalistic questions:

What laws has the defendant broken?
What crime is the defendant charged with?
Is there overwhelming evidence against the defendant?
Would the jury convict?
Are there other explanations for the defendant's behavior?
Did the defendant act maliciously?
Was the defendant acting in a way that a reasonable person might act?
Is someone else guilty—or share part of the responsibility?
Given what the prosecutor is able to actually prove, does it follow that the defendant is guilty of something terrible? Would we apply these rules to everyone?"

Possible Problems

As with many techniques that actively challenge negative thoughts, patients may view this exercise as a naïve attempt to lie to themselves so that they feel better. In some cases, patients may believe that they deserve to criticize themselves and should not defend themselves, because they are really beneath contempt. These sabotaging thoughts should be elicited: "Can you tell me if you have any difficulty with the idea of acting as your own defense attorney?" Some patients believe that they cannot argue against the negative thoughts unless they totally believe the positive side. The therapist can point out that the role of a good lawyer is to take both sides, which allows the jury the opportunity to consider all points of view.

Cross-Reference to Other Techniques

Other relevant techniques include examining the evidence, the point–counterpoint technique, evaluating logical inferences, role playing, and categorizing cognitive distortions.

Form

Form 2.5. (Playing the Role of Your Own Defense Attorney, p. 62).

TECHNIQUE: ROLE PLAYING BOTH SIDES OF THE THOUGHT

Description

In order to modify the negative thought, the patient and therapist can alternate between both sides of the thought. For example, the therapist initially can take the positive or rational position while the patient takes the negative position. After they have role-played these positions, they can switch sides, with the therapist supporting the negative thought and the patient, the positive thought. One advantage of these role reversals is that the patient can observe some highly useful challenges, as presented by the therapist, and the therapist can determine which rational responses work for the patient and which automatic thoughts are difficult for the patient. These role reversals can continue for several rounds.

Question to Pose/Intervention

"Let's take your negative thought and do a role-play. I'll play you in the role of the positive thought—that is, I'll respond in a positive and rational manner. You play the role of the negative thought—you try to convince me that your negative thoughts are really true."

Example

THERAPIST: Let's do a role play. You can play the role of the negative of you as a failure, and I will play you being rational and positive.

PATIENT: [as negative] You and Jane broke up, so you are a failure.

THERAPIST: [as positive] Well, that's all-or-nothing thinking. Are you saying that every single thing about me is a failure?

PATIENT: [as negative] No, but you failed.

THERAPIST: [as positive] You mean, one of my behaviors didn't work out?

PATIENT: [as negative] No, I'm saying that you are a failure as a person.

THERAPIST: [as positive] I'm not sure what it means to be a failure as a person. How could we observe me, in action, as "a failure as a person"?

PATIENT: [as negative] We'd look at how you messed up in the relationship.

THERAPIST: [as positive] You mean, you would look at some of my behaviors?

PATIENT: [as negative] Yeah, OK.

THERAPIST: [as positive] Which specific behavior would you cite?

PATIENT: [as negative] Well, you were critical of her.

THERAPIST: [as positive] OK, so you think that behavior didn't work? Were some of my behaviors positive or neutral?

PATIENT: [as negative] You did do some things that were positive. You were generous to her. You bought her gifts, you made dinner for her.

THERAPIST: [as positive] So some of my behaviors were positive, and some were negative? How could I be a failure as a person if I did some positive things, too?

PATIENT: [as negative] I guess there are negatives *and* positives about you.

THERAPIST: [as positive] You mean, just like every other human being?

PATIENT: [as negative] I guess so.

After the patient and therapist conduct this role play, the therapist can ask the patient which rational response didn't work well with which automatic thought. In the above example, the patient indicated that he'd had a hard time accepting that he had been critical of his girlfriend. He believed that he should never be critical, never make mistakes. This exchange led to an examination of his perfectionism and self-criticism and to an alternative assumption, "I can learn from my mistakes and try to correct them."

Homework

Using Form 2.6 (at the end of the chapter), the therapist can ask the patient to write out positive or rational arguments in answer to his or her negative thoughts and then write out a series of negative responses to these rational arguments. In addition, the patient is asked to indicate which automatic thoughts are still hard to handle and which rational responses do not work well. In the next session these can be examined for their underlying assumptions, such as "I should always be perfect" or "I should never make a mistake."

Possible Problems

Some patients agree with the negative thought and have a hard time arguing against something they believe. The instruction should be to present the kinds of arguments a therapist or friend might make—for example: "You don't have to believe anything right now, we are just trying to get an idea of different ways of thinking." Similarly, patients may say that they have different negative thoughts from those presented by the therapist. The therapist can respond: "You may not have these thoughts right now, but I'd like to see how you would handle them if you did have them."

Another problem with role playing is that some patients may think that the therapist is ridiculing or making fun of them. The therapist can answer: "I am not trying to make fun of you—if anything, I want to help you find some new ways of thinking and feeling. Sometimes the role playing can be annoying; just let me know when you feel that way and we can stop and consider other things to do."

Cross-Reference to Other Techniques

Other relevant techniques include categorizing the cognitive distortions, examining the costs and benefits, examining the evidence, the semantic technique, the double-standard technique, and the point–counterpoint technique.

Form

Form 2.6 (Role Playing Both Sides of the Thought, p. 63).

TECHNIQUE: DISTINGUISHING BEHAVIORS FROM PERSONS

Description

One of the common errors in thinking is to equate a single behavior with the entire person. Thus, if I fail at one behavior, then I am a complete failure. This technique helps patients isolate mistakes or errors and separate these from a global judgment of themselves. In addition, it facilitates patients' abilities to modify particular categories of cognitive distortions: labeling, personalizing, all-or-nothing thinking, and overgeneralization.

Question to Pose/Intervention

"It's important to distinguish between a behavior and an entire person. Sometimes we might say 'I'm a failure,' but the truth is closer 'I didn't do well on that test' or 'I got fired.' Let's look at some of your self-critical thoughts and examine if what you really should be talking about is some of your behavior rather than labeling yourself in such global terms."

Example

THERAPIST: You said that after the exam, you thought that you were a failure. I wonder if we can tell the difference between failing some questions on an exam and being a failure as a person.

PATIENT: But I feel like I am a failure.

THERAPIST: Well, that's emotional reasoning, isn't it? You're saying that your emotions are evidence of your failure as a person?

PATIENT: I know it's not rational.

THERAPIST: OK, but let's look at this idea that "I am a failure." Are there some things that you have done well in your life?

PATIENT: I've taken a lot of courses and passed every one of them. I have friends. I have a boyfriend.

THERAPIST: OK, so those are some successful behaviors. Even on this exam, weren't there 40 questions? Do you think you got some of them right?

PATIENT: Probably most of them. But I really blew it on about five of them.

THERAPIST: Would it be fairer to say that you did well on most of them but didn't do well on a few of them?

PATIENT: Yes, that's more accurate.

THERAPIST: So is this appraisal of not doing well on a *few* of the test questions consistent with thinking that you are a failure as a person, or that you have made some mistakes?

PATIENT: That I've made some mistakes.

Homework

The homework is focused on distinguishing between global labels and specific behaviors. Patients are encouraged to use Form 2.7 (at the end of the chapter), on which they list negative personal labels—for example, "loser," "failure," "worthless"—and then to list relevant positive and negative behaviors. Also, patients are asked to list the negative and positive behaviors they can predict existing in the future—thereby helping them challenge the global labeling—and to articulate their conclusions after looking at the evidence.

Possible Problems

Some individuals are prone to affixing moral judgments on many of their own or others' behaviors. They may think that these judgments are conscientious, ethical, or moral. I have referred to this pattern as "moral resistance" and outlined a number of questions to pose by way of challenging this kind of thinking (Leahy, 2001b). For example, if the patient says "Well, if I did this bad thing, then it means I am bad," we can ask him or her if this rule is applicable to everyone—that is, anyone who ever does anything bad is a bad person. We can ask if this rule promotes human dignity—a question posed by the philosopher Immanuel Kant.

Another typical problem patients demonstrate is making categorical errors in claiming, for example, that "bad people do bad things." Indeed, we can argue that all people do bad things, good people do good things, and bad people do good things. Finally, we also can suggest that terms such as "good person" or "worthless" are not particularly meaningful. We might want to replace these global, value-laden labels with more empirically grounded thinking patterns, such as, "What can I predict about this person's behavior?" For example, the employee who labels her boss as a "bastard" may assume that everything he does will be negative. However, by replacing the global label with pragmatic, empirically-grounded predictions, she will see that her "bastard" boss actually does a lot of positive things—an important realization. The patient can then be asked how she can take advantage of the positives and avoid the negatives.

Cross-Reference to Other Techniques

Other relevant techniques include categorizing negative thoughts, downward arrow technique, examining costs and benefits, and examining the evidence.

Form

Form 2.7 (Evaluating Negative Labels, p. 64).

TECHNIQUE: EXAMINING VARIATIONS IN BEHAVIOR IN VARIOUS SITUATIONS

Description

A frequent error in thinking is to focus on a single instance of a behavior and then generalize it to the entire person. Many of our common language descriptors imply dispositions, traits, or temperaments. For example, we say "He was hostile," rather than stipulating: "I have observed him in 50 different situations, and in this one situation he was 20% hostile, as indicated by his use of critical language." Moreover, when we say "He was hostile," we are attributing the quality of the behavior to the person rather than to factors in the situation. By refocusing on situational factors—such as what led up to his behavior (or what provoked it), what happened after, or the history of his relationship with the other person—we are able to understand his behavior in context. Diffusing our focus beyond the single, given moment in time allows us to see variability in the behavior's frequency and intensity as well as in the situations in which it occurs. This wide-angle focus decreases the likelihood of labeling the person in one-dimensional terms and increases the ability to understand factors—such as provocation or potential consequences—that might support or mitigate the behavior under question.

Question to Pose/Intervention

"When we label someone we are often thinking in all-or-nothing terms. If you label yourself as a 'failure' or 'stupid' (or any negative tag), you are probably ignoring a lot of evidence. Consider the negative label you are using against yourself (or someone else). Now let's think about how much your behavior changes in different situations. Look for various degrees of your behavior. For example, if you label yourself as 'lazy,' try to rate your behavior at different times in terms of *how* lazy you are, from 0% to 100%. Are there some situations in which you are less lazy? Some situations in which you are energetic? What accounts for this variability in your behavior? How is this variation inconsistent with thinking of yourself only in terms of the label *lazy*?

Example

THERAPIST: You said the reason that you don't exercise is that you are "lazy." How lazy do you think you are, from 0% to 100%, where 100% represents totally immobility?

PATIENT: I guess when it comes to exercise, I'd give myself a 95%.

THERAPIST: Are there times when you have exercised?

PATIENT: Yeah, I went to the health club last week, but I hadn't gone for 2 weeks.

THERAPIST: So how lazy were you when you went to the health club?

PATIENT: I guess 0%.

THERAPIST: OK. You work full-time as an executive. What time do you start work, and what time do you finish?

PATIENT: I'm at work at 8 A.M., I finish at about 6 P.M. and then I drive home, which takes about an hour—and, of course, it took an hour's drive in the morning, too.

THERAPIST: So how lazy are you when you are fulfilling this schedule?

PATIENT: Not at all lazy. I'm working all the time.

THERAPIST: And you help out with the kids. You took your son to baseball practice. How lazy were you when you did that?

PATIENT: Not at all.

THERAPIST: So, if you are not lazy in a lot of those areas, then what does it mean to say that the reason you didn't exercise is that you are lazy?

PATIENT: Maybe I was just tired.

THERAPIST: How is that different from saying you are lazy?

PATIENT: It's not as self-critical.

Homework

Using Form 2.8 (at the end of the chapter), patients are asked to list one negative label each day that they apply to themselves or to someone else. Then they should examine how this behavior or quality varies at different times and in different situations. They are asked to examine why their behavior varies in different situations and what this variation says about labeling themselves in these all-or-nothing terms.

Possible Problems

Some individuals cling to their negative labels because they believe that criticizing themselves is both realistic and motivating. They often believe that they need to tell themselves how stupid or inferior they are so that they will not become complacent. The therapist can ask such patients to examine the costs and benefits of the labeling and criticism and to consider the value of increasing self-reward for positive behaviors. Some patients believe that this exercise will "let them off the hook," whereas they would not let themselves go that easily. It is useful for the therapist to point out that patients' variations in behavior may tell them something about what factors encourage positive behavior so that *this* behavior can be increased in frequency. A behavioral experiment could be constructed to help patients examine the advantages and disadvantages of self-reward, over a 2-week period, to see if the negative qualities increase. This exercise is especially useful with couples who believe that holding onto negative labels about their partner motivates the partner to comply.

Cross-Reference to Other Techniques

Relevant additional techniques include categorizing cognitive distortions, the continuum technique, the double-standard technique, vertical descent, cost–benefit analysis, and examining the evidence.

Form

Form 2.8 (Looking for Variations, p. 65).

TECHNIQUE: USING BEHAVIOR TO RESOLVE THE NEGATIVE THOUGHT

Description

Many times the automatic thought is true, and the patient is not distorting reality. Thus challenges to the thought may be insufficient in helping the patient feel more hopeful. However, a nondistorted automatic thought actually can make things more hopeful and the patient less helpless, because the focus then shifts to one of problem solving or problem acceptance and allows the patient the ability to use action to initiate change by acquiring the needed skills, be they social, communication, work-related, or whatever.

Question to Pose/Intervention

"Ask yourself, 'If the negative thought is true, then what can I do to make things better? What are some ways that I can improve my skills, solve the problem, or change the situation?' "

Example

THERAPIST: You sounded pretty discouraged about your job interview.

PATIENT: Yeah. I keep telling you that no one wants to hire me. I just blow the interviews.

THERAPIST: OK, well let's try to role play a scenario wherein I play the role of the person interviewing you, and you can play yourself at the interview. (*Patient and therapist interact, and the patient demonstrates that he acts in a grandiose fashion and blames previous employers.*)

PATIENT: So, how did I do?

THERAPIST: You're right. It turns out that your thought that you blow the interviews is correct.

PATIENT: Oh, great. Now I'm *really* hopeless.

THERAPIST: No. Not really. Actually, this is very good information. Now we have to shift to training you in interview skills. Let's start with examining what this person is looking for in hiring someone.

PATIENT: So, you're saying that my negative thoughts are true?

THERAPIST: In this case, it's great to find out that we can narrow things down to this problem. You can learn better interviewing skills.

The patient and therapist worked on improving his interviewing skills, making a list of *do's* and *don'ts* on interviews and practicing tape recording role plays in therapy. The patient subsequently received a job offer.

Homework

The therapist can explain: "Sometimes our negative thoughts are true. Sometimes someone doesn't like us or something doesn't work out. However, that reality then leads to another set of more positive questions: 'What can I do to solve the problem?' or 'What alternatives are available to me?' Use this form [2.9, at the end of the chapter] to make a list of several things that are bothering you, and then make a list of a number of things that you could do to make matters better for yourself."

Possible Problems

Some patients believe that if their automatic thoughts are true, then things are really hopeless. Consequently, it is essential to point out that cognitive therapy is a form of reality testing or reality therapy in that we examine or evaluate negative thoughts. Thus we remain open to negative thoughts being true. Some patients believe that if the therapist recognizes that a negative thought is true, then the therapist is criticizing them. On the contrary, the therapist can explain that recognizing the truth of a negative thought empowers patients to find ways of making needed changes. However, patients may be so self-critical that they believe that they cannot make these changes. These negative self-statements can be tested out with behavioral assignments: "Let's make a list of simple positive behaviors, and you tell me which of these you think you can do and which you cannot do. Let's look at the costs and benefits of doing each one of these."

Cross-Reference to Other Techniques

Other relevant techniques include graded task assignment, assertiveness training, problem solving, vertical descent, cost–benefit analysis, and examining the evidence.

Form

Form 2.9 (Changing Negative Thoughts by Changing Behavior, p. 66).

FORM 2.1. Defining the Terms

In the left-hand column list the main terms in your automatic thought. In the middle column, define each term. In the right-hand column ask yourself: "Am I using any cognitive distortions? Am I defining things too broadly? Too narrowly? Too vaguely? Am I not allowing for variation—for example, am I demanding that things have to be a certain way to be acceptable? Are there less severe or rigid ways to define these terms? Would other people use a different set of definitions?

Automatic thought: _____

Terms	Definitions	Problems with my definitions
		Conclusions:

FORM 2.2. Cost–Benefit Analysis

After listing the costs and benefits of your belief, circle the most significant ones. Why are these costs or benefits important? Could you challenge your view that these costs and benefits are important? What is an alternative belief—one that is more adaptive? How would you do a cost–benefit analysis on that belief?

Belief:

Costs	Benefits

Result: Costs =   **Benefits =**

Costs – Benefits =

Conclusions:

FORM 2.3. Examining the Evidence

Identify the thought that you are going to evaluate. You might consider testing the negative thought by testing a positive version of the thought—for example, you can test the thought "I'm a failure" by testing the thought "I have had some successes." List the evidence for and against the validity of your thought. Include emotional and irrational "evidence," because this will help us understand how you are thinking about these things. Then weigh out the evidence for and against the validity of your thought, dividing 100 points between the two. Is it 50/50? 60/40? 40/60? Or some other ratio?

Belief: _____

Evidence for . . .	Evidence against . . .
For (%):	*Against (%):*
Subtract: % Against – % For = %	
	Conclusion:

FORM 2.4. Examining the Quality of the Evidence

Identify an automatic you wish to evaluate. Then list evidence that supports that thought. Last, evaluate each piece of evidence for signs of cognitive distortions, such as emotional reasoning, personalizing an event, overgeneralizing, using perfectionistic standards, discounting your positives, filtering out information, mind reading, jumping to conclusions about the future, referring to irrelevant material, or drawing illogical conclusions.

Evidence	Possible problems with its quality or relevance
	Conclusions:

FORM 2.5. Playing the Role of Your Own Defense Attorney

Many times we criticize ourselves but don't take the time to defend ourselves against our negative thoughts. In this exercise you play the role of a lawyer defending yourself against the negative "charges" or criticisms being made against you. Answer each of the questions in this form and examine whether you are being too harsh on yourself.

What "law" was broken? With what offense are you charging yourself? Is there overwhelming evidence?
How would you defend yourself?
Are there other explanations for your behavior?
Did you act with malice or cruelty?
How would a responsible person act?
What is the quality of the case for and against you?
How would a jury evaluate this evidence?

FORM 2.6. Role Playing Both Sides of the Thought

Use *two* copies of this form. With the first copy, you start as the negative thought and argue back with positives. With the second form, you start as the positive thought and argue back with the negatives. Review your answers and then circle those you think are not that helpful to you and the negative thoughts that are still strong.

Negative	**Positive**

Role playing both sides of the thought

Positive	**Negative**

FORM 2.7. Evaluating Negative Labels

In the top left portion of the form write down a negative label of yourself (or someone else) and rate the degree to which you believe this label to be true. Then write out the negative behaviors that are evidence of this negative trait and the positive behaviors that suggest that the person is not always this negative. In addition, list the negative and positive behaviors that you can predict in the future. What conclusions would you draw from this information? Do you still believe that this negative label is as true as you first thought?

Negative Label: _____

Belief (%): _____

Relevant negative behaviors	Relevant positive behaviors

What are some negative behaviors I can predict in the future?	What are some positive behaviors I can predict in the future?

Conclusion:	Rerate the negative label (%):

FORM 2.8. Looking for Variations

Write down the negative label that you are applying to yourself or another person. Now think about what label you would use to describe the most negative end of that scale—for example, "cruel"—and then think about the most positive end of the scale—for example, "kind." Write these ends of the scale in the top right-hand corner of the table. Now write down variations in that kind of behavior in the left-hand column. In the right-hand column, describe the situations in which these different behaviors occur. For example, let's say that you label yourself as "lazy." The other end of the scale is "motivated" or "energized." Write out examples of various degrees of lazy and motivated or energetic in your behavior. Describe the situations. What conclusions would you draw?

Negative label:	Negative end of scale:
	Positive end of scale:
Examples of positive and negative behavior:	Describe the situation:
Conclusion:	What situations are the most positive? Most negative?

FORM 2.9. Changing Negative Thoughts by Changing Behavior

Many times our negative thoughts are true—or, at least, have some degree of truth. When this occurs, it's a great opportunity to think of how you can change your behavior to make things better, or figure out some alternatives that might be better for you. For example, the man who thinks he's not good at job interviews might find out that this negative thought is true. The changes in behavior that he could try could include learning better job interview skills. The woman who laments, "I'm all alone" may be correct a lot of the time. She can learn how to be more assertive, join activities, and also do more rewarding things when she is alone. In this form, list some of your negative thoughts in the left-hand column, and then list some behaviors or activities that you could carry out to help make things better for yourself.

Negative thought	Possible changes in behavior or ways to solve the problem
	Conclusion: **To–do List:** Behaviors When will I do them?

CHAPTER 3

———

Evaluating Assumptions
and Rules

Even if automatic thoughts are true, at times, a fruitful question can then be raised: "Why would that be such a problem?" Using the vertical descent exercise, we examined the implications of rejection for the patient by asking "Why would it bother you if someone did not like you?" and the patient answered, "Because it means that I'm worthless." Recurrent problems of depression, anxiety, and marital conflict often are the result of rigid rules, assumptions, "shoulds," imperatives and "if–then" beliefs. Research on vulnerability to depressive relapse indicates that underlying assumptions of perfectionism and need for approval are activated in negative mood states and by negative life events (Miranda & Persons, 1988; Miranda, Persons, & Byers, 1990; Segal & Ingram, 1994). These underlying assumptions may not seem problematic when things are going well—for example, the man who believes that he is lovable when he has a partner may feel fine when he is in a relationship. However, the threat or actual termination of a relationship may precipitate a major depressive episode, because the underlying assumption (e.g., "I can't be happy if I am alone") and the negative personal schema ("I am unlovable") are activated.

During relatively stable periods, these underlying assumptions may not be apparent. The therapist can examine past episodes of depression or conflict (e.g., "Tell me about a time when you felt really bad. What led up to it?"). Alternatively, the therapist can ask patients to imagine what could possibly happen that would upset them (e.g., the patient answers, "If I did poorly on an exam"). What negative thoughts and assumptions would be activated? These might include, using the examples above: "When we broke up, it made me think I can never be happy because I'll be alone"; or, "If I did poorly on the exam, it would mean that I didn't do my best, which would mean I'm a failure." In this chapter, we examine how the therapist can assist patients in identifying and testing the underlying assumptions and rules that may persist even when patients are feeling well.

TECHNIQUE: IDENTIFYING THE UNDERLYING ASSUMPTION OR RULE

Description

The vertical descent procedure usually leads to the underlying assumptions. These underlying assumptions are the "if–then" statements, rules, "shoulds," "musts," or "have-to's" that are rigid, imperative, and associated with vulnerability to depression, anger, and anxiety. For example, the vertical descent can lead to the following assumptions and rules (or standards):

"If I'm alone, I must be unhappy [or undesirable]."
   Or "If I'm alone, then I'll always be alone."
   Or "People who are single are losers."
   Or "I must have a partner to be happy."
   Or "I can't make myself happy—happiness is only derived from other people."

"If I don't do well at something, then I must be a failure."
   Or "I should always do well at everything."
   Or "I should do better than everyone."
   Or "It's awful to fail at something."
   Or "If I make a mistake, then I should criticize myself."

Depression, anxiety, and anger are associated with a variety of assumptions and rules; the same individual may have several such beliefs activated by a single event. Consider the individual whose supervisor dislikes her, even though she has been an effective employee for years. It is clear from the therapist's perspective that this situation is the result of a personality clash. The patient is terminated from employment but is able to obtain productive work elsewhere. However, this single event leads to the activation of several assumptions:

If I got fired, it means that I failed.
   ↓
If I failed at this job, then I'm a failure as a person.

Or

If I got fired from a job once, then no one will want to hire me [preceding her first interview following her termination].
   ↓
If my boss didn't like me, then I must be alienating everyone.
If people don't like me, then I must be worthless.

In reality, the event of being terminated may often lead to generous severance packages, the opportunity to get away from a stressful work environment, and the chance to pursue new work or training elsewhere. Of course, it may also lead to loss of income, the increased stress of uncertainty in finding a new job, and loss of rewards in the workplace. However, the individual's assumptions, as indicated above, place her at greater risk for depression because they are absolute, rigid, and self-condemning. There is little that is proactive or practical in these assumptions.

Question To Pose/Intervention

"Let's take some of the assumptions and rules that you have just identified. A lot of times we have rules for ourselves or for other people. These rules are often along the lines of 'I should succeed' or 'I must get the approval of other people.' Sometimes we make assumptions that 'If [such and such] happens, then [such and such] else is true.' For example, we might make the assumption 'If I don't succeed, then I am not that worthwhile' or 'If someone doesn't like me, then I must be unlovable.' "

The therapist may wish to use the more comprehensive Dysfunctional Attitude Scale (DAS), which can be scored for various dimensions. The therapist and patient then can examine any extreme responses on the DAS to determine vulnerability to future depression, anxiety, or anger.

Example

THERAPIST: You said that you are upset because you lost your job. I wonder what your thoughts were. Please try to complete the following sentence: "Losing my job bothers me because . . . "

PATIENT: I'll look like a failure.

THERAPIST: And, if I look like a failure, then that would mean . . .

PATIENT: Then I *am* a failure.

With another patient who experienced a breakup with his partner, the therapist inquired as to the meaning of this event for him.

THERAPIST: I know that you are upset because you and Ellen broke up. But let's look at what you are thinking that may add to this distress. "When I think about the fact that Ellen and I broke up, it bothers me because it means . . . "

PATIENT: I'll never find anyone.

THERAPIST: And if I don't have someone, it would mean . . .

PATIENT: I'll be miserable.

THERAPIST: It sounds like you think that you have to be in a committed relationship to be happy.

PATIENT: That's what I think, I guess.

Homework

Using Forms 3.1 and 3.2 (at the end of the chapter), the therapist can ask the patient to try to identify and monitor any "should" statements or rules that might underlie these beliefs. "See if you can identify and keep track of the rules and assumptions underneath those thoughts over the next week."

Possible Problems

Some patients believe that their rules, expectations, assumptions, and judgments are simply facts—that is, they believe, for example, "If you don't make a lot of money, then you are a failure" or "If you are not attractive, then you are ugly." Such patients treat their personal expectations, rules, and values as if they were scientific or objective data. When these rules or expectations are culturally shared—such as the widely held expectations that one should get married or one should be successful—the attachment to them as so-called facts is especially strong. At this stage of identifying the rules and assumptions, the therapist can make clear that the point is not to dispute them but simply to *record* them.

Cross-Reference to Other Techniques

Other techniques of relevance include identifying automatic thoughts, vertical descent, imagery techniques, rational role playing, and examining the costs and benefits.

Forms

Forms 3.1 (Evaluating Assumptions, Rules, and Standards, p. 89); Form 3.2 (Self-Help Form: Monitoring Your Assumptions, Rules, and Standards, p. 90).

TECHNIQUE: CHALLENGING THE "SHOULD" STATEMENT

Description

Many global rules or standards are moral imperatives, such as, "I should always be perfect" or "I should always be successful." Because they are stated as moral imperatives, they often imply a judgment about the worth or value of self or other. For example, "I should always be perfect" might imply "I'm worthless" or "inferior" and "I don't deserve to be happy." Self-criticism, guilt, and shame are common side effects of these moralistic "should" statements. Ellis (1994) has noted that many of these "should" statements are comprised of illogical, overgeneralized, and dysfunctional ideas. Numerous challenges can be lodged against the logic of "should" statements, such as:

> What is the rationale, logic, or evidence that one should do *X*?
> What is the origin of this rule?
> Would this rule be applicable to everyone?
> Could this rule really be a *preference* rather than a tenet?

Cognitive therapy and rational–emotive therapy attempt to deconstruct many of these "should" statements to reveal their illogical, unfair, and pejorative nature.

Question to Pose/Intervention

As indicated above, the therapist might pose a number of cognitive challenges. For example, consider the "should" statement "I should be perfect." Questions to pose might include:

1. What is the evidence that you should be perfect (and what is the evidence that you cannot be perfect)?
2. Where did this rule come from? Who or what authority ordained that you should be perfect?
3. Should *everyone* be perfect? Why would you have a different standard for others than you do for yourself?
4. Would it be more realistic to say that you would prefer to do a better job, rather than insisting on a futile need to be perfect?

Example

THERAPIST: You said that you should have done better on the exam. Why?

PATIENT: Because I'm smart, and I should do the best that I can do.

THERAPIST: What is the best that you can do?

PATIENT: I could get straight A's if I really applied myself.

THERAPIST: But since you are not always getting straight A's, it seems that you are not perfect. Should you be doing things that you might not be capable of?

PATIENT: Maybe if I tried harder, I'd get straight A's.

THERAPIST: What are the costs and benefits of demanding perfection?

PATIENT: The costs are that I feel pressured and disappointed. The benefits—maybe I'll try harder.

THERAPIST: So, how is it working?

PATIENT: I'm miserable.

THERAPIST: What if you had a standard that said "I'll try to do a good job." What would be the benefit of that notion compared to demanding perfection?

PATIENT: Maybe I wouldn't feel overwhelmed.

THERAPIST: Do all your friends get perfect grades?

PATIENT: No. Some of them are barely getting average grades, and some get good grades. No one I know is getting straight A's.

THERAPIST: What do you think of them?

PATIENT: They're doing OK. Maybe I'm tougher on myself.

THERAPIST: What if you applied the same expectations to yourself?

PATIENT: I'd be a lot better off.

Homework

"Select one of your "should" statements. Write it down on this form [3.3, at the end of the chapter], note the degree to which you believe it, the emotion it triggers and the degree to which it occupies you, the costs and benefits, and then challenge the statement by answering the questions.

Possible Problems

Some people believe that challenging their "should" statements will leave them irresponsible or immoral (see Leahy, 2001b) in their behavior. I have distinguished between good and bad "should" statements. Good "should" statements are rules that we would apply to everyone—for example, "You should not rape someone." Patients who object to challenging "should" statements can consider what constitutes a reasonable moral rule—for example, a reasonable moral rule is one that we would apply to everyone and that would enhance human dignity (see Leahy, 2001b). Saying that someone should be perfect in order to be worthwhile implies that everyone is not worthwhile, since no one is perfect. Most people would reject such an absolute and pejorative rule.

Furthermore, the idea that irresponsible behavior would be the outcome of discarding arbitrary and extreme shoulds can be challenged with the evidence: "Do you have perfectionistic standards for everything and always think in the most extreme terms?" Since it is unlikely that anyone is a perfectionist in everything, the evidence will indicate that the individual has not become irresponsible when more reasonable expectations are employed. The double standard is also useful: "If other people are not perfectionistic, then what accounts for the fact that they have not become irresponsible?"

Cross-Reference to Other Techniques

Many techniques are applicable to challenging "should" statements. As indicated, we use the cost–benefit analysis, the double-standard technique, and examine the logic and the evidence. In addition, the therapist might use the techniques of vertical descent, examining rules on a continuum, role plays, and acting against the belief.

Form

Form 3.3 (Examining and Challenging "Should" Statements, p. 91).

TECHNIQUE: IDENTIFYING CONDITIONAL RULES

Description

Let's assume that the patient's underlying assumption is "I am worthless if someone doesn't like me." In order to prevent rejection or negative appraisal by others, the patient may develop "conditional rules"—guidelines and strategies—that will serve to protect him or her from rejection. These might include rules such as "If I give everyone what they want, they won't reject me" or "If I sacrifice my needs to meet others' needs, then I won't be rejected." Conditional rules around the theme of perfectionism might include "If I work all the time, I might do a perfect job" or "If I try something difficult, I will probably fail, so I should avoid any challenges." Conditional rules allow the patient to cope with inadequacies and fears either by compensation—that is, trying to overcome feelings of inferiority by exerting extra effort—or by avoidance of situations that may carry the risk of rejection or failure—that is, avoiding people in order to avoid the possibility of rejection, or avoiding challenges in order to avoid defeat and failure. These ideas were originally developed by Alfred Adler (1964) and later applied to the cognitive model by Guidano and Liotti (1983) and Beck, Freeman and Associates (1990).

Two problems arise in relying on these conditional rules: First, these rules are almost impossible to live up to, and, second, they do not lead to disconfirmation of the underlying assumption. For example, the rule "If I defer to others, I will be liked, and then I won't be worthless" does not allow the person to test out and challenge the underlying assumption or core belief that "I am worthless if someone doesn't like me." For example, the alcoholic patient may believe "I can't survive unless I drink" but does not test out this assumption because he or she does not stop drinking.

Question To Pose/Intervention

"Sometimes we try to avoid worse things that might happen by living in accordance with certain rules. We have already identified your assumption or core belief—'If someone rejects me, then I am worthless.' Now the question we can consider is what guideline or rule do you use to avoid getting rejected? For example, 'In order not to get rejected, I tend to do . . . . '" [Alternatively: 'If I do (such and such), then I won't get rejected,' or 'If I do (such and such), then I won't fail.']

Similarly, sometimes we have rules about what we should avoid, so that bad things won't happen. For example, given your core belief of being worthless, if someone rejects you, you might have certain rules or strategies about how you can avoid any rejection. How would you answer the following question: 'In order to avoid getting rejected, I tend to avoid [what sorts of things or what sorts of people].' [Alternatively: 'In order to avoid failure, I tend to avoid (what sorts of behaviors or tasks).']

Example

In this case, the patient was a highly intelligent woman with perfectionistic standards who felt stuck working in a city job, rather than working in the private sector where there would be more demands and more risks of failure.

THERAPIST: You complain about your current job, but you are reluctant to look for a different job either in the private sector or in the city government. You are reluctant to look for something more challenging. What about challenge makes you uncomfortable?

PATIENT: I'm afraid I might fail.

THERAPIST: And what would that mean to you?

PATIENT: That I'm stupid.

THERAPIST: Are there other things that you have avoided doing or trying because you are afraid you might fail?

PATIENT: Yeah. I didn't go to law school—even though I got accepted.

THERAPIST: So your rule is to avoid doing things that you could fail in?

PATIENT: Right. I guess that's true. I don't want to find out I'm stupid.

THERAPIST: I wonder if there's another way of testing whether you are stupid. For example, how did you do on the SATs?

PATIENT: I did OK. I got in the 95th percentile.

THERAPIST: How did you do in college?

PATIENT: OK. But not as well as I'd like. I wasn't straight-A.

THERAPIST: What kind of grades did you get?

PATIENT: Mostly A's, but I got some B's too.

THERAPIST: If you consider the evidence, does it indicate that you are stupid or not stupid?

PATIENT: Well, I'm not stupid. But I'm not the smartest either.

THERAPIST: Is your assumption that you need to be the smartest in order not to be stupid?

PATIENT: Could be.

THERAPIST: I wonder what the consequence is of that belief?

Homework

The therapist might explain this basic idea and assign related homework in the following manner: "A lot of times we have certain rules that we use so that something bad won't happen. For example, some people have the belief or rule that 'If I worry, then I won't be caught by surprise.' We call this a 'conditional belief'—which is a belief that we think protects or prepares us. Other common conditional beliefs include: 'If I get 100%, then I won't be a failure,' or 'If I impress everyone, then I will be accepted.' Let's get an idea of these types of coping beliefs. Use this form [3.4, at the end of the chapter] to help you identify the conditional beliefs you employ on a regular basis.

Possible Problems

As occurs with the underlying assumptions (discussed above), some patients believe that their conditional beliefs are objective and useful. We emphasize at this point that we are simply collecting information. Later we can evaluate the utility of these conditional beliefs.

Cross-Reference to Other Techniques

Other relevant techniques include identifying assumptions, vertical descent, cost–benefit analysis, examining the evidence, and the double-standard technique.

Form

Form 3.4 (Identifying Conditional Beliefs, p. 92).

TECHNIQUE: EXAMINING THE VALUE SYSTEM

Description

Many assumptions concern one dimension of the individual—for example, an assumption about the necessity of success at work may include only achievement in financial gain. When the patient becomes anxious or depressed about this one dimension, other values are eclipsed. Examining and clarifying the value system can be helpful in placing certain self-deprecatory judgments in the perspective of other superseding values. For example, the patient who focuses excessively on self-worth, as measured by achievement, can be asked to consider additional values such as love, forgiveness, kindness, curiosity, personal growth, fun, and leisure. Forced choices can then be introduced: "If you had to choose between achieving more and giving more love, which would you choose?" The first task is to develop a list of life values, such as the ones just mentioned. Other values a patient may articulate, such as physical well-being, friendship, and religious values, also can be introduced. The patient can then compare the choices and determine which values are higher and which lower in his or her hierarchy. An alternative is to ask the patient to articulate which values he or she would like his or her child or partner to pursue (a variation of a double-standard technique), or which values he or she would like to see adopted by the general public.

Question to Pose/Intervention

"Let's examine a set of different values you might hold as important. Consider the following values: love, forgiveness, kindness, curiosity, personal growth, fun, leisure, self-esteem, religion, cultural/financial/work achievement, physical attractiveness, and approval by others. Let's take the issue you are upset about right now—achieving more at work. If you had to choose between achieving more at work and receiving and giving more love [alternatively, forgiveness, kindness, curiosity, personal growth, etc.], which would you choose?"

Example

THERAPIST: You said it was important to do really well on this project and that now you are criticizing yourself for your performance, which you deem inadequate. Sometimes we place a great deal of value on something—here, you are valuing work achievement. But there may be other things that you value as well. For example, consider love, forgiveness, kindness, curiosity, personal growth, fun, leisure, self-esteem, religion, cultural/financial/achievement, physical attractiveness, and approval by others. (*Writes these down.*) If you had to choose between work achievement and these other values, would any of these other values be more important to you?

PATIENT: Almost all of them. Maybe not leisure—although I really do need to take some time off.

THERAPIST: OK. So all of these other areas are actually more important to you? How about trying love, kindness, and forgiveness on yourself right now?

PATIENT: How?

THERAPIST: By being kind, loving, and forgiving toward yourself for not doing as well as you would have liked to do.

PATIENT: I guess if I did that, I'd feel a lot better.

THERAPIST: Didn't you just say that these are your more important values?

Homework

Patients can be given Forms 3.5 and 3.6 (at the end of the chapter), upon which they identify the value they are upset about—for example, work achievement—and then consider and rank 17 other values. Personal and societal hierarchies are thereby obtained.

Possible Problems

Sometimes what the patient is upset about is the most important value to him or her—for example, work achievement. The therapist can address this circumstance by asking the following questions:

1. If you pursue all of these other values, or any of them, isn't that of some value?
2. Would you apply the same value system to someone you love? Why not?
3. What would most people think of as a more desirable value system?
4. Why would their ranking of values be different from yours?

Cross-Reference to Other Techniques

Other relevant techniques include cost–benefit analysis, the double-standard technique, and vertical descent.

Forms

Form 3.5 (Values Clarification, p. 93); Form 3.6 (A Universal Value System, p. 94).

TECHNIQUE: DISTINGUISHING PROGRESS FROM PERFECTION

Description

Many people hold assumptions or standards that are unrealistically demanding, resulting in a sense of failure and futility. With this technique of aiming for progress rather than perfection, patients can focus on how to improve some aspect of a past performance, rather than struggling to attain an impossible standard. One of my patients, who attended Alcoholics Anonymous meeting, pointed out that this guideline was often mentioned in AA meetings.

Progress can be assessed in numerous ways. For example, the patient who scores a 36 on her first Beck Depression Inventory may complain that therapy isn't working when her BDI score is 22 after 6 weeks—and she is still depressed. Rather than evaluating treatment in terms of the total absence of depressive symptoms, I suggested that she acknowledge the progress she had made, as evidenced by the 14-point decrease in her BDI score. I suggested that we examine what led to this progress so that we could continue building on it and making more progress.

Question to Pose/Intervention

"Examine the advantages of trying to *improve* rather than trying to be *perfect*. If you try to be perfect, you will inevitably be frustrated. In contrast, if you try to make progress, you may feel more in control and hopeful. Are there some areas in which you have made progress? Do you give yourself credit for the progress or only for the perfection? What would be the consequence of giving yourself credit for progress rather than waiting for perfection?

Example

THERAPIST: You are upset right now because you got a lower grade than you expected in the exam. What was your grade?

PATIENT: I got a C. I didn't expect to do well, because I didn't study much. But this grade is a disappointment.

THERAPIST: What thoughts are you having?

PATIENT: I'm a real loser. I probably won't do well in the "real" world.

THERAPIST: Do you think that you could do better on your next test?

PATIENT: I can't imagine doing worse!

THERAPIST: What did you learn about the importance of preparing for the exam?

PATIENT: I guess that I have to study. I guess I'll do better next time.

THERAPIST: So, if you focused on progress and learning, then this might be something to learn from?

PATIENT: Yeah.

THERAPIST: This experience might be an inexpensive lesson in something really important—such as the importance of studying and preparing and not taking your performance for granted. Is this a lesson that could be useful to you throughout your life?

PATIENT: I guess it could.

THERAPIST: So let's focus on what you have learned and how this temporary downturn can motivate you to make progress in the future. It's better than thinking that you're a loser because you're not perfect.

PATIENT: That would be a better way of looking at it.

Homework

The therapist can give patients Form 3.7 (at the end if the chapter) on which to list different areas in which they are self-critical—for example, work or school performance, relationships, health, finances, etc. Then they list the various ways in which they could make progress in these areas—for example, work hard, study more, communicate better, exercise and diet, and save money.

Possible Problems

Some people believe that self-criticism motivates them to work harder. In cognitive therapy we try to focus on problem solving rather than self-criticism, and we point out to patients that diagnosing a problem is not the same thing as solving it. For example, diagnosing myself as 10 pounds overweight is not the same thing as solving the problem by exercising and dieting.

Cross-Reference to Other Techniques

Other techniques of relevance include identifying assumptions, behavioral assignments such as graded task assignment and activity scheduling, problem solving, and cost–benefit analysis.

Form

Form 3.7 (Making Progress Rather Than Trying for Perfection, p. 95).

TECHNIQUE: USING RELAPSE FOR LEARNING

Description

One way to challenge perfectionistic assumptions is to reframe relapse as a learning experiment. The patient with all-or-nothing assumptions about failure and acceptance (or any other standard or value) will view a relapse of a problem as an indication of how hopeless things are. For example, a patient who had decreased her consumption of alcohol to one drink per night had a relapse in which she consumed five drinks. She was highly self-critical and began to think that she was hopeless. However, I proposed that we consider viewing this as a learning experiment—or as a "natural experiment"—in which she could consider how she felt when she did not follow the self-help guidelines (Leahy & Beck, 1988). What she learned from this relapse was that our analysis was correct—(1) she felt worse the next day after a drinking binge, (2) trying to please her drinking friends by drinking with them was not in her interest, and (3) all in all, drinking more than one alcoholic beverage a night was not worth doing. Another way of viewing relapse is to reframe it as a helpful type of pain: "Make pain your friend by recognizing that pain is an essential aspect of learning, at times, and that it is trying to help you recognize what does not work for you."

Question To Pose/Intervention

"Although you are feeling badly that you have had a relapse of your problem, it may be helpful to use this setback as an important learning experience. What have you learned about yourself? What have you learned about what works, and does not work, for you? How could you use the pain and disappointment to guide you in the future?"

Example

A single man was despondent about getting back in touch with his ex-girlfriend, who had significant problems with drinking, mood lability, and reliability. He was now critical of himself because his recent encounter with her reminded him of how bad she was for him.

THERAPIST: It sounds like you are feeling badly about yourself because you saw her again, and you recognized that you were right in the first place to break up with her.

PATIENT: Yeah, but I didn't need to go through this again.

THERAPIST: Well, maybe now you have more information to remind you of what to do the next time.

PATIENT: I already had enough information. She's crazy.

THERAPIST: Well, you might look at what kinds of things you were saying to yourself to entice you to call her again.

PATIENT: Oh, I thought I could have a one-night stand.

THERAPIST: So you thought that you could just be casual about it and not get hurt?

PATIENT: Yeah. Just see her for the sex.

THERAPIST: Perhaps you are not as shallow as you thought you were.

PATIENT: That's a different way of seeing it.

Homework

"When we relapse from the progress we have made, it is a good opportunity to learn something. For example, if you are on a diet and then you overeat and feel bloated, you might start to criticize yourself. But the really valuable point from the experience is to learn what works, and does not work, for you. Using this table [Form 3.8, at the end of the chapter], think about some area that was working for you— for example, diet, exercise, communicating better, self-discipline—and then think about how 'you fell off the wagon.' Rather than criticize yourself, try to identify what worked and what did not work for you."

Possible Problems

Relapse can activate feelings of hopelessness and self-criticism. Common thoughts include "It didn't work, so I may as well give up" and "I'm a failure." This critical response is especially likely with substance disorders, such as drinking, smoking, and binge eating. It is helpful to point out that we can't have a relapse unless we have made improvement in an area. Perfectionistic assumptions about performance often lead to discounting the positive and overgeneralizing the relapse. Useful interventions include viewing the relapse in a temporal context, perhaps using a visual aid such as a sketch of a continuum or a pie-technique, by asking, "How much of the past month have things been better?" or "Where would you put your overall performance for the past month compared to a year ago?"

Cross-Reference to Other Techniques

Relevant techniques include identifying cognitive distortions (e.g., all-or-nothing thinking, fortune telling, discounting positives, overgeneralizing, and negative labeling), looking at progress rather than perfection, identifying the costs and benefits of modifying assumptions, the double standard, and rational role playing.

Form

Form 3.8 (Learning from Lapses, p. 96).

TECHNIQUE: USING CASE CONCEPTUALIZATION

Description

Identifying patients' underlying assumptions and conditional rules is helpful in developing a case formulation or conceptualization (see Beck, 1995; Needleman, 1999; Persons & Miranda, 1992; Tompkins, 1996) which we link the current cognitive assessment of automatic thoughts, core beliefs, conditional beliefs, and personal schemas to developmental issues and current coping styles. For example, the individual who has a personal schema that he is unlovable and that others will criticize and reject him may have the following automatic thoughts:

1. "She thinks I'm a loser."
2. "I am a loser."
3. "When I ask her out, she'll say no."
4. "It's awful to be rejected."
5. "Nothing ever works out."
6. "I'll end up alone."

In addition, he may hold the following maladaptive assumptions:"

1. "You should never let anyone know what you really think."
2. "If you count on people, they will abandon you."
3. "If people really knew what I was like, they wouldn't like me.
4. "You need others' approval to be happy."

Conditional beliefs might include:"

1. "If I am very pleasing and give in, then people will like me."
2. "If I meet everyone's needs, then they won't leave me."

This individual may attempt to cope with fear of rejection either by avoidance (e.g., not approaching people, not disclosing, not asking someone out) or by compensation (e.g., smiling at everything someone else says, engaging in deferring and self-sacrificing behavior). The core belief he holds about himself is that he is defective and unlovable. Reviewing his earlier developmental history might reveal that he was regularly criticized by his father and that his mother threatened to leave the family. In addition, his peers teased him for being smaller than they were.

The case conceptualization could be diagrammed, as in Figure 3.1.

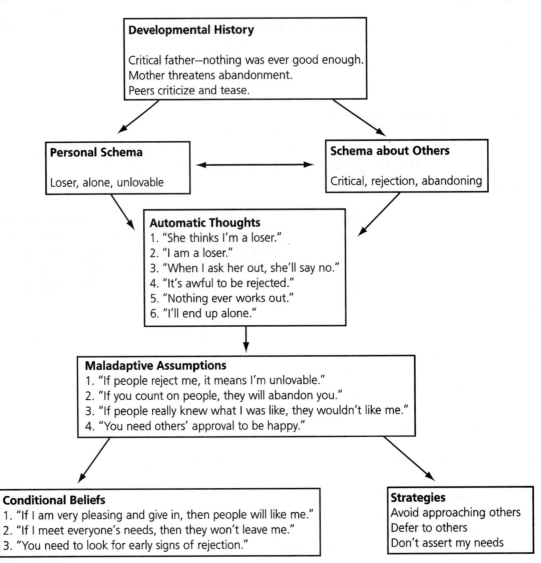

FIGURE 3.1. Diagram of case conceptualization.

Question to Pose/Intervention

The therapist provides case conceptualization in the session, explaining: "It is useful to identify how your thoughts and assumptions are related to each other. I will help you diagram a conceptualization of how your thoughts, feelings, and behavior are related."

Example

THERAPIST: You said that you thought you were a loser because the woman at the party didn't seem interested in you. That's the automatic thought—"I'm a loser." Then you also said that you thought you'd never meet anyone because you don't have much to offer. Let's diagram some of this [*using the schematic in Form 3.9*].

PATIENT: Yeah, that seems to be what I am saying.

THERAPIST: OK. It goes further, though. Your thought that "she didn't like me" then means what to you?

PATIENT: I guess that I'm not lovable.

THERAPIST: Have you had other thoughts like that before? Like, "If I allow people to get to know me, what do I fear?"

PATIENT: Oh, the more they know me the less they will like me. Then they'll leave. They'll find out who the real me is.

THERAPIST: So you seem to feel that people are critical and will reject and abandon you.

PATIENT: Right.

THERAPIST: OK. Let's put that into our chart here.

THERAPIST: Do you try to do things so that people won't criticize you?

PATIENT: Yeah, I generally don't disagree with people. I try to meet everyone's needs before my own.

THERAPIST: Do you avoid anything?

PATIENT: Oh yeah. I avoid approaching new people—starting conversations. I avoid letting people know much about me.

THERAPIST: Now, these ideas that you are unlovable and that people will criticize you, where do you think they come from?

PATIENT: My father was really critical and cold.

THERAPIST: OK. Let's put that in the box for "developmental history." How about your mother, what was she like?

PATIENT: She used to tell dad that she wished she had never married him. She said, "I wish that I could just go away and leave all of you to deal with things. Then you would appreciate me."

THERAPIST: OK. So mom would threaten abandonment. How about the other kids in school?

PATIENT: They'd criticize me because I wasn't as big as they were. I guess they also liked seeing me getting upset. I'd get really upset.

THERAPIST: OK. So if we look at the diagram about your schema you can see that you had a critical father, a mother who threatened you with abandonment, and interacted with kids who would tease you. This made you think that you were a loser, all alone, and that you might not be lovable. That fed into having automatic thoughts about being a loser, getting rejected, and ending up alone. Your assumption is that if people reject you, then you are unlovable. You tried to compensate by either trying to please everyone or by avoiding people if you thought you would be rejected.

PATIENT: That seems to describe who I am.

Homework

The therapist can give patients the case conceptualization developed in the session and ask them to write out thoughts and feelings about it. These might include additional memories or examples or emotional responses to the conceptualization. Patients can add to the case conceptualization on Form 3.9 (at the end of the chapter) any thoughts, feelings, coping styles, assumptions, strategies, or information about childhood experiences that are relevant. Each "box" in the case conceptualization can be utilized for strategies and interventions. Thus, the therapist can later examine effects of developmental history, schemas, assumptions, and beliefs. See the discussion on schema-focused therapy in Chapter 7.

Possible Problems

Although case conceptualization is often a powerful intervention that helps patients make sense of current problems, it may raise concern for some. For example, some patients may believe they are hopeless cases because they were "ruined" by their childhood experiences. These concerns about "fundamental" defects can be challenged by asking patients to consider if they have ever had any beliefs they subsequently changed or learned any new behaviors. Since we are learning and changing daily, knowing that old habits and beliefs were established earlier on may be the first step in changing them now. A good question to ask is, "Since some of the beliefs that bother you now were established when you were 6 years old, would you want to continue believing things you learned as a child?" Another point to add: "When you learned this belief as a child, you did not have the ability to think as an adult. Now you can challenge those ideas with all the benefits of being older and wiser."

Cross-Reference to Other Techniques

All of the techniques described in this book can be helpful in this endeavor. I begin to formulate the case conceptualization from the intake and continue to elaborate on it, with the patient, throughout treatment. This procedure takes the mystery out of therapy and helps patients understand that their problems are comprehensible and potentially manageable.

Form

Form 3.9 (Case Conceptualization Diagram, p. 97).

TECHNIQUE: ENHANCING CURIOSITY, CHALLENGE, AND GROWTH RATHER THAN PERFECTION

Description

Many assumptions are overly demanding and uncompromising in their positions. The individual believes that he or she should be accepted and liked by everyone or excel at every task. As a result, when events are less than perfect, the individual may feel hopeless or self-critical. Dweck and her associates (Dweck, Davidson, Nelson, & Enna, 1978) have found that people can persist more effectively, when confronted with challenging tasks, if they view the task as a learning experience or if they develop curiosity, in contrast to viewing the task as an evaluation or test. Perfectionistic expectations can undermine persistence, since the individual may become discouraged at the first experience of "failure" or "frustration."

Question to Pose/Intervention

The therapist can ask any of the following questions: "What did you learn?," "What could be interesting about this experience?," "How is this experience a challenge?," and "How would you feel if you did better the next time?" More specifically: "If you do poorly on an exam, rather than focus on your score as a final measure of your worth, consider how you could develop curiosity about the subject matter or feel challenged to do better in the future."

Example

THERAPIST: It sounds like you felt discouraged because you did not do as well on the exam as you expected.

PATIENT: Yeah, I was hoping I'd get an A, but I got a B–.

THERAPIST: Which parts of the history test did you do well on, and which parts did you not do well on?

PATIENT: I did well on the essay part—I'm pretty good at pulling things together. But the part on the dates and names—I just didn't know them.

THERAPIST: OK. Let's try to develop some curiosity about why dates might be important in history.

PATIENT: I never thought of it that way. Obviously, you have to know what happens after what.

THERAPIST: How could you develop this task of remembering dates and names into a challenge for yourself?

PATIENT: Maybe I could make up some flash cards and see if I can start learning some of this.

THERAPIST: How would you feel if you did better on this stuff next time?

PATIENT: Like I learned something that I should learn.

THERAPIST: Let's think of that as the next step in your challenge to do better and to learn from this experience.

Moreover, the therapist can ask patients the following: "What is your goal in the situation? Is your goal to succeed at everything? To be accepted by everyone? Could you modify your goal to 'learn how well I can do' or 'meet some new people'?" Often patients' goals revolve around unrealistic standards. By considering new goals, patients are freed to consider more than one way to approach a challenge.

The therapist can use the "Turning Work into Play" form (3.10, at the end of the chapter) to contrast critical thoughts into thoughts about challenge and curiosity. An example is shown in Figure 3.2.

Behavior that I think of critically, in terms of a negative evaluation: Studying and taking the history exam.

Critical Thoughts	Thoughts of Curiosity and Challenge
I'll get a lousy grade.	Let me see how all these events and people fit together.
I'm not good at history.	What's the story being told?
There are some things I just don't know.	I like a challenge. I'll feel great when I do better than I did before.
I'm really stupid when it comes to memorizing things.	I've overcome obstacles before.

FIGURE 3.2. Turning Work into Play: Changing Criticism and Defeat/Disappointment into Curiosity.

Homework

The therapist can ask patients to use Form 3.10 (at the end of the chapter) to consider experiences with which they are frustrated or have felt were failures. Short narratives can be written down, describing what events occurred and what negative thoughts or behaviors resulted. Then patients write down what they learned, what could be done differently in the future, and how they could develop curiosity about the problems to be faced.

Possible Problems

As with the technique of making progress rather than seeking perfection, patients sometimes believe that demanding standards and self-criticism are essential to achieving their goals. The therapist can identify this perfectionistic assumption as in need of evaluation—for example, what are the costs and benefits of an attitude of perfectionism versus one of curiosity and challenge? What evidence is there, for and against, that the experience of curiosity can motivate a person to action? Patients also can be asked what behaviors they engage in simply because they are interested in them?

Patients' curiosity also can be diminished by the excessive self-criticalness, so that they regard the task simply as an obligation or requirement: For example, "I'm not interested in history—I'm taking it only because it is required." The therapist could enhance curiosity in such a patient by asking him or her to speculate about why other people would be interested in history—that is, what makes it interesting to them? Or the patient could be asked if there are any behaviors that were once intrinsically interesting but which have become uninteresting because they were subjected to critical evaluations.

Cross-Reference to Other Techniques

Other relevant techniques include cost–benefit analysis, examining the evidence, double-standard technique, vertical descent, examining the negative filter, and role play.

Form

Form 3.10 (Turning Work into Play: Changing Criticism and Defeat/Disappointment into Curiosity, p. 98).

TECHNIQUE: DEVELOPING NEW ADAPTIVE STANDARDS AND ASSUMPTIONS

Description

We are often reluctant to abandon one belief unless we can come up with an alternative belief that works better for us. Having challenged and rejected maladaptive standards, values, or assumptions, the therapist can assist patients in developing new, more flexible and realistic ones. Often these new statements are expressed as preferences rather than as hard and fast rules. For example, the patient might replace "I should do a perfect job at everything" with a more adaptive standard such as "It's good to have high standards, but it is also good to be able to accept myself no matter how I perform." Or "I'd like to excel, but that's not always possible, so I find satisfaction in what I do achieve." The maladaptive standards usually involve all-or-nothing implications—for example, "I should always succeed"—and are followed by self-criticism or judgment of others. (The words *always* and *never* are easy cues of these types of statements.) New standards, values, and assumptions can be flexible, differentiated, and action-oriented, emphasizing learning, growth, and acceptance rather than judgment, rejection, and quitting—for example, "When I encounter an obstacle, I can engage in productive behaviors to overcome it." These new beliefs can be examined in terms of their costs and benefits, the evidence supporting their helpfulness, and their applicability to others (e.g., "How would you feel if we applied this rule [in contrast to the old rigid assumptions]) to others?"

Question to Pose/Intervention

"A lot of the time we hold assumptions and make rules that we just can't live up to—rules such as 'I should always succeed' or 'I should get the approval of everyone.' We have examined how these rigid rules make life difficult for you. Now let's develop some new rules and assumptions that might be more realistic, more flexible, and more growth oriented. Let's take your old rules and assumptions and come up with some new ones. For example, let's take your rule 'I should always do extremely well' and replace it with a new standard or value: 'I like doing well, but I can also learn from my mistakes, and I can take credit for what I do accomplish rather than measure myself against unrealistic standards.' "

Example

THERAPIST: You felt really bad after the history exam because you didn't get a good grade. Your rule was that "I must get high grades all the time." Let's find a new rule that can empower you by enhancing your curiosity and sense of growth and acceptance.

PATIENT: I guess I could say that I can learn from my mistakes. I could also give myself credit for the parts that I did well on.

THERAPIST: OK. What are the costs and benefits of learning from your mistakes?

PATIENT: The costs are that I might become complacent; I might get lazy and not even try for high grades. And the benefits would be that I stay motivated even when things don't go well. I wouldn't be as self-critical.

THERAPIST: How does that sound to you?

PATIENT: Like I'm better off learning from my mistakes and being challenged.

THERAPIST: What concrete behavior follows from this new formulation? What could you do over the next week to put this new value or standard to work?

PATIENT: I could look at what I did well on and what I still need to work on and I could plan to study. I could set it up as a challenge to memorize some of those dates and names.

THERAPIST: So you could set about making progress rather than demanding perfection?

PATIENT: Right.

In working with another patient, who was overly focused on getting approval from everyone, the therapist asked him to weigh out the cost and benefits of a new assumption. He made the following list:

New assumption: "I'm worthwhile regardless of what others think of me."
Costs: Getting conceited and alienating people.
Benefits: Self-confidence, can take risks, not shy, not dependent on others, more assertive.

Costs: 5%   *Benefits:* 95%   *Costs – Benefits* = –90%
Conclusion: This assumption is better than the assumption that I have to get other people to like me in order to like myself.

Another point to raise in order to evaluate assumptions is to ask patients to consider the following: "Rather than get trapped by your way of reacting, try to identify someone whom you think is highly adaptive. How would this person think and act if this event happened to him or her?" Often other people can serve as role models for adaptive thinking. For example, a single man was concerned about getting rejected if he approached a woman for a date. The therapist asked him to identify someone he thought was confident with woman and to consider how his friend would think of the situation. He was able to identify his friend's adaptive assumption that "It's better to take chances then to play it safe."

Finally, patients can consider the benefits of developing adaptive flexibility: "Examine the benefits of being flexible in your standards and behaviors. What would happen if you allowed yourself some room for error or mistakes?"

Homework

Instruct patients to identify any maladaptive rules and assumptions and then come up with alternatives that are more reasonable (Form 3.11, at the end of the chapter). The guidelines for the new formulations are the following: "The new rule or assumption should be more adaptive, more flexible, fairer, more realistic, and more positive. It should focus on fairness, growth, acceptance, and positive goals. It should be the kind of rule you would use for someone you love and care about." Furthermore, patients should be asked to evaluate the new rule or assumption and propose behaviors that would follow from it (Form 3.12, at the end of the chapter).

Possible Problems

As with any challenge to perfectionism, patients may believe that more reasonable rules are too lenient and that they would run the risk of becoming lax, lazy, and irresponsible. These perfectionistic ideas can be challenged, as indicated above, by looking at the evidence for and against, using the double standard, or carrying out an experiment with the new rules.

Cross-Reference to Other Techniques

Other relevant techniques include cost–benefit analysis, vertical descent, evaluating pro and con evidence, the double standard, and behavioral experiment.

Forms

Form 3.11 (Changing Old Rules/Assumptions into New Rules/Assumptions, p. 99); Form 3.12 (Evaluating and Acting on More Adaptive Rule/Assumption, p. 100).

TECHNIQUE: BILL OF RIGHTS

Description

Patient can be urged to read the Declaration of Independence, focusing especially on the section pertaining to the right to life, liberty, and the pursuit of happiness. All new and old assumptions can be evaluated against these basic rights. The idea is that our rights come from an assumption that a good rule is one that enhances human dignity. The therapist might then explain: "Develop a list of your rights as a person and how you could exercise them. New more adaptive rules and assumptions can be derived from an overarching humane sense of personal rights. These rights could include the following: the right to be free of depression, anxiety, and anger; the right to accept yourself; the right to experience growth, curiosity, and challenge; the right to learn from your mistakes; and the right to accept that some people won't like you."

Question to Pose/Intervention

"As a human being, you would agree that you have certain rights. As the Declaration of Independence states, these include the right to life, liberty, and the pursuit of happiness. Let's come up with your new Bill of Rights. Let's imagine that we would apply these rights not only to you but to each new baby born this year. These would be *human* rights."

Example

THERAPIST: You have been upset because your husband has been drinking, as usual, and criticizing you and telling you that you are stupid. How does this make you feel?

PATIENT: I feel trapped, like I am ready to explode.

THERAPIST: What if we were to come up with your personal Bill of Rights? Let's imagine that we would apply these rights not only to you but to each new baby born this year. These would be *human* rights. What rights would you give yourself?

PATIENT: I'd start with the right not to be battered, not to be criticized, not to have to live with an alcoholic. I have the right to be happy.

THERAPIST: And if it got really really bad and you couldn't stand it any longer?

PATIENT: The right to leave.

THERAPIST: You have a 2-year-old niece. Would you want her to have these rights?

PATIENT: Absolutely.

Homework

Patients can examine some of the problems, rules, or assumptions that have been causing stress and then consider a list of their basic rights. It is useful to have patients use the sentence stem "I have the right to . . . " for each right they identify (Form 3.13, at the end of this chapter).

Possible Problems

People with high, demanding standards or self-sacrificing schemas may believe that they must endure hardship in order to be moral. It is helpful to call attention to the double standard they likely apply by examining the implications of a newborn baby living in a world with these demanding or self-sacrificing rules. Patients also can examine the consequences that have ensued because they have not demanded, or acted upon, their rights.

Cross-Reference to Other Techniques

Other relevant techniques include the double standard, asking others about their ideas regarding human rights (surveying opinions), cost–benefit analysis, vertical descent, and rational role plays.

Form

Form 3.13 (My New Bill of Rights, p. 101).

FORM 3.1. Evaluating Assumptions, Rules, and Standards

It would be useful to examine your typical assumptions, rules, and standards. As you keep track of your negative thoughts over the next few weeks, see if you can identify any "should" statements, if–then statements, "musts," or rules. Write them in the form below. What is your underlying "should" statement? Do you have an underlying assumption such as, "If this happens, then something else must be true"?

Examples of typical assumptions	Endorsement of belief (0–100%)
I must be perfect in everything that I do.	
If I fail at something, then I'm a failure.	
I can't stand failure.	
I must receive approval from everyone to like myself.	
If someone thinks less of me, then I must think less of myself.	
I can't stand it when people think less of me.	
You have to impress people with your personality.	
If I'm not perfect, people won't like me.	
Some people are better than others.	
If I'm not certain about things, then they probably won't work out.	
It's important to have all the information before you make a decision.	
I shouldn't be depressed (angry, anxious).	
Other people should do things my way.	
If I make a mistake, then I should criticize myself.	
If people offend me, then I should get back at them.	
Other assumptions:	

FORM 3.2. Self-Help Form: Monitoring Your Assumptions, Rules, and Standards

My Typical Assumptions, Rules, and Standards	% Belief

FORM 3.3. Examining and Challenging "Should" Statements

Think about one of your typical "should" statements—such as, "I should have done better" or "I should be perfect" or "I should be beautiful." Answer each of the questions in this form. Think about how you could change your "should" statement into a preference—for example, "I would *prefer* to do better" rather than "I *should* do better."

"Should" statement:

Degree of belief (0–100%)

Emotion (and degree 0–100%)

Costs and benefits: Costs:

                             Benefits:

Who established this rule?

Do you apply this rule to everyone? Why not?

Restate this rule as a preference rather than a "should"

What would be a more reasonable expectation?

Re-rate belief and emotion: Belief:

                                Emotion:

FORM 3.4. Identifying Conditional Beliefs

Area of concern	How much of a concern is this to you? (0–100%)	How I try to cope ...
Example: Am I smart? (Intelligence)	95%	In order to be competent, I need to do better than everyone. Or If I avoid really challenging tasks, I won't fail.
Intelligence		
Attractiveness		
Closeness with others		
Trust in self or others		
Laziness in self or others		
Rejection by others		
Being controlled by others		
Being humiliated		
Knowing things for sure		
Being interesting		
Being alone		
Others:		

Examples of conditional or coping beliefs:
In order to be competent, I need to do better than everyone.
In order to be attractive, I need to be perfect in my appearance.
I need to keep control of all my emotions, or I will lose control completely.
If I am cautious, I can avoid rejection.
If I give in to others, then they will like me.

FORM 3.5. Values Clarification

Consider a current value that seems to be bothering you—for example, being financially successful. Contrast this value with each of the values in the left-hand column. Rank all of these values, from 1 to 17, with 1 for the most important. Use a different number for each value In the right-hand column, list some ways that you could pursue these other values.

Current value I am upset about:	How I can pursue values that are important to me?
Love	
Forgiveness	
Family/intimate relationship	
Work achievement	
Friendship	
Financial success	
Self-esteem	
Personal growth	
Physical beauty or attractiveness	
Physical health	
Approval by others	
Kindness	
Fun	
Learning	
Religion	
Cultural endeavors	
Personal freedom	
Others:	

FORM 3.6. A Universal Value System

Values to consider	How I wish the world would rank these values
Love	
Forgiveness	
Family/intimate relationship	
Work achievement	
Friendship	
Financial success	
Self-esteem	
Personal growth	
Physical beauty or attractiveness	
Approval by others	
Kindness	
Fun	
Learning	
Religion	
Cultural endeavors	
Personal freedom	
My current concern (specify):	
Other values:	

FORM 3.7. Making Progress Rather Than Trying for Perfection

Identify some areas in your life that you criticize yourself about—for example, your performance in school or work. Then list some actions that you could take to make improvements in this area—for example, study harder, prepare, work more, learn some skills. List a number of areas of self-criticism and a number of specific actions that you could take to improve those areas.

What I criticize myself about	How I can make progress
	Why would progress be better than pursuing perfection?

FORM 3.8. Learning from Lapses

Consider a behavior that you have been making progress on—for example, exercise, diet, drinking less, smoking less, etc. Write it down in the first column (e.g., "Exercising three times per week"). In the middle column write down what made you lapse from your desired behavior (e.g., "I was too tired to exercise"). In the third column, write down what you learned to make things better (e.g., "I can exercise even if I am tired" or "I can pick up my exercise routine tomorrow"). Lapses or relapses are learning experiences.

The behavior that I am concerned about is: _____

What was working before	What made me lapse	What I learned to make things better in the future

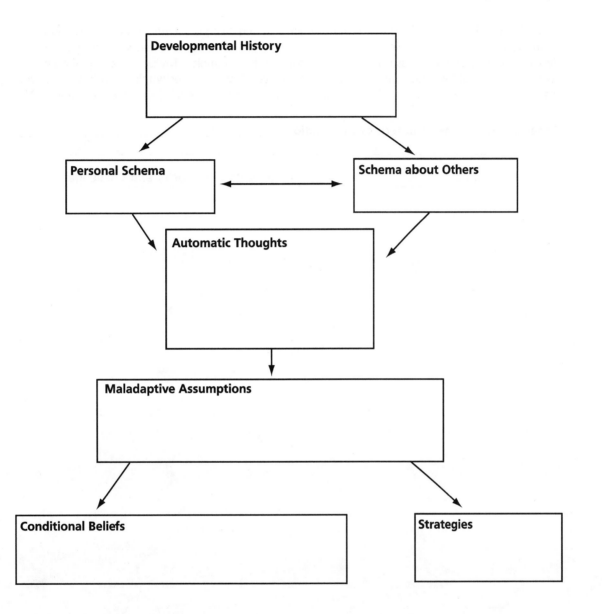

FORM 3.10. Turning Work into Play: Changing Criticism and Defeat/ Disappointment into Curiosity

In the left-hand column write down some examples of negative judgments and criticisms you make about yourself or other people. In the right-hand column write down some ways that you could develop curiosity about the issues in the other column. For example, "My boss is cruel. She doesn't seem friendly at all" is a judgmental thought. Thoughts reflecting curiosity might be "I wonder why that bothers me?" and "I wonder if there are times when she is friendlier? If so, why would that be?"

Behavior that I think of in terms of evaluation: _____

Critical Thoughts	Thoughts of Curiosity and Challenge

FORM 3.11. Changing Old Rules/Assumptions into New Rules/Assumptions

In the left-hand column write down examples of your rules, "should" statements, and assumptions. In the right-hand column, write down more adaptive, practical rules, "shoulds," and assumptions.

Old Rule or Assumption	More Adaptive Rule or Assumption

FORM 3.12. Evaluating and Acting on More Adaptive Rule/Assumption

New Rule or Assumption: _____.

Costs	Benefits	Behaviors to do

FORM 3.13. My New Bill of Rights

It is important to know and exercise your rights. In the left-hand column list the rights you believe you should have. In the right-hand column list the ways that you can pursue these rights. Think of "action plans" for yourself—actions that you could take in the future to make sure that your rights and needs are met.

I have a right to . . .	Therefore I can . . .

CHAPTER 4

Evaluating Worries

Chronic worrying is debilitating—yet many people complain that they have worried all their lives. Worries and fears are characteristic of patients suffering from generalized anxiety disorder, obsessive–compulsive disorder, social phobia, panic disorder, or depression. Simply telling patients not to worry will have little effect; likewise, the technique called "thought stopping," in which the therapist tells the patient to yell "stop" (silently, if necessary) whenever a worry or obsession occurs, is not effective. Indeed, these interventions are close to useless and, in fact, may even increase the worrying by amplifying patients' focus.

The cognitive-behavioral model of worry has been elaborated in recent years by (Borkovec & Hu, 1990; Borkovec & Inz, 1990; Dugas, Buhr, & Ladouceur, in press; Freeston, Rheaume, Letarte, & Dugas, 1994; Mennin, Turk, Heimberg, & Carmin, in press; Wells, 2000, 2002). Worry is a central component of all of the anxiety disorders, with many worriers claiming that their problem has persisted for years (Kessler, Walters, & Wittchen, in press). The various cognitive-behavioral models stress the fact that worriers overpredict negative outcomes, ignore base-rate information, underestimate their ability to cope with negatives, maintain demanding standards of perfectionism and high need for approval, and are intolerant of uncertainty and ambiguity. Intriguing empirical findings suggest that worry actually inhibits the physiological arousal of unpleasant feelings, resulting in both the incubation of worrisome thoughts that rebound later and the apparent short-term reinforcement of worry as a means of emotional suppression (Wells & Papageorgiou, 1995; York, Borkovec, Vasey, & Stern, 1987). Worry is generally experienced in abstract or linguistic form, further "neutralizing" emotional content and inhibiting habituation, since the emotional or arousal component of "worry schemas" is not activated during the process of worrying (Borkovec & Inz, 1990; Wells & Papageorgiou, 1995). Moreover, worriers believe that worry protects against, prepares them for, and prevents negatives, on one hand, while, on the other hand, also believing that worry will result in negative consequences, such as illness or insanity, and that worrying must be controlled or eliminated (Wells, 2000, 2002).

In this chapter we examine a variety of techniques that are helpful in reducing the amount of worry and its negative impact. More detailed descriptions of cognitive-behavioral interventions for generalized anxiety disorder (the disorder most characterized by worry) can be found in Dugas and Ladouceur (1998), Leahy (in press), and Wells (1997a, 1999, 2000).

TECHNIQUE: IDENTIFYING WORRIES

Description

In order to examine and evaluate worries, it is important to categorize the primary modality in which the individual experiences the worries. Some of these worries may be experienced as thoughts (auditory), such as "I worry that I will end up all alone," whereas others may be experienced visually, as images, such as "I see myself in an empty apartment crying."

Question to Pose/Intervention

"Can you tell me what you are thinking when you feel anxious? When you feel worried? Do you ever have visual images or pictures in your mind when you are anxious? Are you making predictions that bother you? Are you thinking that some bad things might happen?"

Example

THERAPIST: You said that you felt really anxious when you were on your way to the party. Can you tell me what was going through your mind?

PATIENT: I thought, "I won't have anything to say—I'll look like a fool."

THERAPIST: Did you have any kind of visual image of what that would be like at the party?

PATIENT: Yeah, I could imagine people laughing at me. I could see them laughing, and I turn away from them, humiliated.

Alternatively, the therapist can inquire:

THERAPIST: Can you tell me what you were worried would happen if you started to talk to someone?

PATIENT: I was worried that I would begin to fumble for words and make no sense.

THERAPIST: Then what would happen?

PATIENT: I'd look like a fool.

Homework

The therapist can ask the patient to write down examples of worries that arise during the coming week, using Form 4.1 (at the end of the chapter). Drawing on the prior interviews with the patient, the therapist can identify examples of these worries that have already occurred during therapy: "We've already identified some examples of your worries. For example, you have told me that you have ruminated on 'What if I fail the exam?' and 'What if I don't pass the course?' You have had worries about meeting new people. Your worries are 'I won't have anything to say' and 'I'll make a fool out of myself.'"

An advantage of this homework assignment is that patients identify specific worries that can later be examined, tested, or challenged. Furthermore, patients begin to realize that there are a limited number of themes and predictions, thereby narrowing the scope of their problem.

Possible Problems

Problems that typically occur include not being able to identify thoughts or worries, confusing worries with feelings or emotions, and not complying with the homework, fearing that writing down worries will make them more "real" and will only increase the intensity of the worrying. Many habitually worried individuals hold the belief that they should "stop thinking" about their concerns or "stop worrying" and that this will decrease their worries. As noted, thought stopping is not a useful technique for depotentiating the habit of worrying. The therapist can examine the patient's possible roadblocks in identifying specific worries: "We find that people often confuse a feeling—such as 'anxious' or 'nervous'—with the actual worry. For example, the worry might be 'I won't pass the test,' and the feeling or emotion in response to that worry is one of nervousness and tension." In response to the idea that writing down worries will make one more worried, the therapist can say: "Some people believe that writing down their concerns will make them more worried and the thoughts stronger. You might recall that we have been writing down your thoughts in our sessions in therapy. Do you think that this activity has made you feel worse, or does it help you get more distance from the thoughts?"

Cross-Reference to Other Techniques

Techniques related to self-monitoring include eliciting, identifying, and categorizing automatic thoughts, mood monitoring, vertical descent, and imagery techniques focused on eliciting automatic thoughts.

Form

Form 4.1 (Self-Monitoring of Worries, p. 136).

TECHNIQUE: EXAMINING COSTS AND BENEFITS OF WORRY

Description

Many people view worry as a form of problem solving, preparation, or protection against possible calamities (see Papageorgiou & Wells, 2000; Wells, 1997a). Indeed, worry *can* be helpful in motivating people to get things done—for example, the worry prior to an examination may be helpful in motivating the student to study for the exam. However, many worries do not serve the function of preparation, motivation, or problem solving. The patient's underlying theory of worry can be explored by evaluating the costs and benefits of worrying.

Question to Pose/Intervention

"What are the costs and benefits to you of worrying? [Alternative: What are the advantages and disadvantages of worrying?] If you worried less, what do you predict would happen?"

Example

THERAPIST: Let's examine the costs and benefits to you of worrying about taking the exam.

PATIENT: OK. The costs are that I am anxious all the time, I can't relax, I feel terrible. I hate exams. The benefits are that I'll be motivated to study.

THERAPIST: If you had to divide 100% between the costs and benefits of worrying, what would it be? 50/50 for costs and benefits? 60/40? 40/60?

PATIENT: I'd say the costs of worrying are a lot more than the benefits. I would give it 75% for the costs and 25% for the benefits.

THERAPIST: So you think you'd be better off if you worried less? What if you worried 50% less? What do you think would happen?

PATIENT: I don't know. I guess I'd worry that I'm not worrying enough!

THERAPIST: Then what would happen?

PATIENT: Maybe I wouldn't do well on the exam.

Homework

Patients can be assigned the task of writing out the costs and benefits of a specific worry, each time they begin to worry, using Form 4.2 (at the end of the chapter).

Possible Problems

Possible problems patients encounter when evaluating the costs and benefits include claiming that there are no benefits to worrying, that they do not consider worrying a "choice," and therefore examining the costs and benefits is not relevant; or that reducing worry might make them irresponsible or careless. We address these issues by asking the following: "Even though you say there are no benefits in worry, people seldom do anything unless they believe—on some level—that it can be helpful. Try not to be rational when you consider this question." The therapist can suggest some possible benefits to worrying: "Is it possible that worrying motivates you, prepares you, or protects you?" We find it helpful to administer the Metacognitions Questionnaire (Form 4.3, at the end of the chapter), developed by Adrian Wells (Wells, 2000), to assess different beliefs about worry. In regard to the issue of whether worry is a choice, we tell patients to forgo deciding that question for the immediate moment and to focus instead on becoming more mindful or aware of worrying as a mental activity. Becoming more aware of something—for example, overeating—can be helpful in gaining control and finally experiencing a sense of choice.

Cross-Reference to Other Techniques

Other techniques that are helpful in identifying the costs and benefits to worrying include identifying automatic thoughts, using vertical descent, self-monitoring of worries, examining the behavioral consequences of worrying, and identifying underlying assumptions.

Forms

Form 4.2 (Costs–Benefits to Worrying, p. 138); Form 4.3 (Metacognitions Questionnaire, pp. 139–141, which allows the therapist to identify a variety of dimensions).

TECHNIQUE: TURNING WORRIES INTO PREDICTIONS

Description

As noted, many worries are expressed in vague or "what if" terms; it is difficult to test out worries that are really rhetorical questions or statements. Consequently, we encourage patients to restate their worries as specific predictions about events in the real world.

Question to Pose/Intervention

"Specifically, what are you predicting will happen? When will it happen? Try to specify exactly what will happen so that we will know whether your predictions are accurate or inaccurate. Can you also predict some positive things that will or will not happen?"

Example

A college student complained of worries about her exams that were coming up in 2 weeks. Her worries were: "I'm not prepared for the exam. There are things that we covered that I don't know. I won't do well on the exam."

THERAPIST: You have a lot of worries about the exam. Let's see if you can rephrase your worries as specific predictions. For example, you said "I'm not prepared for the exam." Exactly what are you predicting will happen?

PATIENT: I won't do well on the exam.

THERAPIST: The exam is in 2 weeks. What do you predict your score will be on the exam?

PATIENT: I don't know. I just won't do well.

THERAPIST: What's an example of a score that reflects "not doing well"?

PATIENT: I guess around 70%.

Homework

Patients can use Form 4.4 (at the end of the chapter) to write down worries as they occur, even if they are "what if" worries. Then they should turn them into specific predictions. The therapist may explain: "After you write down your worry in the left-hand column, then I'd like you to write down the specific prediction you are making. For example, if you worry that you are not prepared for the exam, then write down the specific prediction you just made—for example, "I will get 70% on the exam.""

Possible Problems

As in the worry monitoring described earlier in this chapter, patients may confuse a worry with a feeling. This can be clarified as it was earlier. Another more likely problem is that patients will make a vague rather than specific prediction—for example, "I won't do well on the exam" or "I'll choke on the exam." We urge patients to "act like a good journalist" by asking themselves the "W" questions: "What, where, when: "Exactly *what* will happen, *where* will it happen, and *when* will it happen?" Another problem is that patients may not think past the initial worry—for example, "I'm not prepared"—but focus on how they can solve the problem before it arises—for example, "I need to work really hard." This confusion can be addressed in the session by identifying the string of worries and predictions that follow from the initial thoughts.

Cross-Reference to Other Techniques

The most relevant techniques include identifying and categorizing automatic thoughts, relating a thought to a feeling, and the use of vertical descent.

Form

Form 4.4 (Turning Worries into Predictions, p. 142).

TECHNIQUE: TESTING NEGATIVE PREDICTIONS

Description

In describing this exercise to patients, the therapist might say: "Let's go back over examining your thoughts and predictions. Let's say that you have the thought 'I'm a loser.' What does this thought predict about the future? If it predicts nothing, you would probably agree that it's fairly meaningless. But you are upset with the thought because you think it means something about what's going to happen. For example, you might think 'I'm a loser' and therefore:

- 'I'll never be happy.'
- 'Judy won't talk to me at the party.'
- 'I'll never get another date.'
- 'I'll get fired.'

"Of course, you could be right. But now we have clear predictions that we can test out and see if you are right about being a loser. If your predictions do not come true, you will have to reexamine your negative thought."

However, many times people who have negative thoughts make predictions that are true for everyone. For example, consider the following predictions:

- 'I'll be unhappy.'
- 'Someone won't like me.'
- 'I'll be alone on a Saturday night.'
- 'I'll have problems at work.'

Each of these events is true for almost everyone in the world. To say that these events prove that "I'm a loser" would mean that everyone is a loser. It is important to examine whether the predictions are good *tests* of the idea that is bothering the patient. To be good at testing a belief, the prediction has to differentiate the patient from most other people; it cannot lead to predictions that are true for almost everyone.

Another important aspect of a workable, useful prediction is that it should give us a reasonable time period. For example, the prediction "I'll get fired" should be expanded to specify the date by which this event will happen. Since it is plausible that most people might lose a job sometime during the lifetime, it would be hard to say that losing a job 10 years from now would make the person unique.

Finally, just as we ask patients to predict what will happen, we also ask them to predict what will *not* happen. Examples of predictions of things that will not happen are the following:

- "I won't get a date in the next 3 months."
- "I won't get a raise during the next year."
- "I won't be able to start a conversation with a stranger."
- "I won't be able to finish the project."
- "I won't be able to pay my bills this month."

Using Form 4.5 (at the end of the chapter), patients can list the events they predict will come true and those that will not happen to test out their negative beliefs about themselves or the future. Then they list the actual outcomes.

Question to Pose/Intervention

"Make a list of specific predictions for the next week and keep track of the outcomes. For example, predict the amount of stress you will experience for specific activities and then charts the actual outcome.

Example

For example, a woman is sitting in her apartment feeling lonesome, thinking "I can't believe that I'm alone again! I feel so rotten." These worries or ruminations were addressed in the following manner:

THERAPIST: When you were sitting there thinking about how bad you felt, what were you thinking would happen?

PATIENT: I thought I'd always be alone.

THERAPIST: How could you test that prediction?

PATIENT: I could see if I develop a relationship.

THERAPIST: OK. That would be one way. Could you also keep an activity schedule for a week and see if you spend all your time alone, or if you spend some time with other people?

PATIENT: I already know what I'll find. I spend every day with people at work, and I see my friends at least a couple of times a week.

THERAPIST: So the prediction that you will always be alone isn't true for most days of the week.

PATIENT: But I don't have anyone *special* right now.

THERAPIST: Are you predicting that you never will?

PATIENT: I guess I am.

THERAPIST: OK. We can keep this prediction in mind and test it out in the future. But let's look at the reasons why you think you would never have a relationship . . .

Homework

Homework involves collecting information about specific predictions during the current time frame and testing the predictions against reality. Patients are asked to write down predictions for the coming week about a variety of negative thoughts and worries—for example, "I won't be able to concentrate" or "I'll have nothing to say" or "I won't be able to get any sleep." Then the data are collected and tested against the outcome.

Possible Problems

Testing the predictions derived from worries requires a way to disconfirm the predictions. If patients phrase the worry in terms of possibilities—for example, "It's possible I could have cancer"—then there is no way to prove it is impossible. Another problem: predictions regarding a distant or vague future—for example, "I might go bankrupt some day." In order to set up behavioral experiments to test predictions, it is necessary to position them in the current time frame. Furthermore, some predictions may turn out to be partly true—for example, the outcome of the prediction "I won't be able to sleep" may be "I got 5 hours of sleep."

Cross-Reference to Other Techniques

Identifying automatic thoughts, turning worries into predictions, vertical descent, and mood monitoring are relevant techniques.

Form

Form 4.5 (Testing Negative Predictions, p. 143).

TECHNIQUE: EXAMINING PAST PREDICTIONS AND THOUGHTS

Description

In describing this exercise to patients, the therapist might say: "When you are feeling depressed or anxious, you may get caught up in the here and now of how you're thinking and feeling. You may think *now* 'I'll always be alone' or 'I'll always feel depressed.' But if you were to look back on your negative thoughts in the past, you might find that there is a pattern: You often predict that negative events or feelings will continue indefinitely. By examining the past negative predictions that you have made, you may learn that your pessimism is seldom accurate. Thus *making* a prediction is a lot different from *having a prediction come true*."

Question to Pose/Intervention

"Have you made negative predictions in the past? Have they come true or have they proven to be false? Have you had past negative thoughts about yourself, others, and experiences that have not come true? You were worried about events in the past which you no longer even think about. List as many of these past worries and ask yourself why these are no longer important to you.

Example

Consider the following: Judy recently separated from her husband because she felt she did not love him anymore. Even though it was her choice to separate, actually experiencing the separation triggered thoughts about loneliness that led her to feel depressed. She then predicted that she would never find anyone else to care about and that she would always be depressed.

THERAPIST: You told me that this is your second marriage, and that you also have had a couple of significant relationships besides the two marriages.

PATIENT: Yes. Before Bill there was my marriage to Ted, and I had relationships with Dave and Ed— Ed was before Ted, and Dave was the one I had the affair with last year.

THERAPIST: What was it like for you in the past when relationships ended?

PATIENT: Oh, I always get depressed and feel hopeless. It's just like it is now.

THERAPIST: So could we predict that when relationships end, you'll think "I'll never love anyone again" and "I'll always be depressed"?

PATIENT: Yeah. I keep doing that. Just like now.

THERAPIST: But you did love again, didn't you? After Ted there was Ed, and then there was Bill, and then there was Dave.

PATIENT: I guess it's true. I tend to make these predictions, but then I always have another relationship.

THERAPIST: So what could we predict about you loving again and always feeling depressed?

PATIENT: Well, the pattern is, I will love again, and I will get over my depression.

In addition, it was important for us to examine her belief that the only way she could be happy was by being involved with a man. But helping the patient step back from her current predictions and feelings to realize that she has a recurrent pattern of negative predictions that do not come true was quite helpful.

Another application of this technique is with anxious patients who continually predict that they will have a heart attack or lose control. These people suffer from *panic disorder*—they are afraid of having panic attacks. For example, for 4 years Betsy predicted that she would lose control and pass out on the subway.

THERAPIST: How many times in the past year have you taken the subway or bus?

PATIENT: I try to avoid them, but I'd say about 25 times.

THERAPIST: How about over the last 4 years?

PATIENT: I used to take public transportation more often, so I'd say about 150 times.

THERAPIST: And what percentage of the time did you predict that you would keel over in a faint?

PATIENT: Close to 100%!

THERAPIST: How many time have you passed out?

PATIENT: Never.

THERAPIST: So your predictions have been wrong roughly 150 times—100% of the time?

PATIENT: I guess these predictions aren't coming out true.

Homework

The therapist can explain this next assignment in the following way: "Review some negative events in your life, or events that you thought were negative at the time. List your predictions and thoughts and then list the actual outcomes. For example, a past event might be 'giving a talk,' with the negative prediction or thought 'I'll look like an idiot' or 'I'll freeze up,' and with the actual outcome of 'The talk went, OK, although I was nervous.' You also might have made negative predictions that came true. Make a list of the different negative predictions that you have made in the past, going back as far as you can, then examine the actual outcomes."

Possible Problems

Some patients believe that their negative predictions were not really predictions because they were stated as possibilities, such as "I *might* fail." Review how a worry can be turned into a specific prediction: "Were you really thinking 'I'm going to fail'?" Past worries, even when qualified, should be turned into predictions.

Another problem: The past worry continues—for example, "I might get cancer." This possibility still exists—but it cannot be addressed in that form. These kinds of worries can be restated as "My worry or prediction did not come true this week." Yet another problem: Some patients would rather forget their past events that caused them to worry, believing that to recall them would only make them feel worse. The therapist can point out that examining how past worries about specific events have not come true will add to their new belief that current worries may constitute another set of false predictions.

Cross-Reference to Other Techniques

Related techniques include eliciting, identifying, and categorizing automatic thoughts, mood and thought monitoring, and imagery techniques. In audition, it is helpful to review turning worries into predictions with these patients.

Form

Form 4.6 Examining Past Negative Predictions, p. 144).

TECHNIQUE: REVIEWING THE HANDLING OF PAST NEGATIVE EVENTS

Description

In order to build on a self-efficacy model, we find it helpful to have patients review past problems and how they resolved them. In describing this exercise to patients, the therapist might say: "Many anxious and depressed people predict that outcomes will be negative, and many times they are wrong. But sometimes they are right. Bad things do happen to people. Sometimes they happen even if you do not predict them. The real question is, 'Have you ever been able to handle negative events?' The research on worriers shows that when a negative outcome occurs, worriers actually handle it much better than they thought they would. This is an important finding, for it suggests that part of worrying is underestimating one's ability to cope with negative outcomes. If the worrier believes that he or she can handle negative outcomes, then there will be less provocation to worry."

I often use the following story to drive this point home: "Henry is a business consultant working for a medium-sized company. He and his boss have had a number of conflicts in the past month, resulting in Henry's fear that he will lose his job. Henry obsessed about the idea that he might get fired. We examined his ability to earn a living independently of the company, which was somewhat helpful, but his anxiety still remained. Then we decided to look at his past history of handling negative events.

"It turned out that Henry was fairly skilled in handling negative events in the past, such as difficulties he had in college, finding his first job, dealing with his son's behavioral problems, and building up business leads in a company that was not doing well.

"I told Henry a story that I had heard about another psychologist. The psychologist had a patient who obsessed about getting a sexually transmitted disease. Nothing seemed to help the patient. The therapist and patient reviewed all the things that one could do if he did get a disease, but the patient remained anxious. Then one day the patient came to the office and announced that, indeed, he had contracted syphilis. Much to the patient's and therapist's surprise, the patient responded with excellent adaptive skills to the situation. He obtained the proper medical treatment and quickly recovered.

"A month after I told Henry this story he called me and said, 'Bob, I got syphilis.' At first I had no idea what he was talking about, until he reminded me of the story I had told him. Henry had gotten fired—and now, he said, he felt energized! He had called all of his clients, and most of them were coming away with him into his new consulting company. Just like in the past, he was a survivor.

"In order to examine how you have done in handling negative events in the past, you might use this table [Form 4.7, at the end of the chapter] to list past negative events and ways that you handled them. If you had problems handling negative events in the past, you will benefit from this and other exercises we will explore.

"If you know that you have handled past negative events well, you might want to examine what skills, resources, problem-solving abilities, and other capabilities you brought to bear on these problems or adversities. For example, another patient whom I'll call Kathy, often worried about negative things happening in the future, leading her to believe that she needed to rely on her husband to solve every problem. We examined the problems that she had already faced in her life and resolved—depression, breast cancer, asserting herself with her mother, learning how to drive, overcoming her fear of flying, and negotiating her contract at work. Indeed, as I reviewed with her how resourceful, assertive, and intelligent she was, I realized that she was the kind of person I might call in crisis!"

Question to Pose/Intervention

"Have you made negative predictions in the past that have come true? Have you been able to handle the outcome? Have you faced negative events before? Do you tend to underestimate your ability to handle negative outcomes?"

Example

PATIENT: I just don't know what's going to happen with Ted and me.

THERAPIST: You are worried that your relationship with Ted might end?

PATIENT: Yeah. We're always fighting, and we haven't been intimate in 2 months now.

THERAPIST: You've had some negative things happen to you in the past, haven't you?

PATIENT: Yes. I lost my job 3 years ago, and my mother died last year. I just don't seem to have any luck.

THERAPIST: Have you ever gone through a breakup before?

PATIENT: Oh, yeah. When I was in college, Ed and I broke up. Then 2 years ago I was going out with Glen, and we broke up. It was very upsetting.

THERAPIST: It was upsetting, yes, but you were able to a recover from that breakup. What helped you recover?

PATIENT: Well, I relied a lot on my friends, and then I began to focus a lot more on my work. My friends were terrific.

THERAPIST: If you remember from our talk a few weeks ago, you told me that when you and Glen broke up, you thought you wouldn't meet anyone else.

PATIENT: Yeah, but I did. I met a number of people—some I liked, some I didn't.

THERAPIST: It seems that you were able to recover from the breakup. Maybe you won't break up with Ted, but if you did—perhaps you could think about how you handled some of these other relational situations in the past and harness those skills and resources.

Homework

The homework assignment can be proposed in this light: "If you have been able to handle problems in the past, then you may be able to handle new problems that might arise. I'd like you to spend some time over the next week listing some problems that you have had in the past, related to school, work, family, relationships, finances, health, relocating, making new friends—whatever category is applicable. Use this table (Form 4.7 at the end of the chapter). Write out the kinds of things that you did that were helpful in resolving these problems as well as the kinds of things that were not helpful."

Possible Problems

Many worriers maintain impossible standards of perfectionism. They believe that they should be able to handle negative outcomes at an exceptional level, thus resulting in their observation that when the negative event occurred, they could have done better to cope with it. Because perfectionistic beliefs are a central component of depression, anxiety, and anger, the therapist should examine patients' standards. The cost–benefit analysis and the double-standard technique, as well as examining the evidence as to how self and others compare in coping with negative events, are useful tools for this purpose. Moreover, certain types of negative events may be far more problematic than others. For example, the patient may feel particularly undermined by negative events in relationships but cope better with work problems. The therapist can examine the schemas and assumptions activated in these different categories and can ask the patient to apply skills in one area to the more problematic area (e.g., problem solving, behavioral activation, and communication skills).

Cross-Reference to Other Techniques

Relevant techniques include activity scheduling, problem solving, pleasure predicting, examining the evidence, double standard, vertical descent, and setting up behavioral experiments.

Form

Form 4.7 (Reviewing the Handling of Past Negative Events, p. 145).

TECHNIQUE: LEARNING FROM UNCONFIRMED PREDICTIONS

Description

Some people are able to review their past negative predictions and recognize that they are almost always too negative. For example, Laura had a fear that she would have a panic attack crossing bridges. When she examined her past predictions that she would lose control and crash, she realized that it never happened. However, rather than learning that she was very inaccurate in making predictions, she discounted the past information and said *"But it could always happen!"*

Many anxious people discount the validity of past information because it cannot give them the guarantee about the future on which they insist. They want to rule out both *probability* and *possibility*. The past may be a good indicator of probability, but it says nothing about possibility. Consequently, it is considered irrelevant to the issue of demanding certainty about the future. After all, it is possible that Laura could lose control and crash in her car.

A second reason that people fail to learn that their negative predictions do not come true is that they are so relieved when things turn out well that they do not want to reexamine their distortion in thinking. It is part of the nature of memory processing that we recall events that *do occur* rather than events that *do not occur*. For example, try to recall all the events that *did not occur* yesterday. The question sounds ludicrous—but, in some ways, it is relevant to the pattern of making a lot of negative predictions that do not come true but failing to note the absence of these unwanted occurrences.

A third reason people fail to learn from past experience is that they develop *exceptions to the rule*, which we refer to as *discounting*. For example, Gary predicted that Paula would reject him at the party. However, when he spoke with her, she was quite friendly. Gary discounted this unexpected reception by saying "She was just *acting* friendly. She's a phony." Thus Gary could not learn from the experience because his belief could not possibly be disconfirm.

A fourth reason that people might not learn from past experience is that they are heavily invested in their negative belief. Perhaps they think that their negative belief protect them in some way, or they just have a hard time acknowledging that they are wrong. In some cases, patients get into power struggles with the therapist—or with other people—and believe that they will "lose face" if they admit that they are wrong.

Question to Pose/Intervention

"Are you able to learn from your past negative predictions? Think back about your negative predictions from the past. Did some of them not come true? When you think back about the fact that some of them did not come true, what do you make of it? Do you discount this evidence of incorrect predictions? Do you think that somehow your new negative predictions must be valid?"

The therapist can examine, with patients, their tendency not to learn from past experience by asking them to list evidence from the past that seems to contradict the negative thoughts in the present and to consider the following points:

1. They need guarantees that are not feasible in the "real" world.
2. They do not reexamine occurrences that contradict their belief.
3. They discount the evidence of incorrect predictions.
4. They demonstrate a need to maintain their belief and to be right.

Example

THERAPIST: You are thinking now that the discoloration on your face is a sign of skin cancer. Have you made these kinds of predictions before?

PATIENT: Yeah. It's always something. Last year I thought I had AIDS. A couple of months ago I thought that I had a brain tumor.

THERAPIST: So you have made a lot of predictions that haven't come true. What is the evidence that this discoloration is not skin cancer?

PATIENT: The doctor looked at it and said it's nothing to worry about. I've had this on my face a lot of other times.

THERAPIST: So what do you make of the doctor's verdict?

PATIENT: She could always be wrong.

THERAPIST: That's true. And if she could be wrong . . . ?

PATIENT: Then I shouldn't accept what she says—what *any* doctor says—unless I can be certain.

THERAPIST: And if you accepted what your doctor said but you did not feel certain?

PATIENT: I would always regret it, if it turned out to be skin cancer.

THERAPIST: Is your thought "I should continue worrying and checking until I can be certain"?

PATIENT: That's it.

Homework

The patient is asked to engage in a point–counterpoint. This exercise involves giving a rational response to the current negative thought (e.g., "I might have AIDS"), then challenging the rational response, and, again, challenging the negative thought. An example of this process is shown in Figure 4.1.

Possible Problems

One problem is that patients may claim that they cannot think of any challenges to the rational response. They may agree with the therapist. In this case, the therapist should attempt to modify the task into a role play, in which the therapist plays the negative counter to the rational response. This addition may reveal automatic thoughts and assumptions that patients cannot challenge adequately.

Cross-Reference to Other Techniques

Examining the costs and benefits, role playing both sides of the thought, examining the evidence, examining the logic, and using the double standard are all relevant tools.

Forms

Form 4.8 (Point–Counterpoint, p. 146); Form 4.9 (Learning from Disconfirm Predictions, p. 147).

Automatic Thoughts	Rational Responses
I might have AIDS.	I haven't engaged in any unsafe sexual behavior.
You can never be completely sure how one might get it.	You can't be completely sure about anything, but the probability is almost zero.
But you could be wrong.	I could be anything, but it's not worth worrying about every possibility. It is highly improbable.
Improbable isn't good enough. You have to be sure.	Why do I have to be sure?
So that I will never have any regrets.	What's so bad about regrets? It's impossible to live life and never have regrets.

FIGURE 4.1. Point–Counterpoint

TECHNIQUE: DISTINGUISHING BETWEEN PRODUCTIVE AND UNPRODUCTIVE WORRY

Description

Many people who worry will resist considering—let alone accepting—the idea that worrying is useless. Indeed, worrying *can* be a helpful catalyst for preparation and a deterrent to negative outcomes. Since many worriers believe that worrying is helpful in solving problems (Borkovec, Alcaine, & Bear, in press; Nolen-Hoeksema, 2000; Wells, 1997, 2000), the therapist must address the issue of what is "productive" and what is "unproductive" worrying (Wells, 1997). The goal of therapy is not for patients to eliminate all worrying but to learn to distinguish useful from useless worrying and how to turn worries into solutions. The therapist might use the following explanation.

"Let's imagine that you are beginning a 700-mile drive. You might begin the journey with productive worries such as 'Do I have enough gas? Have I checked the oil and coolant? Do I know the way? Have I given myself enough time to get there?' These are useful worries because they are prudent; they are focused on events or problems that have a reasonable probability of being relevant to your trip, could reasonably cause you a problem if left unexamined, and, most importantly, *lead you to solving a problem.* In contrast, suppose your train of thought went in the following direction: 'What if I have a heart attack while I'm driving? What if the tires explode on the highway? What if I get kidnapped? What if I leave for the day and my wife runs off with someone?' Each of these worries describes something that is *possible* but *highly improbable*, is stated in catastrophic terms, and describes something over which you have very little control.

"I distinguish between productive and unproductive worries as the difference between a 'to do' list and a 'what if' list. A 'to do' list leads to a set of reasonable actions that I can take. For example, I can check the gas, oil, and coolant, get a map and contact the Automobile Club to get an estimate of how long the trip will take. This is a list of prudent actions. In contrast, worries about heart attacks, exploding tires, kidnapping, and infidelity do not lead to a 'to do' list. Thinking about these 'what ifs' only leads to a sense of doom and helplessness. These are unproductive worries.

"Not all 'what ifs' are unproductive, however. Some 'what ifs' can be translated into a 'to do' list. For example, 'What if my computer crashes and wipes out the CPU? My document would be lost!' This worry could be translated into a problem-solving question: 'What could I do to secure my files on the computer?' The 'to do' list mentality leads to the productive action of backing up the files in the hard drive on a disk."

Unproductive worries are typically phrased in nonconfirmable ways, such as "I can't believe that this is happening" or "I feel so lousy I can't stand it." These ruminations lead to, deepen, and maintain depression (Nolen-Hoeksema, 2000). They can be rephrased by raising the following questions: "Can I change my statement to a prediction?," "What is the problem that needs to be solved?," and "What would be a possible solution to the problem?"

Question to Pose/Intervention

"Some worries are productive, and other worries are not productive. A productive worry is a concern about something that is plausible—something that a reasonable person might think about. For example, if you were driving from New York City to Washington, DC, it would be productive to ask yourself 'Do I have enough gas?' and 'Do I have a map?' Productive worry leads to a 'to do' list of actions that I can take. In contrast, unproductive or useless worries are about very unlikely events—things that a reasonable person would not worry about. A lot of times, these worries don't lead to anything that you can do. Worries that are unproductive include, for example, 'What if I get a flat and my car spins out of control?' or 'What if my engine blows up?' or 'What if someone runs into me?' "

Example

THERAPIST: You said that you are worried about the exam. We went over some of these worries—for example, the worry that if you blow the exam, then you won't get into law school and you won't be able to get a job. Those worries led to worries about not making a living and then being a failure.

PATIENT: Yeah, I have a whole string of worries.

THERAPIST: Some of these worries are what we would call "unproductive worries." They are worries that aren't plausible right now and that you can't really do much about. For example, the worry that you might end up as a failure, without any job, is not something you can do anything about today. You can't go out and get a job today because you're in school.

PATIENT: I have a lot of worries like that—like "What if my boyfriend leaves me?" or "What if I get sick?"

THERAPIST: Do any of these worries—about doing poorly on the exam, not getting into law school, ending up with no job, and failing in life—lead to a "to do" list—for today and this week?

PATIENT: I guess the only thing is preparing for the exam.

THERAPIST: OK. Let's make a list of things to do to prepare for the exam. When you have the other unproductive worries, you can write them down in your "list of unproductive worries" and put them in a drawer.

PATIENT: What you're saying is that I should only focus on things that I can do something about?

THERAPIST: That's right. We'll narrow ourselves to the productive worry and turn it into a "to do" list.

PATIENT: That sounds more manageable.

Homework

Patients can be asked to monitor their worries and then check off whether each is productive or unproductive. Productive worry is worry that others would find plausible or reasonable and that leads to a specific action. A more detailed table (Form 4.10, at the end of the chapter) is provided that requests patients to ask themselves a series of questions about their worry, such as "Is this worry something with a very low probability of occurring? What prediction am I making? What is the problem that needs to be solved? What specific actions can I take? Do these actions seem reasonable? Am I worrying over things about which I have little or no control?"

Possible Problems

Some patients respond that they know that all of their worries are irrational. However, not all worries are entirely irrational or without benefit—for example, worrying about an upcoming annual medical examination or bills due is preferable to ignoring such tasks. We wish to indicate to patients that some worries can quickly be turned into a useful "to do" list. Other patients may confuse "possible" worries with "plausible" ones. For example, it is possible that a tire will blow out on the highway and the car spin out of control. However, the only "to do" list for this worry is to make sure the tires are inflated and that normal speed limits are observed. Individuals who claim they need certainty to feel safe can examine the costs and benefits of demanding certainty and consider why they are willing to tolerate many uncertainties on a daily basis but demand certainty for the current situation.

Cross-Reference to Other Techniques

Other relevant techniques include identifying automatic thoughts, vertical descent, mood monitoring associated with thoughts, and cost–benefit analysis.

Form

Form 4.10 (Productive and Unproductive Worries, p. 148).

TECHNIQUE: ASSIGNING WORRY TIME

Description

Worries seem to preoccupy an inordinate amount of time for some people, leading them to worry at work, at home, and when they are trying to fall asleep. One technique that is useful in addressing chronic worrying is to establish "stimulus control" over worries—that is, to restrict worrying to a specific time and place (i.e., stimuli), thereby decreasing the association of work, home, and bed with worrying. Furthermore, creating this specific "worry time" helps worriers recognize that they can exercise some control over worrying, even if it only means delaying it a couple of hours. Finally, by assigning a specific time for worrying, worriers come to recognize the limited and finite nature of the content of their worries—that is, they generally worry about the same types of things. This recognition helps reduce the overwhelming sense that they are worrying about *everything*.

The therapist explains that a specific time and place should be chosen for worrying, that the patient should limit the time during which the worrying occurs but to worry intensely during this time. If worries occur earlier or later during the day, the worrier should jot them down on a piece of paper and save them for worry time. No other activity should be engaged in during worry time, and the patient should be encouraged to write out the worries, making no attempt at this point to challenge or resolve them. A specific duration should be set—for example, 30 minutes—and worrying should cease at the time limit but not before.

Question to Pose/Intervention

"Sometimes people feel that their worrying is out of control and that they are worrying all of the time. I'd like you to plan to set aside 30 minutes each day to engage in your worry. Write down all of your worries. If you have a worry during another time during the day, just write it down on a piece of paper and set it aside until your worry time."

Example

THERAPIST: Sometimes people feel that they are worrying all of the time. They feel that they have little control over when, or how much, they worry. Is that how you feel?

PATIENT: Yes. I just can't get these worries out of my head. I'll find myself worrying when I am on the bus or sitting at home alone.

THERAPIST: How does all that worrying make you feel?

PATIENT: Like I have no control over my worries. Then I try to tell myself to stop worrying, but that doesn't do any good.

THERAPIST: I'm going to suggest something that might sound a little odd to you. It's called "worry time." What we suggest is that you set aside some time every day to focus on nothing else but your worries. If you have a worry earlier in the day, just write it down and assign it to yourself during the worry time.

PATIENT: Won't this make me worry more?

THERAPIST: Almost everyone thinks that. But we find that you end up limiting most of your worrying to the worry time and end up worrying *less*.

PATIENT: It seems odd that assigning myself worry time would make me worry less. I thought I was trying to get *rid* of my worries.

THERAPIST: Well, we're not really trying to get rid of your worries. We are trying to get more control over the worries.

PATIENT: When should I do this?

THERAPIST: Plan a regular time every day—a long time before you go to bed. Don't do the worry time when you are in bed. Just write out the worries during that time.

PATIENT: OK. I'll try doing it at 5:30, when I get home from work.

Homework

The therapist can explain the assignment as follows: "Assign 30 minutes each day during which to worry intensely. Write down all of your worries, noting how anxious you are before you start the worry time and how anxious you are after the 30 minutes. Please use a time long before you go to bed. Sit down at a table—not on your bed—and write out all of the worries that come to mind. If you have any worries earlier in the day, write them on a piece of paper and put them off until the worry time. When you have done this exercise for a week, look back at your worries and see if there are some common themes that keep repeating themselves. You can use this form (4.11, at the end of the chapter).

Possible Problems

Sometimes worriers find that they cannot fill entire time period with worries. This "problem" suggests that the worrying is limited—as does the recognition that the worries are similar in content. Intensive worry time serves the purpose of providing stimulus exposure unmediated by neutralization (i.e., by trying to resolve the worries—similar to the type of exposure used when treating people with obsessions and compulsions. Presumably, worriers try to neutralize their feared images by trying to find solutions (Borkovec et al. in press). In contrast, worry time compels them to focus on their worries without neutralization, thereby leading to habituation of the worry pattern.

Cross-Reference to Other Techniques

Worry time involves identifying automatic thoughts. Other techniques that may be related include monitoring thoughts and feelings, vertical descent, imagery techniques, and categorizing automatic thought distortions.

Form

Form 4.11 (Worry Time, p. 149).

TECHNIQUE : EXAMINING IF THE THOUGHT IS TESTABLE

Description

Many people label themselves or make predictions that are based on thoughts or statements that can never be proven false. For example, in the previous section I described how terms such as "worthless person" or "good for nothing" are not even definable: We don't even know what we are talking about when we use those terms. Ironically, we can get ourselves upset over something that is meaningless.

Patients should look at their thoughts as hypotheses or statements about what they think the facts are. Consider the follow statements asserted as "facts":

"Bill is six feet tall."
"I will fail the test."
"It's going to rain tomorrow."
"She won't talk to me."
"No one likes me.

We can "test" the truth of each of these statements by collecting information—by making observations about what is true or false. We can measure Bill's height, we can see how I do on the test, we can look outside tomorrow to see if it rains, we can observe whether she talks to me, and we can collect information about whether people like me. These are *testable thoughts that can be either true or false*.

Some thoughts stated as facts, however, are not testable. We say that they are not open to *disconfirmation*; they are not "falsified" (Popper, 1959). If there is no possible way to disprove a statement, then the statement is meaningless. Here are some examples of statements that are not open to disconfirmation:

1. "No matter what I do, I am worthless."
2. "Angels exist."
3. "There are spirits that control us."
4. "It's possible that I could go crazy."
5. "I need to know for sure."

Consider how each of these statements could be disproved—or not.

1. If "no matter what I do I am worthless", then how can I disprove this? Since you discount all evidence of behavior as indicating you're worthwhile, then you are stating *as an axiom*—as a statement that cannot be challenged—"I am worthless." You are simply saying "I am worthless and there's nothing you can say that can change that belief."
2. The statement "Angels exist" also is not open to disconfirmation. We could confirm it only by observing angels, but since angels are generally unobservable, the fact that we don't observe them proves nothing. We can't possibly disconfirm the idea that "Angels exist."
3. The same thing is true about unobservable "spirits" that control us. We can't observe them, so we can't disprove any possible influence over us.

4. The statement "It's possible that I could go crazy" also cannot be disproved, since the possibility exists for everyone.

5. We all do many things—for example, drive to work, eat lunch, start conversations—about which we don't know for sure what's going to happen next. Still, we do them. But the belief of needing to know something *for sure* cannot be disproved. It's a preference, an emotion, a "need" or a "want," and there is nothing to prove or disprove.

The criterion of "falsifiability" is important because it allows us to test out the truth of statements. Science is based on taking statements and testing them against the facts. If thoughts cannot be tested, then the thinker can never find out what is true and what is false. From the scientific point of view, such thoughts are meaningless because they cannot be tested.

Question to Pose/Intervention

"Is there any way that your worry could be tested? Is it at all possible to disprove your worry? When you make a prediction that something bad will happen, how will we know if you are right or wrong?"

Example

THERAPIST: You are saying that you are worried you won't do well at the party.

PATIENT: Yeah, I think that I'll screw up.

THERAPIST: When we are worried and we make predictions, we often find ourselves expecting that something will not work out. How will you know if there are some things that do work out? What could count as some positive outcomes?

PATIENT: I guess if people talk to me and smile at me?

THERAPIST: OK. That would be one way of showing that your negative prediction might be inaccurate. How else?

PATIENT: If I had a good time.

THERAPIST: How would we know if you had a good time?

PATIENT: If I met some people, had some conversations, and didn't freak out.

THERAPIST: OK. So let's write those down as possible outcomes to see if your prediction is wrong.

Homework

The therapist can explain the assignment as follows: "Using this table [Form 4.12, at the end of the chapter] consider the thoughts that bother you—'I'm a loser and I'll fail'—and indicate how you could test out their truth or falsity. What would you need to observe or know to conclude that you are a loser or that you have failed? How would you know that you were not a loser and had not failed?"

Possible Problems

Some worriers predict their own worry and emotions—for example, "I'll go to the party and worry and feel nervous." This kind of prediction becomes circular—"I'll worry because I'm anxious." The therapist should ask the patient to predict positive events involving behaviors displayed by self and others—for example, "I will talk and smile at someone" or "Someone will initiate a conversation with me." In other cases, worriers may discount the positive outcomes, pointing out that this is no guarantee of future positive outcomes. In this case, the demand for certainty can be addressed though "uncertainty training," as described later in this chapter.

Cross-Reference to Other Techniques

Relevant alternatives include distinguishing thoughts from facts, testing predictions, the semantic (definition) technique, and examining the evidence.

Forms

Form 4.12 (Making Thoughts Testable, p. 150).

TECHNIQUE: SELF-FULFILLING PROPHECIES

Description

When we try to explain why negative events occur, we may often overlook our own role in their existence. Avoidance, procrastination, and coercion are three types of behavior that foster self-fulfilling prophecies. The avoider eschews interactions with people and explains her lack of relationships by claiming there are few good people available. The procrastinator claims that it will make him anxious to work on the project, not realizing that the reason that he is generally so anxious when working on these projects is because he's put them off until the last minute. The coercive or punitive spouse complains about his wife's coldness, not recognizing that his criticisms have led her to withdraw.

Question to Pose/Intervention

"Are your problems the result of how you yourself make your predictions come true? Have you behaved as if your thoughts were true and therefore not had the opportunity to find out that you are wrong? For example, you have assumed no one would like you, so you don't interact with people or you leave as soon as you feel uncomfortable. As a result, you have few opportunities to challenge your negative thoughts."

Example

Consider a young woman who claims that it is difficult to meet a man. She says that she goes to parties, but men do not seem to pursue her.

THERAPIST: What are your thoughts before you go to the party?

PATIENT: I think "I'll never meet a man."

THERAPIST: If a woman were going to show an interest in meeting a man, how would she show that interest?

PATIENT: I don't understand.

THERAPIST: Would she look at the man, look in his eyes when she meets him, smile at him, compliment him, ask him questions?

PATIENT: Well, I can't do that!

THERAPIST: You mean "I don't do that." If you did that, rather than looking down and withdrawing the second you feel the man is not interested—if you stuck with it—what would happen?

PATIENT: I'd get rejected.

THERAPIST: Could it also be that the man might respond positively, smile back, ask you about yourself, maybe even ask you out?

At this point, the patient recognized that her shyness and avoidance might actually be the reason why men were not pursuing her. I told her to monitor the number of times men smiled and looked at her and to look back, smile, and ask them about themselves. The outcome for her over the next 2 months was an increase in the interest directed toward her by the men she met.

Now consider a businessman who procrastinated on his taxes until the week before they were due, resulting in excessive pressure to get the information to his accountant. His thought was, "Every time I think of doing my taxes, I get anxious because I think it'll be so unpleasant." Consequently, he delayed until the last minute. The therapist asked: "Is doing your taxes the event that is unpleasant? Or is doing your taxes *at the last minute* the unpleasant event?" Since he had never tried doing his taxes early, he could not distinguish between the two and had concluded that delaying an unpleasant task would be the better option. This was a self-fulfilling prophecy.

The question such patients need to ask is: "Could my behavior [or lack of a certain behavior] be the cause of what I'm complaining about?"

Depressed individuals often complain to their friends and focus excessively on the negative. Then they complain that people do not like them. If the belief is "I have no friends" or "People do not like me," the question could be: "Am I doing something that could be alienating to people?" Some patients see this question as a criticism. The therapist can explain that the question and answer could empower them by directing them to focus on the behavior that needs to be changed—such as, decrease complaining and negative focus.

Homework

The purpose of the homework assignment is to help the patient recognize that negative predictions often lead to negative outcomes. These are "self-fulfilling prophecies." The therapist can ask the patient to list a number of negative predictions from the past or from current experience. The therapist can then ask the patient to identify what is likely to make these negative predictions come true. For example, how will the patient's procrastination, avoidance, lack of trying, giving up, or even hostile and aggressive behavior lead to confirming these negative predictions. The form for self-fulfilling prophecies can be used as a homework assignment.

Possible Problems

Self-critical patients often view the fact that they have a role in their own problems as further evidence of their failure. They may believe that the therapist is blaming the patient. The therapist should validate these concerns and focus on "fixing the problem rather than fixing the blame." Examining the costs and benefits of recognizing one's role in the problem and examining alternative ways to behaving—for example, acting against one's negative predictions—may be helpful.

Cross-Reference to Other Techniques

Other techniques that are useful include graded task assignments, activity schedules, examining alternatives, problem solving, double-standard technique, and rational role-plays.

Form

Form 4.13 (Identifying Negative Predictions, p. 151).

TECHNIQUE: FLOODING UNCERTAINTY

Description

Worriers often complain about the *possibility* of the dreaded event—for example, "Well, it's possible the plane *could* crash . . . I *could* get AIDS at the dentist's office . . . I *could* go crazy . . . I *could* lose all my money." It is *not* possible to eliminate possibility—although many worriers certainly try to do so. The therapist should focus on how the patient can estimate *probability*, given the information available and given what we know about the base rates of various human experiential categories in the real world. Thus it is possible that one could get AIDS from a dentist, but the probability is so low that it approaches 0%. It is also possible that a plane taking off from Chicago could crash, but, again, this probability is remote.

Question to Pose/Intervention

"A lot of time we worry about things that are possible but are not really that probable. For example, it is possible to have a heart attack when anxious, but what is the probability? If we worried about everything that is possible, then we would worry about *everything*. For example, it's possible that you could walk out on the street and someone could think you are Satan and attack and kill you. But what is the probability of such an event happening? We get information about probability by looking at how often something generally happens in the real world. Sometimes we refer to information about probability as the base-rate. For example, what base-rate (or the percentage) of people who have headaches also have brain tumors? We would talk to all the people who have headaches—which is just about everyone—and ask how many of these people also have brain tumors. The answer would amount to a very small percentage.

Example

The patient reported that he had a headache and that he was worried he might have a brain tumor that was the cause of the headache. He had recently heard of someone in the news who had a brain tumor.

THERAPIST: What is the evidence that you have a brain tumor?

PATIENT: I have a headache. Isn't that one of the signs of a brain tumor?

THERAPIST: How long have you had a headache?

PATIENT: For a couple of hours.

THERAPIST: What makes you think that this is a brain tumor?

PATIENT: I heard about this guy who died from a brain tumor—they said he had headaches.

THERAPIST: How many people in New York City have headaches in any given year?

PATIENT: I'd imagine over half.

THERAPIST: How many of those headaches are caused by brain tumors?

PATIENT: Almost none.

THERAPIST: So, if you were to estimate the probability that someone who has a headache also has a brain tumor, what would it be?

PATIENT: It's possible, though, isn't it? Even if it's a very low probability? I could be that unlucky one in a million.

THERAPIST: Are you trying to rule out all probability and have absolute certainty?

PATIENT: I know, it's impossible. But I wish I had certainty.

THERAPIST: What are the costs and benefits of demanding certainty?

PATIENT: The cost is that I'm anxious a lot. And the benefits—I don't know, maybe that I can catch something wrong sooner.

THERAPIST: But you live with uncertainty every moment of the day. How do you manage that?

PATIENT: I just accept a lot of things that are beyond my control.

THERAPIST: What if you accepted this headache in that way?

PATIENT: I might be better off, but I also might overlook a symptom of a serious condition.

THERAPIST: What's the probability that you have a brain tumor?

PATIENT: Almost 0%.

THERAPIST: If you want to eliminate possibility, then you might spend all your time worrying. What if you simply focused on things that seem plausible or that have some probability? For example, what is the probability that if you don't pay your credit card bill on time, you will get penalized?

PATIENT: 100%.

THERAPIST: That's a probability that makes sense. There is no certainty in an uncertain world. What would be the advantages and disadvantages of accepting that you can never know a whole lot of things for certain and to accept uncertainty as a human condition?

PATIENT: I'd be better off. I keep driving myself crazy by demanding certainty. I guess I think that if I try to achieve certainty, then I'd be less anxious—but it only makes me more anxious.

THERAPIST: Exactly.

After the patient established that certainty is impossible, the therapist asked him to repeat this sentence for 10 minutes, "No matter what I do, I can never achieve certainty." After an initial increase, his level of anxious arousal decreased.

Homework

Patients are asked to write down examples of worries that involve a demand for certainty—for example, worries about health, finances, relationships, or work. Each worry is recast as "I am not sure if X will happen"—for example, "I am not sure if I have cancer." Then patients are asked to write down the costs and benefits of demanding certainty in order to resolve or depotentiate this particular worry.

Finally, patients are asked to repeat the worry that has been restated in terms of "I am not sure . . ." for 15 minutes each day.

Possible Problems

Some patients fear that repeating their worry as a statement of uncertainty will make them more anxious. This thought flooding should be done within the session the first time to demonstrate that the anxiety will decrease. Some patients may need more than 15 minutes—and they should be instructed to continue repeating their thought until the arousal has decreased by half. Patients may interrupt the effect of flooding by repeating the thought in a rote or mechanical way or by distracting themselves with other behavior or stimuli. Doing so may interfere with the habituation process. These "safety behaviors" should be eliminated.

Cross-Reference to Other Techniques

Other relevant techniques include cost–benefit analysis, acceptance training, double-standard technique, and vertical descent.

Form

Form 4.14 (Flooding Yourself with Uncertainty, p. 152).

TECHNIQUE: TIME MACHINE (SELF)

Description

Often we believe that what is happening to us now will continue to disturb us forever. We get engulfed in the field, caught up in the moment, and find it difficult to escape our emotions and our current perspective. At times, we focus entirely on what is directly in front of us in that moment, failing to realize that our thoughts and feelings will change. When we are caught up in the moment, we cannot imagine variations in how we will feel at another time and in a different situation. Decentering would involve stepping back and observing how feelings and experiences change.

The purpose of the time machine technique is to foster perspective on a current problem. Patients can use this exercise either to go back into time or to go forward in time. The therapist asks patients to imagine that they are placed in a time machine that will take them back to the past or into the future of their own lives.

Question to Pose/Intervention

The therapist can ask the patient to recollect pleasant past memories: "Go back in time and recall very pleasant experiences." Notice how your mood changes when you think of past positive experiences.

"You are very worried about this right now, but I wonder how you will feel about this a week from now, a month from now, a year from now, 5 years from now. What would be some reasons why you would be less upset about this in the future? You may feel engulfed in the moment right now. What other events (unrelated to this event) will transpire over the next day, week, month, and year that will lead you to disregard this event?"

Example

THERAPIST: You are very upset about not doing well on your job. You told me that your boss criticized your performance on the job last Tuesday. Let's go into the time machine and go back to a time when you were feeling happy. Perhaps it was a time during your childhood.

PATIENT: I can picture myself sitting on the porch with my parents. It's summer and we're drinking lemonade. It's warm outside, but we're sitting in the shade and it's cool.

THERAPIST: How are you feeling in this memory?

PATIENT: I feel relaxed. I have a feeling of well-being.

Going back into time to a pleasant memory is helpful in getting patients to recognize that they can escape from this one moment that bothers them and experience pleasurable and peaceful feelings. The next step is to place patients into a time machine that goes forward into the future to a time when they will no longer care about what is happening now.

THERAPIST: Now, I want you to imagine that you are going forward into the time machine to the future. Let's imagine that it's a month from now. How do you think you'll feel about your boss's criticism of your work last Tuesday?

PATIENT: I can't imagine I'd care that much. But I'd still think of it.

THERAPIST: How about 6 months from now? How would you feel?

PATIENT: I probably wouldn't care.

THERAPIST: How about a year from now?

PATIENT: I'd probably have forgotten about it.

THERAPIST: Now, that's interesting. I wonder how many things have bothered you in your life—things that you felt were devastating at the time—which you don't care about now, and can't even recall them.

PATIENT: Probably almost every one of them.

This exercise is helpful in getting patients to understand that the immediate reaction to a situation may be the most disturbing, but that its negativity wears off with time.

Homework

The therapist can explain this assignment as follows: "One way of changing your worries is to put them in perspective—that is, to imagine how you would feel about these concerns in the future. We can call this the "time machine" method, since you will imagine yourself going backward or forward in a time machine. Ask yourself how you would feel about this concern at different times in the future. What would be some reasons why you would feel less bothered by this worry? Would you have found that other things valuable to you—and things that you simply enjoy—would overshadow these things that you are worried about? Use the table [Form 4.14, at the end of the chapter] to write down your different worries and then indicate how you would feel about these things at different times in the future.

Possible Problems

Some patients who feel hopeless may believe that they will feel worse in the future. For example, the patient going through a breakup may believe that he or she will feel increasingly lonely in the future. The therapist should inquire as to what positive actions could be taken to handle loneliness—for example, activity scheduling, becoming proactive in pursuing contact with people, engaging in challenging and interesting behavior, such as taking a class or joining a hiking group. Alternatively, the therapist can ask the patient if he or she had experienced losses before and how was he or she able to make progress in regaining a satisfying social life. Often, the worried patient may underestimate his or her ability to handle problems that arise but may be able to recall coping competently in the past.

Cross-Reference to Other Techniques

Other relevant techniques include the double-standard technique, problem-solving techniques, rational role plays, vertical descent, and examining the evidence.

Form

Form 4.15 (Time Machine, p. 153).

TECHNIQUE: TIME MACHINE (OTHERS)

Description

Just as gaining distance in time can help us feel better about what is currently happening, we can imagine that others also will care less about what is happening as time passes. For example, the socially anxious patient believes that people will notice his or her anxiety and remember it, resulting in the impression that he or she is weak and inadequate. In fact, of course, people seldom remember other people's anxiety (since it is usually irrelevant to what is important to other people).

Question to Pose/Intervention

"You are worried what other people are thinking about you, but people often stop thinking about things after a short period of time. Can you imagine yourself in a time machine that goes forward a week, a month, a year in time, and now you are learning what people are thinking about. If you are concerned with how others think of you, put them in our time machine and ask yourself how they will feel about your concern 1 week, 1 month, 1 year from now. Are they thinking about you and your performance? Or are they thinking about something else?"

Example

This exercise was used with a young executive who feared that people would notice his anxiety at a meeting and that they would form a lasting, negative impression of him. His automatic thoughts were "They'll see I'm anxious, think I'm weak, and word will get back to my boss. It could have terrible consequences." Simply eliciting these automatic thoughts reduced his anxiety slightly, since he realized the unlikelihood of this sequence of events. However, we continued to examine his mind-reading assumptions that people were thinking about his anxiety by using the following version of the time machine:

THERAPIST: OK. Let's imagine you're at that meeting. Who will be there?

PATIENT: Probably six executives from the other companies. I'm the only one representing my company.

THERAPIST: Now let's imagine that someone named John is at this meeting. He's from Company X. He sees that your face is flushed and he thinks "That guy is anxious!" How would that make you feel?

PATIENT: More anxious!

THERAPIST: Alright. Now, one of your assumptions is that people are thinking about your anxiety a lot. Let's see if that makes sense. I want you to describe to me, hour by hour, what John might be doing after the meeting ends.

PATIENT: Well, I don't really know, but I would imagine the meeting will end at about 11 A.M., and he'll probably call his office, then go to lunch.

THERAPIST: Is he thinking about your anxiety at lunch?

PATIENT: I can't imagine he would.

THERAPIST: Then what happens?

PATIENT: He finishes lunch and drives back to the airport, where he waits for his plane. Then he gets on the plane.

THERAPIST: Is he thinking about your anxiety?

PATIENT: No.

THERAPIST: Then what happens?

PATIENT: He's probably doing work on the plane. Maybe having a drink. Then, after a couple of hours, the plane lands and he gets his car and goes home. Then he sees his family . . .

THERAPIST: Are there things that John might be worried about or thinking about during the day?

PATIENT: He might be thinking about whether the meeting went well for him or whether he has any problems on his job. He might wonder about his marriage or his health. There could be a million things.

THERAPIST: Does it seem likely that he's thinking about your anxiety?

PATIENT: No, he has other things on his mind. It's funny. It seems kind of conceited of me to think he'd think about my anxiety.

THERAPIST: Well, it's probably not conceited, because it actually makes you feel badly when you think these things. But imagine if your automatic thoughts were true. Here's what it might look like. John is at the meeting, noticing your anxiety. He gets lost going back to the airport because all he can think about is your anxiety. He can't get any work done, because he's thinking about your anxiety. His wife feels he's ignoring her because when he gets home he just thinks about your anxiety. Far-fetched, isn't it?

PATIENT: I can't imagine that would ever happen.

THERAPIST: So, if he noticed that you were anxious, how long would he think about it?

PATIENT: Possibly 10 seconds.

Homework

The therapist can explain the assignment as follows: "Using this table [Form 4.16, at the end of the chapter], write out the kinds of things that you are worried about—especially how you think you appear to others and what they might be thinking of you. Then ask yourself, if you were in a time machine, what would they think about this in the future at the various times that are listed. What things—other than your behavior—would they think about.

Possible Problems

Patients may think that people form rigid negative beliefs about them, based on their current behavior or performance. For example, a man feared that if he lost his erection with a woman, she would form a long-lasting negative belief about him. This fear was examined in several ways: "Predict how she will feel about this lost erection 1 week, 1 month, and 1 year from now. If you continued to see her, would there be other times when you would have rewarding sex with her? Are there other things that she would learn about you? Even if she did form a negative view of you—and she held this a year from now and you no longer saw her—how would this be a problem for you?"

Cross-Reference to Other Techniques

Relevant techniques include turning worries into predictions, identifying and monitoring automatic thoughts, and vertical descent.

Form

Form 4.16 (Why Others Won't Care Later about My "Negative" Behavior, p. 154).

TECHNIQUE: NEGATION OF PROBLEMS

Description

Therapy often seems to serve the function of raising problems, with each session focusing on "what's gone wrong." Of course, we want to help people solve their problems, but it also may be useful to place events in perspective by recognizing that some problems that seem like insurmountable are really minor inconveniences or, in fact, not problems at all. This exercise, "negation of problems," is (obviously) not meant to serve the purpose of denial or repression; rather, it is used with other cognitive therapy techniques to help patient understand that their problems are not necessarily roadblocks that prevent progress. By examining how something is "not really a problem," patients put things in perspective. This focus also draws patients' attention to how problems can be solved and reduces rumination on the problem.

Question to Pose/Intervention

"You are worried that something might go wrong. Let's see if you can come up with some reasons why this is not a problem. Imagine that this thing happens—whatever it is. Can you think of some reasons why this might not be a problem—even if it did happen? You might want to think about how you could solve the problem, put it in perspective, or even ignore it."

Example

In this technique, patients are asked to restate each "problem" using this sentence stem: "This is not a problem because . . . "

THERAPIST: Right now, you've been feeling pretty low because you're out of work and you're looking for a job. You've had some hopeless thoughts that we've gone over, and it seems that you're now able to see some possible solutions. Let's try this: I'll start by restating the problems that have bothered you, and you respond, "This is not a problem because . . . "—and then you tell me what the solution is. For example, if I said "You think it's a problem because it's raining outside," you might respond with "That is not a problem because I have an umbrella." OK. Let's start with "You don't have a job right now . . . "

PATIENT: This is not a problem because I know I can get a job.

THERAPIST: Yeah, but there are a lot of people looking for jobs.

PATIENT: That's not a problem because I have an excellent resume. I have a lot of experience.

THERAPIST: You have no structure to your day.

PATIENT: That's not a problem because I can spend my day on my job search and I can exercise and see friends.

THERAPIST: But some people might think less of you because you don't have a job right now.

PATIENT: That's not a problem because my friends and family are supportive, and I don't have to care about what other people may or may not think.

The value of negating problems is that it mobilizes patients to minimize the negativity in the semantic structure of their responses. They immediately respond with the idea that it is not a problem and then provide a more positive perspective or a solution.

Homework

The therapist can ask patients to list some things that they are worried about and then come up with as many reasons as possible why these worries are not really problems. Negation of the problem can include listing solutions, placing it in perspective, arguing that it does not interfere with other valued goals, or other logical and empirical challenges. Form 4.17 (at the end of the chapter) can be used to expedite this exercise.

Possible Problems

As with any technique that attempts to minimize a problem, patients may experience it as invalidating and dismissive. The therapist can inquire as to these feelings and suggest to patients that this is an experiment in thinking, rather than a final description of facts. Double-standard techniques and rational role play can be utilized to help patients put things in perspective. Listing all of the behaviors that are still available—even if this "problem" exists—can help put it in perspective.

Cross-Reference to Other Techniques

Other relevant interventions include problem-solving techniques, use of the continuum, rational role play, use of the time machine, double-standard techniques, and examining alternative assumptions that are more adaptive.

Form

Form 4.17 (Negation of "Problems", p. 155).

TECHNIQUE: FEARED FANTASY WORRY

Description

People often worry because they are trying to avoid having an image or thought that is very upsetting to them (Borkovec & Hu, 1990; Borkovec & Inz, 1990). For example, an individual may worry that he is spending too much money or that he is not earning enough. He thinks of all of the ways that he could tighten his budget. But if we utilize the vertical descent technique, we will learn that he has an ultimate fear of becoming destitute and ending up as a street person. All of his cognitive energy is deployed in trying to prevent this terrifying thought from occurring. Similarly, an individual may lie in bed worrying that she will not get enough sleep, focusing all of her mental energy on her physical and cognitive arousal, further disrupting her sleep patterns (Harvey, 2001a, 2001b). But what if these patient *practiced* their feared fantasy worry? What if they practiced holding the image for long periods of time, of ending up on the street impoverished or not getting enough sleep ever again? This paradoxical flooding of the feared fantasy should result in habituation to the worst fear, thereby short-circuiting the worries that precede it.

Question to Pose/Intervention

"A lot of the time we worry because we are afraid that something even worse might happen. For example, you might be worried that you will not get to sleep in the next hour. But if we dig deeper we might find the worry that you will get absolutely no sleep and will feel exhausted tomorrow. I'm going to ask you to try to identify that 'worst fear'—the worry that you fear most. Then I want you to practice repeating this worry, over and over, until you become bored with it."

Example

THERAPIST: You are worried that you will lose more money. Try to tell me what this would mean to you. If I lose more money, then . . .

PATIENT: I will go broke.

THERAPIST: OK. So your real fear is not just losing money but going broke. We find that a lot of the time, people worry about things and they come up with all kinds of ways of avoiding that image or that thought.

PATIENT: Well, I try to get reassurance from people. I ask my wife what she thinks, and she tells me that things will work out.

THERAPIST: But the real problem is being able to accept going broke. It's hard to live with having that thought. That's what you have to practice—the thought of actually going broke.

PATIENT: It's too upsetting.

THERAPIST: Let's see. What are some reasons why you *won't* go broke?

PATIENT: I have lots of other investments, and I have a job and my wife has a job. I won't go broke.

THERAPIST: But let's practice the image and the thought of going broke. What image or picture comes to mind of you going broke?

PATIENT: I see myself as homeless, with no money.

THERAPIST: OK. Close your eyes and get this image really clear in your head. Now repeat "I will go broke and end up homeless."

PATIENT: "I will go broke and end up homeless."

THERAPIST: How anxious do you feel—from 0–100%?

PATIENT: About 80%.

THERAPIST: Keep repeating this . . .

PATIENT: (*Repeats the thought and the image for 10 minutes, and his anxiety drops to 5%.*) I'm feeling bored with this.

THERAPIST: That's because you can tolerate having the thought that you will go broke.

Homework

The therapist asks patients to use vertical descent ("What would happen next that would bother you?") until the worst fears are identified. These are then listed and their costs and benefits estimated. Next, patients form a visual image of the worst fear and the statement that goes with it (e.g., "I will die from cancer"). Patients then focus on the image and repeat the statement for 15 minutes.

Possible Problems

Some patients believe that repeating a feared fantasy will make them feel worse. This exercise can be set up as an experiment within the session: "Let's see how your anxiety changes the longer you hold the image in your mind." Many worried patients find this process to be counterintuitive, because all their effort has been focused on escaping their negative images through worry and reassurance seeking. Another problem can be patients' belief that the worst fantasy is a plausible reality—for example, some people *do* go bankrupt. In this case, the worried patient can be assigned the homework of collecting information on how people cope with negative life events—for example, how do people cope with bankruptcy, divorce, or cancer? Coping models are helpful in reducing the anxiety about worst possible outcomes.

Cross-Reference to Other Techniques

The therapist can ask patients to examine past worries and outcomes the costs and benefits of worrying about the worst possible outcome, the evidence for and against these worries, the ability to solve problems, should they arise, and the double-standard technique.

Form

Form 4.18 (Feared Fantasy Worry, p. 156).

TECHNIQUE: ACCEPTANCE

Description

In presenting this exercise, the therapist can say: "Rather than trying to control and change everything, perhaps there are some things you can learn to accept and make the best of. For example, perhaps you won't be perfect in your job, but you could learn to appreciate what you can do. Rather than criticize yourself for having a problem or catastrophic the problem, start with 'I accept that I have a problem with, for example, depression, and now I will try to find a solution to that problem.'"

Question to Pose/Intervention

"We learn to accept a lot of things in life. If you live in Vermont in the winter, you learn to accept the cold. If you live in Miami in August, you learn to accept the heat. Think about practicing a detached acceptance of what is going on. Act as an observer—someone who does not necessarily need to act. How would you describe what is going on without passing a judgment on it or recommending an action? Are there any advantages you might have as an detached observer? What would happen if you decided to be a detached observer and watch these events just go by?"

Example

THERAPIST: Many times we worry about things we feel we need to control. But what if we were to aim for accepting and observing instead of worrying? When we accept and observe, we do not judge, we do not control. For example, if it is cold outside in January, we can observe it and accept it. No doubt we would wear warm clothing, but it is a reality with which we live. What if you were to aim for accepting the things that you currently worry about?

PATIENT: I don't understand.

THERAPIST: Well, let's take your worry that your aches and pains are a sign of terminal cancer. Even though your doctor tells you that all you need is exercise, you still worry that you might die. Accepting your aches and pains means to observe them but not judge them. It means to simply describe. It means not interpreting, just recording. How would you describe your legs?

PATIENT: I feel a little tension in my left leg. A small pain. Sort of like a little needle, but then it goes away at times.

THERAPIST: How does your foot feel?

PATIENT: I noticed it doesn't feel unusual. I can feel my toes more in my shoe. I can feel a little warmth on the bottom of my foot.

THERAPIST: How about accepting eventually dying? What would that look like?

PATIENT: I can see myself as a dead body. I can see that I am not moving. I am not breathing. I stand back and see myself.

THERAPIST: How does that feel to stand back and observe?

PATIENT: I feel a little nervous at first, but there's a sense of calm as well.

Homework

The therapist can explain this assignment as follows: "We worry about many things in life that we really cannot control ultimately. One technique that is useful, if we are uneasy in these ways, is to practice acceptance. You already practice this acceptance in many areas on a day-to-day basis. You accept the fact that you are hungry, need to sleep, have to pay your bills, go to work, get stuck in traffic, or that it is hot or cold. You don't protest or worry about these things. Acceptance can involve becoming an observer who does not judge or interpret or control. The observer sees and accepts. Let's look at some of the things that you worry about and see how you could learn to accept them. Use this table [Form 4.19, at the end of the chapter] to make a list of your worries and write down a description of what has actually happened—just the "bare bones" of it. Avoid making any predictions, interpretations, judgments, or solutions. Simply describe the event or situation. For example, let's say you lost money in your investments. Write down exactly what happened. Then estimate the costs and benefits of simply *accepting* this. Try to be passive, to feel no protest, just acceptance."

Possible Problems

Many worriers pride themselves on preventing bad things from happening. Acceptance is the ability to accept what *may* happen. The therapist can help patients examine the costs and benefits of *solving* versus *accepting*. It is often helpful to have patients examine all the things they accept on a daily basis.

Cross-Reference to Other Techniques

Other relevant techniques include uncertainty training, double standard, rational role play, vertical descent, and identifying automatic thoughts.

Form

Form 4.19 (Practicing Acceptance, p. 157).

FORM 4.1. Self-Monitoring of Worries

Write down the date and time of each of your worries, noting the situation that give rise to each worry, your emotion or feeling (e.g., anxious, sad, helpless, self-conscious), and the specific content of your worry (e.g., "I'll get into an argument" or "I won't know what to do").

Date/ time	Describe situation	Emotion or feeling	Specific worry

FORM 4.2. Costs–Benefits to Worrying

Specific worry	Costs	Rate costs	Benefits	Rate benefits	Costs–benefits

FORM 4.3. Metacognitive Questionnaire

This questionnaire is concerned with beliefs people have about their thinking. Listed below are a number of beliefs that people have expressed. Please read each item and say how much you generally agree with it by circling the appropriate number. Please respond to all the items. There are no right or wrong answers.

		Do not agree	Agree slightly	Agree moderately	Agree very much
1.	Worrying helps me to avoid problems in the future.	1	2	3	4
2.	My worrying is dangerous for me.	1	2	3	4
3.	I have difficulty knowing if I have actually done something, or just imagined it.	1	2	3	4
4.	I think a lot about my thoughts.	1	2	3	4
5.	I could make myself sick with worrying.	1	2	3	4
6.	I am aware of the way my mind works when I am thinking through a problem.	1	2	3	4
7.	If I did not control a worrying thought, and I let it happen, it would be my fault.	1	2	3	4
8.	If I let my worrying thoughts get out of control, they will end up controlling me.	1	2	3	4
9.	I need to worry in order to remain organized.	1	2	3	4
10.	I have little confidence in my memory for words and names.	1	2	3	4
11.	My worrying thoughts persist, no matter how I try to stop them.	1	2	3	4
12.	Worrying helps me to get things sorted out in my mind.	1	2	3	4
13.	I cannot ignore my worrying thoughts.	1	2	3	4
14.	I monitor my thoughts.	1	2	3	4

(continued)

		Do not agree	Agree slightly	Agree moderately	Agree very much
15.	I should be in control of my thoughts all of the time.	1	2	3	4
16.	My memory can mislead me at times.	1	2	3	4
17.	I could be punished for not having certain thoughts.	1	2	3	4
18.	My worrying could make me go mad.	1	2	3	4
19.	If I do not stop worrying thoughts, they could come true.	1	2	3	4
20.	I rarely question my thoughts.	1	2	3	4
21.	Worrying puts my body under a lot of stress.	1	2	3	4
22.	Worrying helps me to avoid disastrous situations.	1	2	3	4
23.	I am constantly aware of my thinking.	1	2	3	4
24.	I have a poor memory.	1	2	3	4
25.	I pay close attention to the way my mind works.	1	2	3	4
26.	People who do not worry have no depth.	1	2	3	4
27.	Worrying helps me cope.	1	2	3	4
28.	I imagine having not done things and then doubt my memory for doing them.	1	2	3	4
29.	Not being able to control my thoughts is a sign of weakness.	1	2	3	4
30.	If I did not worry, I would make more mistakes.	1	2	3	4
31.	I find it difficult to control my thoughts.	1	2	3	4
32.	Worrying is a sign of a good person.	1	2	3	4
33.	Worrying thoughts enter my head against my will.	1	2	3	4

(continued)

		Do not agree	Agree slightly	Agree moderately	Agree very much
34.	If I could not control my thoughts, I would go crazy.	1	2	3	4
35.	I will lose out in life if I do not worry.	1	2	3	4
36.	When I start worrying, I cannot stop.	1	2	3	4
37.	Some thoughts will always need to be controlled.	1	2	3	4
38.	I need to worry in order to set things done.	1	2	3	4
39.	I will be punished for not controlling certain thoughts.	1	2	3	4
40.	My thoughts interfere with my concentration.	1	2	3	4
41.	It is alright to let my thoughts roam free.	1	2	3	4
42.	I worry about my thoughts.	1	2	3	4
43.	I am easily distracted.	1	2	3	4
44.	My worrying thoughts are not productive.	1	2	3	4
45.	Worry can stop me from seeing a situation clearly.	1	2	3	4
46.	Worrying helps me to solve problems.	1	2	3	4
47.	I have little confidence in my memory for places.	1	2	3	4
48.	My worrying thoughts are uncontrollable.	1	2	3	4
49.	It is bad to think certain thoughts.	1	2	3	4
50.	If I do not control my thoughts, I may end up embarrassing myself.	1	2	3	4
51.	I do not trust my memory.	1	2	3	4
52.	I do my clearest thinking when I am worrying.	1	2	3	4
53.	My worrying thoughts appear automatically.	1	2	3	4

(continued)

		Do not agree	Agree slightly	Agree moderately	Agree very much
54.	I would be selfish if I never worried.	1	2	3	4
55.	If I could control my thoughts, I would not be able to function.	1	2	3	4
56.	I need to worry in order to work well.	1	2	3	4
57.	I have little confidence in my memory for actions.	1	2	3	4
58.	I have difficulty keeping my mind focused on one thing for a long time.	1	2	3	4
59.	If a bad thing happens which I have not worried about, I feel responsible.	1	2	3	4
60.	It would not be normal if I did not worry.	1	2	3	4
61.	I constantly examine my thoughts.	1	2	3	4
62.	If I stopped worrying, I would become glib, arrogant, and offensive.	1	2	3	4
63.	Worrying helps me to plan the future more effectively.	1	2	3	4
64.	I would be a stronger person if I could worry less.	1	2	3	4
65.	I would be stupid and complacent not to worry.	1	2	3	4

FORM 4.4. Turning Worries into Predictions

Worry	**Specific Prediction** (specifically, what will happen and when will it happen?)

FORM 4.5. Testing Negative Predictions

I predict . . . will happen.	Actual outcome . . .

FORM 4.6. Examining Past Negative Predictions

It is useful to look back at your negative predictions in the past to see if you have a bias toward negative fortune telling. Think back about situations (i.e., activating events) when you made negative predictions. For example, you might have gone through a breakup and predicted "I'll never have another relationship" or "I'll never feel happy." Write down your prediction from the past in the second column and write down what actually happened in the third column.

Past Activating Event	Prediction/Thought	Actual Outcome

FORM 4.7. Reviewing the Handling of Past Negative Events

All of us deal with negative events from time to time. Perhaps you do not think that you can handle negative situations that well. Think back about negative experiences that you have had and identify ways that you were able to cope. What did you eventually do to make things better? Also, identify some problematic or unhelpful ways of coping—for example, drinking, isolating yourself, pursuing no-win relationships, procrastinating, or just complaining. Finally, examine your current problem and identify some possible effective ways of coping and some ineffective ways of coping.

Past Negative Events	How I Coped	Unhelpful Ways of Coping

Current Problem That I Worry About	How I Could Cope Effectively	Unhelpful Ways of Coping

FORM 4.8. Point–Counterpoint

Start with the automatic thought and then challenge it with a rational response. In turn, challenge the rational response. Keep going back and forth—challenging your previous response.

Automatic Thoughts	Rational Responses

FORM 4.9. Learning from Disconfirmed Predictions

Describe some past evidence that contradicts current negative beliefs and how or why you do not use this information to invalidate your current belief. Examine if some of the reasons listed are reasons why you do not learn from past negative predictions.

Past evidence against belief	Why I didn't learn from this
	• Need for infeasible guarantees • Don't bother reexamining instances that contradict my belief • Discount the evidence • Need to maintain my belief and to be right
	Other reasons . . .

FORM 4.10. Productive and Unproductive Worries

We all worry about something some of the time. The question here is whether your current worry is productive or unproductive. Productive worry is worry that leads to concrete, specific action. It is worry about something that is plausible or has a reasonable probability of occurring. Unproductive worry is simply worrying about what is possible—what *could* happen—but about things that are very, very unlikely.

My current worry: _____

Question	Answer
Is this something with a very low probability of occurring?	
What prediction am I making?	
What is the problem that needs to be solved?	
What specific actions can I take?	
Do these actions seem reasonable?	
Am I worrying about things over which I have little or no control?	
Is this a productive or unproductive worry?	
Why or why not?	

FORM 4.11. Worry Time

Write out your worries using the form below. Is there a pattern or a common theme? Do these worries seem realistic?

Time/Date:	Duration (minutes):
Place:	
Anxiety at start of Worry Time (0–100%):	Anxiety at end of Worry Time (0–100%):

Worries:

Common themes in my worrying:

FORM 4.12. Making Thoughts Testable

Thought	How could I test it?

Note: Is there anything wrong with how your thoughts are stated? Are they really testable? Could we really collect information that could weigh against your thought?

FORM 4.13. Identifying Negative Predictions

In the left column list your negative predictions (e.g., "No one will talk to me at the party"). In the second column, list all the things that you do that make your prediction "come true" (e.g., "I don't talk to people" or "I act like I'm afraid"). In the right column, list things that you could do to act against your negative prediction—for example, what you would do if you believed the opposite of your negative prediction (e.g., "I'd introduce myself to people" or "I'd ask people about themselves").

My negative predictions	How I make these predictions come true	Alternatives that can disprove my negative predicitons

FORM 4.14. Flooding Yourself with Uncertainty

In the left-hand column, write down the thought that you will repeat to yourself—for example, "It's always possible that [something terrible] could happen to me." In the middle column, note that you have repeated the thought in 3-minute intervals. In the right-hand column, note your anxiety level, from 0–100%. Keep repeating the statement over and over, until your anxiety has been reduced by half. Thus, if your highest level is 80%, then repeat the thought until the anxiety is less than 40%. Keep repeating the thought for at least 15 minutes, regardless of your anxiety level.

Thought to be repeated	Time: Exposure	Anxiety (0–100%)

Possibility: _____

Costs of accepting that it is possible: _____

Benefits of accepting that it is possible: _____

FORM 4.15. Time Machine

How I'll feel about what's bothering me now in . . .	Why I would not feel as bad about this
1 week	
1 month	
6 months	
1 year	
5 years	

FORM 4.16. Why Others Won't Care Later about My "Negative" Behavior

My negative behavior	Other things that the person will do or think about that have nothing to do with me

FORM 4.17. Negation of "Problems"

Problem	Why It's Not a Problem

FORM 4.18. Feared Fantasy Worry

First identify your worst fears behind your current worry and estimate the costs and benefits of those worst fears, then focus on the image of the very worst fear and repeat to yourself the statement that goes with it for 15 minutes. At 3-minute intervals, estimate and record your level of anxiety.

Identify your worst fears behind your current worry	Cost of worrying about this	Benefit of worrying about this
Repeat the feared image and the statement that goes with it	**3-minute intervals**	**Anxiety (0–100%)**

FORM 4.19. Practicing Acceptance

The thing I am worried about is:	
Costs and benefits of acceptance:	Costs:
	Benefits:
Things I accept daily that could bother me if I let them:	
Why I accept these things:	
Describe, in some detail, what is actually happening that is causing the worry (do not judge, interpret, or predict):	Detached Observer:
Conclusion:	

CHAPTER 5

~

Information Processing
and Logical Errors

$\mathbf{C}$ognitive theory proposes that anxiety and depression are maintained and augmented by distortions in information processing. As we will discuss in Chapter 7 on eliciting and modifying schemas, the cognitive model suggests that individuals selectively attend to and recall information consistent with preexisting beliefs. In this chapter, we focus on errors in information processing that result in selective confirmation of negative beliefs, and we examine typical logical errors that lead individuals to go beyond the current information to draw negative conclusions.

TECHNIQUE: LIMITED SEARCH

Description

One of the hallmarks of depressive and anxious thinking is the habit of seeking information that is consistent with the negative concept and overlooking or discounting for any information that is inconsistent with the negative concept. This cognitive pattern is one of schematic processing—that is, the individual with this schema selectively attends to, searches for, remembers, values, and recognizes, information consistent with its particular underlying or composite beliefs or concepts. Cognitive psychologists refer to this particular pattern as "confirmation bias." In lay terms, it is looking only for information that is consistent with our beliefs. Thus, if we believe that people with blue eyes are nasty people, we will notice any information that confirms the belief and then stop looking. In the search process, we may ignore any information that is inconsistent with that belief (see Simon, 1983).

The therapist might explain this concept as follows: "We are going to explore something called 'limited search,' which is a quality of information processing that limits your awareness and focus to proving that your depressive or anxious thought is true. For example, let's suppose that your negative thought is 'I'm a failure.' In order to confirm that thought, you might focus only on information that shows your failures. Once you get hold of evidence that you have failed, you stop looking for any other information—especially information that shows that you have succeeded. Consequently, you say to yourself 'See, I've failed'—as if you have proven, beyond any doubt, that you are a failure.

"Compare this highly selective process to the search function on your computer. What if I asked my search function to find any mention of the word *failure*. It would then find numerous places in the text where the word *failure* appears. If I possess a limited search schema, I might conclude that all I'm writing about is failure. Depressive and anxious thinking, driven by biased information processing, is almost always characterized by a limited search schema. When you are anxious, you might wonder, 'Is it possible that I could make a mistake?' Since it is always *possible* to make a mistake, the answer would be 'Yes,' which would lead you to stop looking for more information and quit now! Limited search leads to limited behavior."

I use the following explanation for professionals: "Consider the following example, taken from an elementary course in statistics in which we examine chi square. Let's say you notice that there are 15 examples of blondes who are intelligent and then conclude that blondes are intelligent. However, you might want to ask other questions: 'Are there blondes who are not intelligent? Are there brunettes who are intelligent? Are there brunettes who are not intelligent? How about other people?' You then come up with the following table:

	Blondes	Brunettes	Bald
Intelligent	15	30	10
Not Intelligent	15	30	2

"Much to your surprise, you learn that, in this sample, half of the blondes are intelligent, as are half of the brunettes. In fact, there are twice as many brunettes who are intelligent, but only because the brunettes are twice the number of blondes in the sample. Most interesting to those who are not bald, an overwhelming number of bald individuals are intelligent, even though they are the fewest in the sample.

"Most people do not examine all the possibilities of the chi square or of sampling bias. For example, if you are depressed, you might emphasize the fact that you failed at something and conclude that you are a failure, even though it would be useful to look at the following table, which argues against your conclusion:

	Self	Others
Tasks Failed	3	30
Tasks Succeeded	57	70

"In examining the table, you might observe that you did fail at 3/60 tasks (5%), whereas others failed at 30/100 tasks (30%). The search for information may be so limited that you see only the cell in which you have three failures and conclude that you are a failure. However, a more complete and accurate search might lead you to examine the possibility that you also succeeded on 60 tasks and that the 'norm' is 30% failure (much higher than your 5% failure rate).

"Consider the following example, imagining it occurring in your own practice. Let's say that you have just heard that a patient is terminating therapy. Your first thought is, 'I didn't help that patient.' You then feel awful. However, what if you looked at your entire caseload for the past year and found that 80% of your patients do not terminate prematurely. You would feel better. And what if you find out that for other therapists, only 40% do not terminate prematurely. You would feel compassion for your colleagues but better for yourself. (Of course, the numbers could work against you if the outcome were different.)"

Question to Pose/Intervention

"To determine if you are engaging in a pattern of limited search, you might ask yourself the following questions: 'What information is consistent with my negative view? What information is inconsistent with my negative view? How do others do at this task? In addition, consider the costs and benefits to you of limiting you search to the negative. Lastly, given that you are predicting a negative outcome, what positive or neutral outcomes could you also predict?'"

Example

THERAPIST: You said you are feeling really bad right now because you did poorly on the chemistry exam. What did you get?

PATIENT: I got 75%. That's failing for me. And I also got a 70% on the other quiz in the course.

THERAPIST: What do you conclude from these grades?

PATIENT: I'm really an idiot.

THERAPIST: What is your average grade so far?

PATIENT: I'm averaging about an A– in about 25 courses.

THERAPIST: So you were focusing only on the grades from these two tests?

PATIENT: Yeah.

THERAPIST: What's the average grade in your school?

PATIENT: About B-level work. I'm doing better than average.

THERAPIST: When you do a very limited search and focus only on these two tests you didn't do well on, you ignore all the other information. Are you aware of this?

PATIENT: I was just looking at these tests.

THERAPIST: What if you looked at all the tests that you and your classmates take. What would you conclude?

PATIENT: I'm doing fairly well.

THERAPIST: Sometimes, when we are depressed, our thinking is so biased that we focus only on the negative, and we don't look for any positive information. Perhaps the glass is both half empty *and* half full.

Homework

The therapist can ask patients to list disappointments and negative thoughts about their performance on some task or problem. Then they are instructed to look for additional evidence that refutes those thoughts and evidence for and against the idea that others do well or poorly on these tasks.

Possible Problems

Some patients argue that this more exhaustive search for information is just rationalization about negative behavior that is real—"After all, it is a fact that I didn't do well." The therapist can indicate that it is also fact that other facts exist—and that a more accurate picture can be drawn only if all the information is used. Perfectionistic patients may protest that their "failure" on a single task is intolerable. In response, antiperfectionistic challenges can be utilized, such as "Exactly what will happen as a result of not doing well?" and "What will remain the same?"

Cross Reference to Other Techniques

Other useful interventions include challenging dichotomous thinking, thinking along a continuum, and the double-standard pie and semantic techniques.

Forms

Form 5.1 (Using All the Information, p. 179); Form 5.2 (Self-Help Form: A More Comprehensive Search for Information, p. 180).

TECHNIQUE: IGNORING BASE RATES

Description

To determine the risk in any given action, we generally ask ourselves, "What are the chances that this might not work out?" But how do we get the information to assess the odds? Kahneman (1995) and Kahneman and Tversky (1979; Tversky & Kahneman, 1974) have indicated that most of us place undue emphasis on information that is recent, salient, and personally relevant. We ignore abstract information about "base rates"—that is, the frequency distribution of events in the entire sample under consideration. For example, in considering how dangerous it is to fly, anxious travelers, hearing of a plane crash that day on the news and watching the burning wreck of the airplane, immediately conclude that the airplane they are due to board the next day is likely to crash. They have ignored the base rate—that is, that air travel is considerably safer than any other means of traveling the same distance. Because the information on the news is recent, salient (burning wreckage), and personally relevant (flying tomorrow), its impact is greater than the abstract information conveyed in statistical tables.

We ignore base rates all the time. For example, American women are likely to overestimate their weight compared to others, and almost all Americans believe that they are middle class, regardless of their economic position. Tversky and Kahneman (1974) found that most people use irrelevant information to "improve" their estimates of the likelihood of an event. Similarly, anxious travelers will place great emphasis on any noises onboard the airplane when estimating the perceived danger posed.

Many people who are depressed or anxious believe that their psychiatric problems are unusual, even though national surveys reveal that half the population has experienced a psychiatric condition. In evaluating an individual's ability to assess performance or judge the risk posed by certain behaviors, it is useful to examine first which base rates the individual is employing—knowingly or unknowingly.

Question to Pose/Intervention

"When something unpleasant happens, we often only focus on the negative in the moment, and we ignore how often something like this happens, in general, to everyone else. For example, a person might fear that headache means that she or he has a brain tumor—but we would want to know what percentage of people, in general, who have headaches also have brain tumors. We call this information 'base rates.' It tells us how often something is generally true. Let's take the area you are worried about. Consider how base rates are relevant to your fear of flying. How often do airplanes crash? What percent of the time is a crash occurring in the real world?"

Example

PATIENT: I'm really afraid of flying next week. I just saw that there was a near-miss at the airport.

THERAPIST: Near-misses are scary, but what did that lead you to believe?

PATIENT: Flying is dangerous. There was that airplane that blew up last year over Long Island.

THERAPIST: It sounds like you are focusing on two very newsworthy stories. Are you concluding that these events indicate that flying is now dangerous?

PATIENT: I guess I am.

THERAPIST: If we wanted to know if flying were dangerous, shouldn't we examine the number of people killed per miles traveled? Or, perhaps we could examine the number of flights that take off that end in a crash.

PATIENT: I guess that would be the logical thing to do.

THERAPIST: Well, first, we know that flying is far safer per mile traveled than all other means of transportation.

PATIENT: Yeah, I've heard that. But it's still frightening to me.

THERAPIST: Did you know that 65 million passengers flew in and out of O'Hare Airport in Chicago last year and no one was killed?

PATIENT: That's interesting.

THERAPIST: Or that you could fly, round-trip every day, for 45,000 years on a commercial airline before your "number" came up?

PATIENT: It sounds safer than I thought. But how about that crash off Long Island?

THERAPIST: What makes it newsworthy is that an airplane crashed. Do you think they'd want to interview the 65 million passengers who landed safely at O'Hare and ask them about how they felt about nothing happening?

Homework

The therapist can elicit patients' estimates of base rates by asking "What percent of the time does X occur?" or "What per cent of the population has X?" These figures can be extrapolated into conclusions that the patient may find difficult to defend. For example, the patient mentioned above claimed that the chances were 1% of any plane crashing. Since several hundred planes would be arriving or leaving New York every day, we would then conclude, given her "guesstimated" base rate, that several planes would crash every day in New York. This percentage was untenable to her.

Patients can use Form 5.3 (at the end of the chapter) to examine estimates and base rates. Patients write down their prediction—for example, "The plane will crash"—and then their estimate of the percentage of times their feared outcome occurs, in general—for example, 1%. Similarly, the form can be used to make a needed comparison, For example, the patient who believes that he is poor writes that statement in the left-hand column (i.e., "I'm poor") and in the right-hand column notes his estimate of the average income in the population. The therapist can use a normal distribution curve to illustrate where patients believe they place in comparison to others.

Possible Problems

Problems include the demand for certainty—"I could be the one!" This kind of demand directs the therapist to examine the costs and benefits of demanding certainty versus the value of acceptance and to practice flooding (see Chapter 4). Another problem involves patients' impression that this intervention is invalidating. The therapist can explain that the purpose of this exercise is to examine all the information in order to achieve a valid interpretation of events.

Cross Reference to Other Techniques

Other relevant techniques include examining costs and benefits, evidence, conducting an exhaustive search, examining overgeneralization and applying decatastrophizing, and double standard.

Form

Form 5.3 (Estimates of the Likelihood of Events, p. 181).

TECHNIQUE: EXAMINING THE LOGIC

Description

Much of depressive and anxious thinking is characterized by illogical conclusions. Consider the following:"

"I am single, therefore I am unlovable."
"I failed at the test, therefore I'm a failure."
"Since bad things *can* happen, they *will* happen."
"If Bill doesn't like me, then I am worthless."
"If good things happen to me, then something bad is likely to follow."

Illogical conclusions often are prefaced by "because" or "therefore." Much of depressive thinking begins with an observation of a fact and then draws a negative conclusion that does not logically follow from the fact. Logical errors include:

Extrapolating from a single instance to a universal generalization
Overidentifying a behavior with the entire person
Confusing possibility with necessity or probability
Believing that all events are interdependent with one another (i.e., a good event must be compensated by a bad event).

Examples of challenging illogical thinking include:

- *Examine internal contradictions*: "Do you hold two thoughts that are self-contradictory? For example, 'I should be perfect, but I don't want to criticize myself' or 'I'd like to meet as many people as possible, but I never want to be rejected.' "
- *Reduction ad absurdum*: "Look at the logical implication of your beliefs—is it absurd? For ex-

ample, 'If I'm single, then I'm unlovable.' Implication: 'All people who are married were once single; therefore, all married people are unlovable.'"

- *Challenge recursive self-criticism*: "Examine whether you are locked in an inescapable loop of criticizing yourself for being self-critical. For example, 'I think I'm a loser because I'm depressed, and I'm depressed because I think I'm a loser.'"

Questions to Pose/Intervention

The therapist can ask patients the following questions:

- "Given these facts, what conclusion are you drawing?"
- "Are any other conclusions possible? Is it at all possible to imagine another outcome?"
- "Could someone else imagine another outcome different from your prediction/conclusion?"
- "Are you confusing a possibility with a necessary outcome? With a probability?"
- "Has what you thought could never happen, ever actually happened?"
- "When you predict that one event will cause another event, how does it actually cause the other event? Is there a physical force involved? Is there any communication between events?"
- "Would you apply your conclusion to everyone [every situation]?"

Example

Consider the following example:

THERAPIST: You said that you think you are worthless because you are single. Would you agree that everyone who is married was once single?

PATIENT: Yes. Of course.

THERAPIST: So, from your logic—that is, if you are single you are worthless—then it follows that everyone who is married got married to a worthless person, and they were both worthless until they got married.

Or, consider the following:

THERAPIST: You said that since it is possible that the elevator could crash, then it probably will crash.

PATIENT: I know it sounds foolish, but that's how I think.

THERAPIST: Is it possible that an extraterrestrial could land on your head?

PATIENT: I guess it's possible, but I've never seen one.

THERAPIST: You've never seen an elevator crash either. But both events are possible. The question is, "How *probable* are these events?"

PATIENT: I don't know. With the extraterrestrial, very improbable. I don't know about the elevator crashing.

THERAPIST: Well, how often have you heard of an elevator crashing?

PATIENT: I've never heard of it.

THERAPIST: Would it be reasonable to think that it is improbable—very improbable?

PATIENT: Yeah, I guess so.

THERAPIST: What would happen if you thought that everything that was possible was probable?

PATIENT: I'd worry all the time.

Homework

The therapist can use Form 5.4 (at the end of the chapter) to help patients assess common distortions in conclusions. This form can be explained as follows: "We all make common mistakes in how we reason or how we draw conclusions. I'd like you to examine some of the negative thinking that you have and identify some problems with this thinking. For example, imagine you go to a party and someone is not friendly to you. If you are really negative, you might conclude, 'No one likes me.' The error in your thinking is that you are drawing a conclusion about everyone from an experience with a single person."

Possible Problems

Some patients claim that their negative conclusions are really accurate. The homework exercise is aimed at examining the logic of inferences or conclusions. We also can examine the empirical validity of these thoughts by considering the evidence for and against the thought or by examining the underlying assumption (e.g., "I should get the approval of everyone").

Cross-Reference to Other Techniques

Other relevant interventions include identifying the underlying assumption, double-standard technique, examining the conditional rules, and evaluating the evidence for and against the validity of a thought.

Form

Form 5.4 (Examining Logical Errors, p. 182, which the therapist can use and modify—or not give it to the patient if it seems too difficult to handle).

TECHNIQUE: LINKING UNRELATED EVENTS AND SEEING PATTERNS THAT ARE NOT THERE

Description

Almost all of us have, at some time, linked two events that are actually unrelated to one another and concluded that one is a cause of another. Whether we call this magical thinking, superstitious thinking or simply human nature, we are generally searching to identify causes of events that may or may not be within our control. The tendency to see patterns that are not there is part of schematic processing and helps reduce the information overload that affects all of us. Moreover, as noted, many individuals are driven toward confirmation bias in their thinking, looking for evidence that will confirm their negative views. Illusory correlations, categorical statements, and the perception of patterns and trends that are not there may contribute to feelings of anxiety and depression—even when there is ample evidence, potentially available, that is countervailing. The therapist's task is to dispute these illusory correlations and false patterns.

Often we believe that two events are related to each other simply because we have observed that

Event 1 occurs with Event 2 some of the time. For example, we may be anticipating taking a plane to Florida, leaving New York next Saturday. We hear on the radio that an airplane has crashed at Kennedy Airport. We recall that another airplane was hijacked from Kennedy 3 months ago. The conclusion that we draw is that there is a high probability that another plane will crash or be somehow waylaid near Kennedy Airport. This is the illusion of correlation—we attribute a significant predictable relationship between two events when, in fact, there may be no predictability.

People who are anxious are prone to this illusion of correlation, often resulting in magical thinking: "I wore that red tie when Susan broke up with me. It must be bad luck to wear that tie." Or the individual might think: "When I'm in an elevator, I need to check for sounds that signify danger. I've been doing that for years now and no elevator I've been in has ever crashed."

The problem with illusory correlation is that the pattern of relationship in which we established a belief may not exist. For example, if we are trying to predict whether the elevator will crash, then we would want to know how likely is it that the elevator will crash when we are not checking for odd sounds. Thus, the obsessive "checker" might conclude "The elevator didn't crash because I was checking." If we want to know how dangerous it is to fly from JFK Airport, we need to know how many planes took off and landed safely. In other words, we need to look at the probability of an event in the presence and absence of another event.

Question to Pose/Intervention

"You are concluding that because two events occur in time, one is a cause of the other. Imagine if you went into a house and noticed that there were ashtrays everywhere. Would you conclude that ashtrays cause people to smoke? Or suppose you recognized that Mary wore a red dress on Mondays. Would you conclude that wearing a red dress caused the work week to begin? Think of some of the things that you are linking together as a cause of each other. For example, you said, 'I noticed that a plane crashed; therefore planes must be crashing a lot now.' In order to test whether one thing is a cause of another, we have to examine the many times in which one thing does not occur while another thing does. For example, if you had a fear of flying, you might think flying was dangerous because you read a recent story about a plane crash. However, how would you account for the millions of times people fly when planes do not crash?"

Another way to word this explanation: "You seem to think that these two events are related to one another. For example, you think that generally when X happens, Y will follow. Perhaps you even think that one is a cause of another. However, in order to test out this possible correlation, we need to know how likely is Y to happen when X does not happen."

Example

The patient was a professional investor who worried about the volatility of his stocks.

THERAPIST: You are concerned about your compulsion to watch the screen several hours a day, to see if your stocks have gone up or down. Let's explore why you do that.

PATIENT: I guess my thought is that I can catch something earlier.

THERAPIST: Is there a risk of trading too frequently in your stocks because you are anxious?

PATIENT: Definitely. I've lost a lot of money that way.

THERAPIST: What happens with your stocks when you are away from the desk?

PATIENT: They do whatever they will do. I'm no worse off. I remember worrying about going away on vacation, and when I returned, my stocks were actually up.

THERAPIST: So you have the illusion that watching stocks keeps them from going down and that you can catch something early?

PATIENT: Yeah.

THERAPIST: Would you be willing to limit the time that you screen-watch? Let's see, over the next month, if your stocks go up or down when you are watching versus not watching.

PATIENT: OK.

This patient decreased his screen-watching time, which he spent looking for illusory correlations and patterns that were not there. Needless to say, his decreasing viewing had no effect on the direction of his stocks, but it did help decrease his panic-driven trading practices.

Another example of illusory correlation or false pattern recognition is the following:

THERAPIST: You seem to think that there is a lot of danger in flying. You just heard on the news that a plane crashed at JFK Airport.

PATIENT: Yes, I can remember back in September when those planes were hijacked.

THERAPIST: That's true. That was a terrible tragedy. Are you thinking it's dangerous to fly?

PATIENT: Yeah. The planes are being blown up or crashing. It seems to be happening a lot now.

THERAPIST: What do you base that conclusion on?

PATIENT: Well, the plane crashed recently, and then the two planes were hijacked in September.

THERAPIST: Do you think the recent crash was related to the hijacking?

PATIENT: No, they said it was some kind of technical problem. Something about weakness in the structure of the plane.

THERAPIST: So these events are unrelated?

PATIENT: Yeah.

THERAPIST: How many planes take off and land at JFK in a month?

PATIENT: Thousands.

THERAPIST: How about in a year?

PATIENT: Tens of thousands, I'd guess.

THERAPIST: How do you explain that all the other planes landed safely? Is there a pattern there?

PATIENT: Oh—you just have to be on the wrong plane.

THERAPIST: That would be unlucky. But is there really a pattern of crashes, if these two events are unrelated and almost all of the other planes landed and took off safely?

PATIENT: I guess there really isn't a *pattern* per se.

THERAPIST: And what do you make of seeing a pattern to crashes that are not related to each other? You were linking the terrorism with the mechanical failure.

PATIENT: Yeah. I guess they really aren't related.

THERAPIST: It's kind of like a coincidence?

PATIENT: That's right.

Homework

The therapist can have patients record examples of patterns or correlations that they perceive may be contributing to their worry or depression. For example: "I get worried because I think that [X pattern] is occurring," or "I feel worried because I think that A will cause B." Behaviors such as checking, monitoring, avoiding, or exertion of effort to forestall a perceived calamity can be monitored. The therapist can ask patients to consider counterexamples to these patterns or correlations: "Are there exceptions to these rules or patterns? Are there times this does not occur?" The goal with the homework is to facilitate a more differentiated perspective, so that patients begin to acknowledge "Sometimes this is not true."

Possible Problems

There may be some patterns that *are* correlated and need to be addressed. For example, the patient may notice that her new boyfriend is drinking more on the weekends and that when she asserts herself, he is cruel and condescending. It is important to view the intervention as a means whereby we collect information. Patients often come up with examples to support their unfounded correlation: "I know a man who . . ." or "I saw several examples of . . ." These confirmation-biased examples often contribute to strengthening the belief.

Cross-Reference to Other Techniques

Other relevant techniques include evaluation of the evidence, examining probabilities, semantic technique, examining the quality of the evidence, behavioral experiments, and evaluating rules for disconfirmation.

Form

Form 5.5 (Seeing Patterns That May Not Be There, p. 183).

TECHNIQUE: CREATING FALSE DICHOTOMIES

Description

Typical of much of depressive thinking is the view that only two choices exist for the person, neither of which is attractive, resulting in the feeling of being trapped and helpless. For example, a woman who was unhappily married and engaged in an affair with another married man believed that she had to choose between these two unappealing relationship alternatives. It did not occur to her that there might be numerous other alternatives—other than these two men—that could be more attractive (e.g., more suitable men, friends, spending time alone).

The key to the effective negotiation of problems is the creative exploration of a third, fourth, even fifth alternative. Rather than getting stuck in one position—for example, "Either we do exactly what you want or we do exactly what I want"—we might examine several other alternatives that meet both our needs. For example, a manager at a company was upset that she was passed over for a promotion. She indicated that she was so angry that she wanted to go into her boss's office, tell him he was a jerk, and quit on the spot. We examined the costs and benefits to her of this course of action and then explored what her long-term goals might be at the company. She readily identified these goals as increased responsibility, respect, and financial reward. First we identified her false dichotomy: "Either I tell him off or I'm a doormat." Then we created an alternative: "Let me explain to him how I can be helpful in making this company grow." After rehearsing her plan to present her boss with this third alternative—how she could be helpful—she met with him, impressed him with her business acumen and diplomatic skill, and secured a promotion for her in another part of the company. Several years have passed since that experience. She still works at this company, has substantial financial rewards, and feels secure in her position. By sidestepping a false dichotomy—either clobbering the person or passively acquiescing—she was able to construct a better option for herself.

Other examples of false dichotomies include:

"I'm a winner or loser, a failure or a great success, poor or rich."
"I've got to choose between these two jobs . . . lovers . . . places to live."
"I've got to do it now or never."
"I've got to keep this job because I'll never get another one."
"It's either John or Bill—and I don't like either one that much."

Question to Pose/Intervention

"You may be viewing things in all-or-nothing terms. We call this dichotomous (all-or-nothing/black-and-white) thinking. For example, you might say 'I am always failing' or 'I am always getting rejected.' The important point is to look at all the shades of gray and all of the evidence that suggests that things change and things vary. Try to look for evidence that goes against the all-or-nothing thinking. Look for examples of when things are going a bit better for you."

Example

THERAPIST: You said that you are a complete failure and that you are always messing up. I guess that a complete failure is someone who never gets anything done?

PATIENT: Right. I'm a loser.

THERAPIST: OK. This sounds like all-or-nothing thinking—black and white. Let's see if there are any shades of gray. Are there any things that you have done right in the past year?

PATIENT: Yeah. I took a class on accounting and did OK in it. And I lost 10 pounds. That was good.

THERAPIST: Do your friends like you?

PATIENT: Yeah, they think I'm a pretty good friend. I listen and I can be fun. I have a sense of humor when I'm not depressed.

THERAPIST: OK. So this all-or-nothing thought, "I'm a complete failure", doesn't seem to hold up to the facts?

PATIENT: Yeah. But I got a B on an exam and I was hoping for an A.

THERAPIST: So you discount the B? Is your all-or-nothing thought "If I don't get an A, then I'm a complete failure"?

PATIENT: I guess. I know it sounds irrational.

THERAPIST: Why?

PATIENT: Because I get different grades. I do very well on some things and sort of well on others.

THERAPIST: Maybe that's the way to think about things . . . shades of gray, variation.

PATIENT: I'd feel better if I did.

Homework

The homework is focused on identifying all-or-nothing thinking. Examples include thoughts that use the following language: *all, total, complete, always, never, and the most*. The patient should record examples of all-or-nothing thinking on Form 5.6 (at the end of the chapter), then note examples of when the thinking is not true, and lastly, rewrite the all-or-nothing statements beginning with the sentence stem, "Sometimes I . . . "

Possible Problems

Some patients contend that the evidence of their worthlessness, or that nothing works out, is overwhelming. They will challenge this exercise as a mere rationalization. The response to this position acknowledges that there may be a lot of evidence to support the negative but points out how important it is to examine evidence of when things *are* better—" . . . so that we can figure out why things work when they do." For example, a patient complained that her relationships with men "never work out." When we examined the evidence of better relationships she'd had with men, we noticed that these relationships involved single men who were not depressed. This insight was useful in helping her avoid future no-win relationships.

Cross-Reference to Other Techniques

Other relevant techniques include looking for variations in a belief, examining the evidence, role playing both sides of the thought, distinguishing behaviors from persons, and distinguishing progress from perfection.

Form

Form 5.6 (Challenging False Dichotomies, p. 184).

TECHNIQUE: REDUCTIO AD ABSURDUM

Description

A common technique that is used to challenge an argument is to carry the logic of the argument to an absurd conclusion. Doing so can take several entertaining forms. One form is to take the structure of the argument and examine how a parallel argument would be absurd.

For example, consider the following:

1. Some people who make mistakes are stupid.
2. I made a mistake.
3. Therefore, I am stupid.

A parallel form of argument would be:

1. Some animals have four legs.
2. I am an animal.
3. Therefore, I have four legs.

Or:

1. Some horses have brown eyes.
2. I have brown eyes.
3. Therefore, I am a horse.

Another way of reducing an argument to absurdity is to look at the illogical implications of the statements. For example, many single people believe "If I'm single, then I'm unlovable." To reduce this thinking to an absurdity, consider the following: "All people who are married were once single. Therefore, all married people are unlovable." Consider the following thinking:

1. I haven't finished yet.
2. Therefore, I will never finish.

The absurd implication of this is:

1. Everyone who has finished once had not finished at a prior time.
2. Therefore, everyone who has finished will never finish.

Question to Pose/Intervention

"We can examine the logical implications of your thoughts. Let's see if your reasoning leads to reasonable ways of viewing things. Let's write down your different thoughts and the reasons that you give for them and see what this would lead us to if we carried your thinking forward. Consider the following thought: 'If I'm single, then I'm unlovable.' This belief leads to the following implication 'All people who are married were once single' and conclusion 'All people who got married were unlovable.' Maybe you have some illogical thoughts that we can examine."

Example

THERAPIST: You said that you are worthless and that's why you want to die.

PATIENT: I seem to fail at everything.

THERAPIST: What do you mean by *worthless*?

PATIENT: Someone who hasn't achieved a lot.

THERAPIST: What is *a lot*?

PATIENT: Someone who isn't very successful or rich.

THERAPIST: So are you saying that people who are not successful and rich are worthless?

PATIENT: I guess so. It sounds so judgmental.

THERAPIST: If we carried your reasoning forward, we might say that people who are worthless don't deserve to live.

PATIENT: Well, that sounds very elitist.

THERAPIST: And then we could conclude that we should kill anyone who is not successful and rich?

PATIENT: Oh, I wouldn't go that far.

THERAPIST: Why not? The Nazis did. They murdered old people, handicapped people, and retarded people.You see, if we carry this judgment to its logical conclusion, then we should get rid of all people who aren't successful and rich.

PATIENT: That would be inhuman.

THERAPIST: How could you be more humane toward yourself?

Homework

Using Form 5.7 (at the end of the chapter), the therapist can ask the patient to identify several negative thoughts and the underlying implications of these thoughts, if carried to the extreme. For example, the patient who says "I've failed and I don't deserve to live" can be asked what the implications would be if we used this reasoning for everyone—that is, everyone who fails at something should die.

Possible Problems

Some patients believe that their irrational conclusions are valid. The exercise does not address the validity of the thought but rather its implications were it generalized. Thus the issue is not whether the thought is "true" or "logical" but what the implications of this thought would be as a general principle or process of reasoning. The therapist can explain: "We are not examining whether or not your thought is true or false. We are only examining what it would look like if we applied this reasoning to everyone else."

Cross Reference to Other Techniques

Other relevant techniques include challenging "should" statements, examining costs and benefits, examining the value system, and developing new adaptive assumptions.

Forms

Form 5.7 (Reducing Thoughts to Absurdity, p. 185).

TECHNIQUE: EMOTIONAL HEURISTICS

Description

A common feature of anxious and depressive thinking is to base estimates of reality on one's current emotional state. For example, Finucane, Alhakami, Slovic, and Johnson (2000) have found that inducing anxious arousal leads individuals to increase their estimates of risk and danger for unrelated events. This outcome suggests the underlying emotional reasoning of "I feel anxious, therefore, there is danger." Emotions are not a good indicator of external events. In examining emotional heuristics, we ask patients to consider how emotions might affect thoughts—a causal direction (emotions → thoughts) that might seem odd to some cognitivists. Mood induction techniques, in which patients learn how to create a specific mood, can be used to modify the emotional heuristic. For example, if the patient is utilizing emotional reasoning or if his or her thoughts are emanating from a negative mood, the mood can be modified by inducing a positive mood. Using the Velten technique, for example, patients either repeat positive words or recall positive imagery until a positive mood is experienced, and then they examine the current problem in the new mood state (Snyder & White, 1982; Velten, 1968).

Question to Pose/Intervention

Emotional Reasoning

"When we are worried or anxious or depressed, we often use our emotions to guide us. So you might think 'Things are really bad' because you are feeling sad or anxious. This is called 'emotional reasoning.' Examine what you are worried about and ask yourself if you are using your emotions to guide your thinking. Is there an alternative way of viewing things?"

Emotional Heuristics

"Sometimes your mood directly affects how you think. For example, you might feel sad, and this sadness produces a lot of negative thoughts. Your experience of the world is colored by your sad mood. In order to examine this pattern, we ask you to do three things. First, write down your current negative mood and any negative thoughts you are having. Second, repeat positive words for 10 minutes, until you begin feeling better. Third, now try to think of the current situation from the vantage point of your new, more positive mood. Write down these new thoughts, especially any positive or constructive thoughts that you might have."

Example

Emotional Reasoning

THERAPIST: You said that you are feeling really upset about flying next week. How would you describe this feeling of "being upset"?

PATIENT: I'm really jittery. I can't get my mind off of the fact that I'll be flying, and the plane might crash. I feel really tense. I can't sleep.

THERAPIST: So that's how you know you're upset—you feel jittery and tense and can't sleep. When you think about flying, how do you relate your fear of flying to feeling jittery?

PATIENT: I feel really tense, afraid, so I think "It's going to be really dangerous."

THERAPIST: It sounds like you are using your fear and your tension as evidence that the flight will be dangerous.

PATIENT: Yeah, whenever I feel really tense, I think that something bad is going to happen.

THERAPIST: But is your tension and anxiety really evidence that something bad is going to happen?

PATIENT: No, it's just my feeling.

THERAPIST: What if you ignored the way you were feeling and you asked yourself, "Is there any really strong evidence that this flight will be dangerous?"

PATIENT: I don't have any evidence that it will be dangerous.

Emotional Heuristics

THERAPIST: You've been feeling really down recently, and now that you and Nancy have broken up, you are flooded with negative thoughts and feelings. Sometimes when we feel really down, our negative mood just triggers lots of negative thoughts.

PATIENT: Yeah, I've been thinking that I'll never meet anyone quite like her. Never be happy again.

THERAPIST: OK. Let's try an experiment. I'd like you to close your eyes and try to relax. We're going to work at creating a positive feeling. I want you to open your eyes and read these words. Try to concentrate on the positive feelings these words evoke. (*Gives patient the Velten cards.*) How are you feeling?

PATIENT: Better. A lot less sad than before.

THERAPIST: Let's look at how you think about this breakup with Nancy. Any positive or neutral thoughts?

PATIENT: Well, maybe it's for the best. We tried, but we're just very different from each other.

THERAPIST: Can anything good come from this breakup?

PATIENT: Maybe I can meet someone who is more my type.

THERAPIST: How does that thought feel?

PATIENT: Better. Like there's some hope.

THERAPIST: Does this shift tell you anything about how changing your mood changes your thinking?

PATIENT: Yeah. I feel less sad reading these words, and now I'm thinking . . . in a way, I'm thinking about things in a more positive light.

THERAPIST: So, what we learned is that our feelings can affect how we think about things.

Homework

Using Form 5.8 (at the end of the chapter) the therapist can ask patients to (1) examine some of the negative beliefs they are holding at the present time (e.g., "No one likes me," "I'll always be alone," or "I can never do anything right") and (2) consider the emotions that are associated with those beliefs (e.g., anxiety, depression, sadness, anger, loneliness). Lastly, the therapist can ask patients to examine how they would view the current situation if they were feeling "especially good" or "especially optimistic."

Possible Problems

Some individuals may have a difficult time imagining feeling differently from the way they currently feel. Highly anxious or sad patients may be enveloped by their negative mood. The therapist can help patients induce a positive mood by use of relaxation exercises and positive imagery. This imagery can be used to guide patients to a more positive set of memories of past happiness or calmness. This induced positive or relaxed emotion then can be utilized to challenge the emotional heuristic characterizing the current situation.

Cross Reference to Other Techniques

It is often useful to utilize distancing techniques such as the double standard, placing things in perspective, or looking at the current situation from "the balcony." In addition, the time-machine technique, examining the costs and benefits, and examining the evidence for and against the validity of the belief are useful.

Form

Form 5.8 (Mood Induction and Alternative Thoughts, p. 186).

TECHNIQUE: RECENCY EFFECTS

Description

A common "rule of thumb" (or heuristic) is to place greater emphasis on recent information than on averaging information over a longer period of time. Recent events are often viewed as more representative than baseline or repeated events. For example, the individual who hears about a recent plane crash may conclude that planes are now very dangerous; an individual whose relationship has ended may feel rejected and conclude that this recent "rejection" is likely representative of all relationship outcomes in the future.

Question to Pose/Intervention

"You seem to be placing a lot of emphasis on what has been happening recently. For example, you noticed that [X] happened recently, and now you are thinking that [X] is going to continue to happen. Let's step outside of the current situation and take a longer-term view of things. How many times in the past [year] has [X] *not* happened? How many times has [X] actually happened?"

Example

THERAPIST: You are afraid to fly next week because, you said, there was a plane crash last week.

PATIENT: Yeah, I think that flying is dangerous.

THERAPIST: Do you think that flying feels more dangerous to you this week than it did 2 weeks ago—before that crash?

PATIENT: Yeah, of course!

THERAPIST: It seems that you think the recent crash reflects how dangerous flying is. But how many planes have taken off in the past year and arrived safely at their destination?

PATIENT: Thousands, I guess.

THERAPIST: So if one plane out of thousands crashes, what is the likelihood of the next plane crashing?

PATIENT: Very small.

THERAPIST: Sometimes we emphasize recent events more than makes sense. In order to figure out how dangerous flying is, you need to look at *all* the flights over a long period of time. Imagine that you are playing roulette, and you play 100 times and lose each time. But now, on the next throw, you win. Would you conclude that you are having a winning streak?

PATIENT: No.

THERAPIST: You would guess that the next game of roulette is more likely to be similar to the first 100 games—each of which you have lost.

PATIENT: That makes sense.

THERAPIST: So the recent event is not the only one to consider—you need to consider all of the prior events.

Homework

Homework is focused on contrasting recent events that are perceived negatively with earlier events that may contradict the recent ones in their outcomes. The therapist asks patients to list the recent events or experiences that are troubling, then to list as many prior events—especially events in the distant past—that are not consistent with the current events or experiences. (Form 5.9, at the end of the chapter, can be used.) Alternative, more positive thoughts are thereby elicited. To counter recency effects on the estimates of current danger (e.g., the patient who believes that airplanes are unsafe because there was a recent plane crash), valid base-rate information can be obtained. For example, the patient who has a fear of flying can consult the Internet at *www.airsafe.com* to learn how many millions of passengers fly on each airline safely.

Possible Problems

Due to the recency effect, patients may recall more negative events that are consistent with their negative automatic thoughts than positive ones. For example, a patient who did poorly on an exam recalled prior experiences of not achieving his goals and of being rejected as a failure. The therapist can ask such patients if there were any times in the past when they passed the exam, accomplished a goal, or achieved anything that was at all pleasurable. At times it is helpful to have patients bring in their curriculum vitae or résumé.

Cross Reference to Other Techniques

Other relevant techniques include examining the evidence, reviewing the quality of the evidence, viewing probabilities in a sequence, and examining the costs and benefits of worrying. In addition, uncertainty training—such as exposure to uncertainty thoughts—can be helpful.

Form

Form 5.9 (Examining the Recency Effect, p. 187).

TECHNIQUE: ARGUMENTS BASED ON LOGICAL FALLACIES

Description

Aristotle identified a number of common fallacies in arguments or logical deduction. Many people use authoritative hearsay as proof of truth, claiming that something is true because someone in authority says it is true. For example, it is common to hear statements beginning with "My father always said . . . " or "My boss says . . . " or "My therapist says . . . "Another example of a fallacy in arguing is to refer to convention—that is, "Everyone does this"—as proof or evidence. Related to this fallacy is the argument baaed on prior examples—for example, "This is how it was always done." These arguments do not prove that something is currently correct, logical, practical, desirable, or moral. Lots of authorities have claimed very incorrect things—such as claiming the earth is the center of the solar system. Similarly, the fact that someone else does something a certain way does not mean it will be useful for you to do it that way. Indeed, there may be a variety of ways of doing something, and one should consider tradeoffs, preferences, and the opportunities currently available. Another fallacious argument is the *ad hominem* (i.e., against the person) argument: "The only reason he believes [such and such] is because he is a terrible person." These *ad hominem* arguments attack the character of the person rather than establish the validity of the argument. For excellent discussions of logical fallacies, see Diane Halpern, *Thought and Knowledge: An Introduction to Critical Thinking* (2003), and Irving Copi and Carl Cohen, *Introduction to Logic* (1994).

Question to Pose/Intervention

"A lot of times we hold negative beliefs because we are responding to ideas or arguments that are not valid, though they carry the weight of authority or convention. For example, someone powerful or deemed an 'expert' asserts that something is true. Or, the argument is based on the assertion (which is really an unsubstantiated assumption) 'That's what everyone does.' Similarly, arguments may be based on prior behavior—for example, 'That's what was done in the past,' or the argument is no more than an attack—for example, 'Only an idiot would do this.' Think about why you believe some of the negative things you believe. Then ask yourself if you are basing your judgment on authority, convention, approval, fear of personal attack, or simply that things were done a certain way before."

Example

THERAPIST: You said that you feel ashamed that you are gay. Why is that?

PATIENT: Other people look down on gay people.

THERAPIST: Everyone?

PATIENT: Well, not everyone. But my father always criticized gays, and the Bible condemns them.

THERAPIST: It seems that you are basing your shame on need for approval, authority, and convention. Did you ever hear about Galileo?

PATIENT: He was an astronomer.

THERAPIST: Right, and the Catholic Church condemned him because he claimed that the earth was not the center of the solar system. He claimed that the earth turns. But the Church authorities—and almost everyone else—criticized him. Were they right or was Galileo right?

PATIENT: Well, Galileo was right.

THERAPIST: OK. So think about the fact that you are gay, and that you feel ashamed because of the authority and disapproval of your father. Is he really knowledgeable about these areas?

PATIENT: No.

THERAPIST: And when you say that being gay isn't what everyone is, does that mean it's wrong? Not everyone is left-handed. Not everyone likes chocolate.

PATIENT: No. It's a personal thing. It's something you're born with.

THERAPIST: So if we reject arguments based on authority or winning approval or what some other people want, then we are left with your personal orientation.

Homework

Using Form 5.10 (at the end of the chapter), the therapist can ask patients to list all of the arguments that fuel their self-criticism or negative beliefs. For example, if the patient has negative beliefs about being gay, resulting in shame, these negative beliefs should be listed. Similarly, if the patient has demanding expectations of self—for example, "I should succeed at everything I try"—then the negative beliefs underlying these expectations are listed. Then patients list as many arguments as they can think of that support their negative beliefs. For example, arguments that "support" the negative beliefs that one should not be gay might include arguments based on conventional perspectives (e.g., "Most other people are not gay"), authority (e.g., "My father thinks it's bad"), ad hominem (e.g., "People who are gay are defective"), emotion, form of ridicule, popularity, etc. Then patients list why these arguments are illogical. For example, the argument that convention determines right and wrong is illogical, since conventions are always changing and there is a wide range of behavior in society. Ad hominem arguments are invalid because denigrating a person's character does not invalidate the point of view with which you disagree.

Possible Problems

Some individuals have a difficult time analyzing the errors in logical thinking in these fallacious arguments. For example, long-held beliefs in convention ("Most people think that people who do X are Y") are difficult to dislodge. The therapist can help patients analyze the logical errors in these arguments by examining how such arguments would apply in different circumstances. For example, arguments based on convention are dislodged by illustrating the prior conventions of slavery and anti-Semitism. Ad hominem arguments are dislodged by pointing out all the famous people who were vilified (Jesus, Moses, Buddha, Lincoln, etc.).

Cross Reference to Other Techniques

Related techniques include cost–benefit analysis, double standard, rational role play, and reductio ad absurdum.

Form

Form 5.10 (Fallacies in Arguments: Analyzing Negative Beliefs, pp. 188–189).

FORM 5.1. Using All the Information

Negative thought: _____

Evidence this thought is true of me	Evidence this thought is true of others	Evidence this thought is not true of me	Evidence this thought is not true of others

FORM 5.2. Self-Help Form: A More Comprehensive Search for Information

Developing More Complete Information		
	Self	Others
Failure		
Success		

Questions to Ask Myself about My Search for Information	
Question	Answer
What information is inconsistent with my view?	
How do others do on this task? Do they fail, too?	
What are the consequences to me of limiting the information that I consider?	
Is there any pattern to my excluding information?	
Am I always looking for the negative?	

FORM 5.3. Estimates of the Likelihood of Events

Prediction or Negative Belief	What is the likelihood that this is true in the population? (0–100%)

FORM 5.4. Examining Logical Errors

Examples of logical errors: Drawing conclusions that do not follow, confusing possibility with probability, confusing a behavior with a person, linking two independent events, making self-contradictory statements (e.g., "I have a lot of success, but I'm a failure"), basing self-worth on what someone thinks.

Negative Thoughts	Errors in My Thought

FORM 5.5. Seeing Patterns That May Not Be There

Many of us see patterns in events that may not be completely accurate. For example, someone might say "Everything is going badly for me," not recognizing that there are many things that have been going well. Or someone might think that one event or action is a cause of another; for example, "Every time I try to have a conversation with anyone, it ends up badly." It is important for us to examine whether these patterns exist in reality or mostly in our mind. Try to come up with examples that disprove your thought that there is a pattern or that one thing is always a cause of another thing.

Pattern that I see	Evidence against this pattern

FORM 5.6. Challenging False Dichotomies

Sometimes we use all-or-nothing thinking which creates false dichotomies. Examples of this type of thinking are "I am either a winner or a loser" or "I always get rejected." In the left-hand column, write down some examples of your all-or-nothing thinking (your false dichotomies). In the middle column, write down examples of when this thinking is not true. In the right-hand column, rewrite your negative black-and-white statement by saying something positive as well as negative—for example, "Sometimes I do well and sometimes I don't do well." If your negative thinking concerns a choice ("It's either A or B"), then come up with at least one alternative.

Example of all-or-nothing thinking (false dichotomy)	Examples of when this thinking is not true	"Sometimes I . . . "

FORM 5.7. Reducing Thoughts to Absurdity

Look at the logical implication of your belief—is it absurd? For example, the implication of the thought "If I'm single, then I'm unlovable" is "All people who are married were once single."

Current negative thought	Why it would be absurd to think this way

FORM 5.8. Mood Induction and Alternative Thoughts

In the left-hand column, write down your current negative thoughts; in the middle column list your negative feelings or emotions. Then try this mood induction experience:

Mood Induction: Close your eyes and try to form an image of a positive and relaxing scene. Relax all of your muscles and breathe slowly. When you have a positive scene in mind, try to think of some positive words. These words might include *relax*, *calm*, *warm*, *kind*, *safe*, etc. After you have formed this positive image and feel calm and relaxed, try to think of the current situation in the most positive light—think of it from the point of view of your positive feelings. Then open your eyes and write down your positive thoughts while in this positive mood.

Current Negative Thoughts	Current Negative Feelings	Alternative Positive Thoughts While in Positive Mood

FORM 5.9. Examining the Recency Effect

In the left-hand column list any recent events that have triggered your negative thoughts (e.g., poor performances, accidents, rejections, disappointments, etc.). In the right-hand column list events that are not recent but that contradict these current experiences. For example, the person who says "I just did poorly on the exam—I'm really dumb" may be basing these negative thoughts solely on a recent experience and would therefore list all the examples in the past of positive performances on exams.

Recent event or experience from which I may be overgeneralizing	Prior events that contradict this

FORM 5.10. Fallacies in Arguments: Analyzing Negative Beliefs

Look at these examples of mistakes and errors (fallacies) in thinking. All of us engage in these fallacies at some point. Now examine some of your current negative thoughts and see if any of them fit any of these fallacies in reasoning. Can you think of how you might correct these fallacies? What is wrong with your reasoning?

Logical Fallacies	Examples of Fallacies in Negative Beliefs	Examples of My Use of this Fallacy	What Is Wrong with This Thinking?
Attacking the person	He's wrong because he's a bad person.		
Appeals to authority	My father thinks it's wrong.		
Convention	That's the way it's always been done.		
Emotion	I feel upset when I think that, therefore it's wrong.		
Fear	Terrible things will happen if you believe that.		
Pity	You shouldn't do that because it will make someone else unhappy.		
Fear of ridicule	If you do that, everyone will think you're a loser.		
Popularity	It's what everyone does.		
Begging the question	You shouldn't do something other people don't like. Therefore, it's wrong to do it.		
Post hoc	I must have been an idiot—it didn't work out.		

(continued)

Logical Fallacies	Examples of Fallacies in Negative Beliefs	Examples of My Use of this Fallacy	What Is Wrong with This Thinking?
Gambler's fallacy	I must have a string of good luck. [Alternative: My luck will turn because I just lost a lot.]		
Guilt by association	He must be a bad person since he hangs out with that guy.		
Lack of imagination	I can't think of any reasons that he did that—he must be crazy.		
"No true Scotsman"	No real man would do that—he did that, so he's not a real man.		
Relativistic fallacy	Everything is relative. Anyone can have a point of view. There is no reality.		
Slippery slope	If you make a mistake, everything will fall apart.		
Correlation means causation	I noticed that a lot of people who do X are like that. He did X, therefore he is like that.		
Small sample	My two friends had a bad experience with Internet dating, therefore it's a bad idea.		
False forced choice	I've got to choose between Susan and Carol.		
Confusing a preference with a necessity	I'd like to be rich, therefore I should be rich.		

CHAPTER 6

—

Putting Things in Perspective

Negative thoughts may be partly true. For example, it may be true that the person made mistakes, did not do as well as others on the test, or that money was lost in the stock market. The problem with dealing with these negative events arises when they are viewed in the most extreme way imaginable. For example, the individual who loses 30% of his portfolio in the stock market may view this as signifying that he has no money left or that he will not be able to live the life he wants to live. Evidence of the interaction because life events and cognitive style is provided in numerous studies (see Ingram et al., 1997). In this chapter we review a number of techniques that can help patients put things in perspective. It is important to note that the word *rational* is derived from *ratio*—which means perspective or proportion.

TECHNIQUE: PIE CHART

Description

Self-criticism is a central component of depression and anxiety. When a bad event happens, we might believe that we are 100% to blame. The woman going through a divorce blames herself entirely for the end of the relationship, and the woman seeking a job blames herself 100% for not getting the job offer. The person personalizes the entire problem, and causality is assigned in all-or-nothing terms.

One intervention that is useful in challenging all-or-nothing thinking is the pie chart, in which the individual is asked to consider a pie with different-size pieces in it that represent different degrees of responsibility for an event. The patient then indicates all of the possible causes for the event and how large a piece of pie should be ascribed to each cause. He or she then considers the remaining cause—self—and ponders how this "slice of the pie" reflects his or her degree of responsibility.

190

Question to Pose/Intervention

"Let's consider a pie with different pieces in it. (*Therapist draws circle with different segments.*) Now I want you to consider all of the different causes for this event [the event that bothers the patient and for which he blames him- or herself]. Each piece of the pie represents a possible cause of the event. How big a piece of pie is represented by each of these causes? How much of the pie is due to you?"

Example

For example, a woman working in an office where excessive demands are placed on her to get the job done criticized her work performance, labeling herself a "failure." Her assumption was "I should get the entire job done, and if I don't, it's entirely my fault." We decided to list possible contributing factors to the job problems, assigning various percentages of causality to each, with the condition that the total must be equal to, or less than, 100%:

Limitations in computer software	10%
Staff do not provide me with enough information	10%
Unreasonable expectations of senior staff	30%
Lack of technical and personnel support	45%
Lack of my effort	0%
Lack of my ability	5%

We then converted these ratios into a pie chart (Figure 6.1).

Homework

The therapist asks patients to think about the bad event or outcome for which they are blaming themselves (or someone else). The therapist can explain: "I want you to consider all of the possible reasons why this [bad event] happened, including your role and the role of other people or the importance of

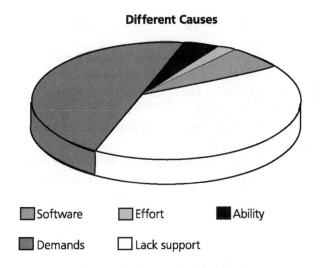

FIGURE 6.1. Example of a pie chart.

the situation. Also consider the role of 'bad luck.' Now look at this copy of the pie chart [Form 6.1, at the end of the chapter] and divide up the pie into the different causes or elements. How much of the pie is left over for self-criticism?"

(A variation of this exercise can be used to challenge labeling. For example, patients can be asked to list the negative label for self—for example, "I'm stupid"—then list all of their other qualities and behaviors. A pie chart can be used to divide up the various components of patients' self-concept.)

Possible Problems

Patients may have difficulty identifying other possible causes of the event, especially if they are blaming themselves exclusively. The therapist can ask patients to consider taking the role of their own defense attorney, who is required to come up with new ways of viewing the situation so that they are not blamed entirely. What would the defense attorney say? The therapist can also offer suggestions of possible causes—for example, the other people involved may have engaged in certain negligent behaviors, it was a bad choice, the patient had bad luck, the patient did not try as hard as he or she could, etc. Another problem arises if patients believe that this reattribution is just another set of excuses for themselves—that is, they believe they are "morally obligated" to blame themselves entirely. The therapist can use the double-standard technique to examine the severity of the judgment.

Cross-Reference to Other Techniques

Other relevant techniques include point–counterpoint, examining the evidence, cost–benefit analysis, use of the continuum, looking at the issue from the balcony, and rational role play.

Form

Form 6.1 (Pie Chart Exercise, p. 213).

TECHNIQUE: CONTINUUM

Description

Much of depressive thinking is dichotomous—all-or-nothing—thinking: either "I'm a loser or a winner;" either "I'm brilliant or stupid." This black-and-white thinking can be examined using the continuum technique. The purpose of this technique is to help the patient think in terms of degrees or variations rather than all-good or all-bad. Often the depressed, anxious, or angry individual responds to events as if they were catastrophic. Rather than view an event as an inconvenience or a frustration, the individual thinks that the world is coming to an end and things cannot be tolerated as they are. The continuum technique requires that the individual view the event along a scale from 0% to 100%, where 0 corresponds to the absence of anything negative and 100 corresponds to the worst possible outcome imaginable—for example, the Holocaust. Patients are asked to consider how bad they feel about the current event, place this evaluation along a 100-point scale of possible bad outcomes, and then consider other points on the scale. Each point along the continuum, in 10-point increments, is identified, and a corresponding event is associated with that point. Typically, patients have difficulty identifying events or outcomes that are lower in the scale of negative outcomes, especially points along the scale below 75%, illustrating the tendency to view things in all-or-nothing terms. Patients are then asked to reevaluate the outcome, assigning a new point value and indicating why it is not as bad as it seems.

Question to Pose/Intervention

"You said that this event was pretty bad. Just how bad do you feel, from 0 to 100%, where 100% represents the worst feeling you can imagine—something like the Holocaust—and 0% represents the absence of anything negative? I am going to draw a line with markers for each 10-point increment.

```
_____

 0     10    20    30    40    50    60    70    80    90   100%
No negatives                                 ↑              Holocaust

                                         Current event: _____
```

You have assigned the current event a 90% bad rating. Now let's look at some of the other points on the scale. Let's take 95%. What would be something that could happen to someone that would be 95%? 80%? 70? 60? 50? 40? 30? 20? 10? Are there some points that are hard to fill? Why would it be hard to fill out points below 60%? Are you looking at what is happening right now in extreme terms? Would you think of changing where you place this event on the scale? What are some reasons why it is not as bad as you thought it was?"

Example

THERAPIST: You said that you are upset because Roger never called you back. You went out with Roger twice. You seem very upset right now. I wonder, from 0% to 100%, where 100% represents the most upset you've ever been, how upset you are, right now, thinking about this?

PATIENT: I'd say about 95%. I'm really angry and hurt.

THERAPIST: OK. That's pretty bad. Now let's imagine that Roger never calls back. Where would you put that possibility in terms of bad things that could happen—from 0% to 100%, where 100% represents the Holocaust?

PATIENT: I'd give it about 75%. I'm always getting rejected.

THERAPIST: OK. Let's draw out a scale from 0% to 100%—we call this a continuum. Now, 100% represents the Holocaust, and 75% represents Roger not calling you. Let's see, what would you put at 90%?

PATIENT: I guess being physically assaulted.

THERAPIST: OK, what would you put at 85%?

PATIENT: Getting injured but recovering.

THERAPIST: 60%?

PATIENT: I don't know. Losing my job.

THERAPIST: 50%?

PATIENT: My friend getting angry at me over nothing at all.

THERAPIST: 40%?

PATIENT: This is getting kind of monotonous. I don't know. Feeling overweight—like I've gained 5 pounds.

THERAPIST: Do you have a hard time filling in points below 50%? I wonder why.

PATIENT: I guess most things aren't too bad. Most things are under 50%.

THERAPIST: Do you really believe that Roger not calling you is 75% as bad as the Holocaust? Or almost as bad as being assaulted?

PATIENT: Probably not. It just feels that way.

THERAPIST: Your feelings are really important, but it might be important to look at this event in perspective. For example, why is this not really as bad as losing your job?

PATIENT: I need my job to pay my bills. I don't need Roger.

Homework

The therapist asks patients to consider examining some of their negative labeling, catastrophic thinking, and all-or-nothing judgments/conclusions: "I want you to think about some of the things that really upset you this week or about which you're worried in the near future—things that got—or get—you really anxious, depressed, or angry—and pick one on which to focus. Think about how bad this event or situation feels and what your automatic thoughts are about it. Now write down what is bothering you—let's say, you're giving a talk next week, and you think that someone won't like it. How bad does this—someone not liking your talk—feel from 0% to 100%? Use this form [6.2, at the end of the chapter]. It illustrates what we call a "continuum," and it runs from 0% to 100%, where 0% represents the absence of anything negative, and 100% represents the Holocaust. Where would you put this event (someone not liking your talk) on this scale? Then fill in every 10-point marker on the scale with an event or situation that you would rate at that degree of negativity."

Possible Problems

Some patients may view the continuum technique as invalidating, perhaps even resenting the comparison to something so catastrophic that it would automatically diminish the grievousness of their problem. In this case the therapist should ask patients to consider the costs and benefits of viewing things as terrible or awful. Some people believe that they need to catastrophize events, lest their needs are dismissed as trivial. The therapist can examine the origins of this invalidation schema through schematic work (see Chapter 7). Another common problem is that patients get frustrated filling in the points below 60%—and the therapist may be hesitant in pushing for completion of the form. We have found that persisting in filling in every 10-point increment on the scale, down to 10%, is "helpfully frustrating," since it drives home for patients the extremity of their initial ratings.

Cross-Reference to Other Techniques

Other relevant interventions include cost–benefit analysis, categorizing cognitive distortions (catastrophic thinking, emotional reasoning, labeling, all-or-nothing thinking), constructing alternatives, and double-standard technique.

Form

Form 6.2 (The Continuum Exercise, p. 214).

TECHNIQUE: DOUBLE STANDARD

Description

We are often far more rationale and fair in evaluating other people than in evaluating ourselves. The double-standard technique asks patients to consider the implication of applying their current judgments to other people. For example, if the patient believes that she is a failure because her relationship did not work out, she can be asked if she would judge someone else (e.g., a friend) similarly if his or her relationship did not work out. A variation is to ask the patient if other people, looking at the situation, would judge the patient to be a failure. The patient is invited to consider that she may have one standard for herself (a very severe one) and another standard for others. The question is posed: Why should she be more severe on herself than she would be on other people? In addition, she is asked to consider why other people would be less severe in judging her than she is in judging herself: Why are different standards used in judging self and other, and different standards that other people would have for the patient? These questions suggest that the patient should consider what standards would make sense if they were applied to everyone.

Question to Pose/Intervention

"If you had a girlfriend who was going through this same situation, how would you judge her? Is there some reason why your judgments would be less severe for others than for yourself? Is there some reason why you have a double standard—one that is very critical of yourself but very understanding of others? How would other people look at this situation? If they are less critical of you than you are of yourself, why would you have a more severe standard for yourself than others would have for you? Why would others be more understanding of you than you are of yourself?"

Example

THERAPIST: You said you think that you are a failure because you are having a hard time separating from George. What if you had a girlfriend who was going through what you are going through? What would you think of her? Would you think she was a failure?

PATIENT: No, I'd probably be very supportive of her.

THERAPIST: What kinds of supportive things would you say?

PATIENT: I'd tell her that she was having a hard time because, understandably, she was very attached to her husband.

THERAPIST: It sounds like you have a double standard. You're more critical of yourself than you are of your friend. Why is that?

PATIENT: I guess I expect more of myself.

THERAPIST: What would happen if you expected the same of yourself that you expect of others?

PATIENT: I'd feel a lot better.

As noted, an alternative is to ask patients how others would judge them. This allows patients to recognize that others likely would have less demanding standards for them than they (i.e., patients) would have for themselves.

THERAPIST: How would your best friend, Fran, judge how you are reacting to this separation?

PATIENT: I don't think she would judge me. She'd probably think I was just being a human being. She knows I have a lot of good things going for me.

THERAPIST: Like what sort of things?

PATIENT: Well, she knows that I am a decent friend. I'm smart, reliable. I care about my friends.

THERAPIST: Is there some reason your friends are less critical of you than you are of yourself?

PATIENT: I guess I have higher standards for myself than others have for me.

Homework

Using Form 6.3 (at the end of the chapter) patients are asked to list several self-critical thoughts and to consider (1) the advice they would give a friend who had a similar problem, and (2) why they hold a double standard that is far more self-critical.

Possible Problems

One problem that occurs with perfectionistic patients is that they believe they should hold themselves to standards that are higher than those for other people. For example, a patient with a high income thought she was a failure because she was not earning as much as a colleague. When she was presented with the double-standard technique, she agreed that she held herself to higher standards but believed she was capable of more than others. We find it helpful to distinguish between "higher" and "highest" standards, since many perfectionistic people believe that 100% is the only standard. Such patients can examine the implications and the evidence of what would happen if they aimed for 80%, 90%, or 100%—and to examine what they give up by requiring themselves to pursue the highest standard.

Another problem arises when patients firmly believe that others would be critical of them. This problem leads to two questions. First, are patients correct in their predictions about others? This issue can be tested by canvassing friends for their opinions—for example, "What would you think about me if I lost my job?" Second, patients can consider the range that exists among people. Perhaps some friends *are* highly critical, and those friendships may need to be reconsidered. For example, a woman with bipolar disorder told several friends about her condition. One of her friends became wary and critical, which led the patient to reconsider whether this person was a true friend.

Cross-Reference to Other Techniques

Role play against the thought and examine cognitive distortions costs and benefits, evidence, logical distortions, and evaluate the assumptions.

Form

Form 6.3 (The Double-Standard Exercise, p. 215).

TECHNIQUE: LOOKING AT IT FROM THE BALCONY

Description

Fisher and Ury (1991) describe a technique in negotiation that requires the participants to stand back and look at the interaction from a balcony. Selman (1980) described this technique as a form of role-taking ability—"systemic role-taking"—in which individuals examine their interactions with others from a third-person point of view. Often we get locked into interactions that seem increasingly frustrating. The goal of this exercise is to facilitate a more larger perspective that may transcend the immediate situation.

Question to Pose/Intervention

"If you were to step back from the current situation and observe yourself as if you were looking down from a balcony, what would you see or think?"

Example

THERAPIST: You and Carol have been arguing about sharing chores at home. Both of you work hard in your jobs, and you both feel that household chores should be shared. Let's look at this current argument, in which you got really upset with Carol when she asked you to wash the dishes after she cooked dinner.

PATIENT: It wasn't that she "asked" me —she ordered me.

THERAPIST: OK, so the way that she said it bothered you. What did it make you think?

PATIENT: She doesn't respect me.

THERAPIST: How did you feel about that thought?

PATIENT: I felt really angry. I stormed out.

THERAPIST: OK. That's one interpretation—that she was ordering you—and your response was pretty strong. Sometimes we get caught up in the situation, and we have a hard time seeing it from another point of view. Try closing your eyes right now and imagine that you are someone standing on a balcony about 50 feet above you and Carol in the kitchen. You can hear everything. How would you describe what happened from your point of view on the balcony?

PATIENT: Carol was cooking dinner for a couple of hours, and she was pressured for time. I was acting like I was in a lousy mood at dinner. I was kind of curt with her.

THERAPIST: OK, from your vantage point on the balcony, what happened next?

PATIENT: Carol and I were finishing the meal, then clearing the table, when Carol said, "Be sure to wash the dishes."

THERAPIST: OK, from your point of view on the balcony, how did that seem?

PATIENT: Normal. Like she had done a lot more than I had that night, and I was in a pissy mood.

THERAPIST: From the balcony, all we can see is what you and Carol said and did. We can't see your pissy mood.

PATIENT: Right. So I was probably overreacting.

198   COGNITIVE THERAPY TECHNIQUES

Homework

Patients are asked to list several interactions or problems that are bothering them and to imagine looking down on these from a balcony (Form 6.4, at the end of the chapter). How would they see each situation from the distance and perspective of the balcony? What would be the advantages of this added perspective?

Possible Problems

Some people get caught up in their emotions and have difficulty standing back and viewing things from another perspective. Taking another perspective can be enhanced by mood-regulation techniques, such as practicing relaxation via slow breathing or calming imagery prior to taking the more distant perspective. Another problem is that patients continue to view and experience the event as if they were one of the actors in the event. This identification with the scene being viewed can be reduced by having patients describe only the physical details and behaviors they are observing, rather than inferring the personal traits or motivations of the participants being described. For example, patients can write down the dialogue they hear.

Cross-Reference to Other Techniques

Other relevant interventions include the double-standard technique, examining the evidence, cost–benefit analysis, examining alternative interpretations, time machine (self and others), and role playing against the thought.

Form

Form 6.4 (View from the Balcony, p. 216).

TECHNIQUE: CONSTRUCTING ALTERNATIVES

Description

George Kelly (Kelly, 1955) proposed "constructive alternativism" as a method for modifying rigid thinking. This approach involves considering multiple perspectives and actions that are possible, given the current situation. Anxious, depressive, and angry styles of thinking are often characterized by a rigidity or inflexibility that locks patients into one response—often a maladaptive one. Constructing alternatives allows patients to consider various other thoughts and actions that might mitigate their current response.

Consider the individual who is taking a test and believes that he is going to do poorly on it. Using this method, he would consider a number of reasons why he might do well, why the test results are not essential to his survival, and what actions he can take if he does score poorly on the test. This framework places the test in perspective as a minor inconvenience rather than a life-changing evaluation.

Question to Pose/Intervention

"Let's imagine that this negative outcome you are dreading [fearing] does happen. What kinds of thoughts could you have and actions could you take that might lead to some positive outcomes for you? What could you still do? What alternatives are available to you? What are some short-term and long-term plans of action for you to carry out?"

Example

THERAPIST: You are concerned that you and Ken might break up. How does this make you feel?

PATIENT: I feel really hopeless because I rely on him so much.

THERAPIST: Well, we never know what will happen, and it is always possible that the relationship could come to an end. If it did, we might want to examine some things that you could do for yourself to feel better.

PATIENT: It seems like I could never be happy without him.

THERAPIST: What kinds of enjoyable activities did you engage in before you met Ken?

PATIENT: Well, I like my work, and I like my friends. I saw my friends more often, and I enjoyed hiking and skiing and exercising. I haven't been going to the health club as much. I've gained weight in the last 2 months, worrying about this relationship.

THERAPIST: OK, so those could be some things you might do again. What other things would you be freer to do if Ken were not around?

PATIENT: I really like this guy Phil, whom I met at work. We flirt a lot.

THERAPIST: You might be able to follow up with Phil on something. Are there some negative things with Ken that you wouldn't have to worry about anymore?

PATIENT: I wouldn't have to worry about fighting and arguing and breaking up and what he's doing or thinking. It's a drag sometimes.

THERAPIST: OK, so these are some alternatives that you would have available if Ken were out of the picture?

PATIENT: I guess that's true. Things wouldn't be all bad. In fact, some things might be better.

Homework

Using Form 6.5 (at the end of the chapter), the therapist can ask patients to describe the current troubling situation and their negative thoughts about it. Then instruct patients to consider the various alternative behaviors and opportunities that are available to them. How do these alternatives compare to their current negative focus?

Possible Problems

Patients may believe that their perspective is the only "true" view. The therapist can introduce the idea that there are many potential and actual truths—that is, there are many different angles or pieces of information or behaviors available. Consider the person going through a divorce. There are a number of "truths" in this complex situation: for example, far less time with the former spouse, less time with children, financial strains, freedom to pursue new relationships, giving up on something that is not working, clarifying goals, and learning how to have better relationships. Each is "true," but no single one is the entire truth.

Cross-Reference to Other Techniques

Other relevant techniques include vertical descent, examining the evidence, double-standard technique, continuum, time machine, problem solving, and role play.

Form

Form 6.5 (Considering Alternatives, p. 217).

TECHNIQUE: SETTING A ZERO POINT FOR EVALUATION

Description

Many depressed individuals compare themselves to a perfect person who is able to accomplish everything at a 100% peak level—and with very little effort. They seldom consider the entire range of normal, and less-than-normal, performance. Often perfectionistic individuals compare themselves to the best they've ever performed. By reversing this pattern and setting a zero point for evaluation, patients are required to focus on *all* of the things that they do as a "positive."

Question to Pose/Intervention

"You seem to compare yourself to the best you've ever done or the best that others have done. But what if you measured yourself against a zero-point evaluation? What have you done, or what do you have, that is better than zero?"

Example

For example, a retired manager who had experienced some success in his work and who was respected in his community would compare himself to people who were extraordinarily wealthy and famous. His focus was on what he did not have rather than what he did have. This focus reflected his dichotomous, all-or-nothing thinking and precluded any appreciation of what he did have.

THERAPIST: You seem to think about other people who have millions of dollars and who are famous. Do you ever compare yourself to the poorest person in your community?

PATIENT: No.

THERAPIST: Let's imagine that you were to compare yourself to a homeless person. What does that person have, compared to you?

PATIENT: Well, I've seen homeless people on the streets, of course. I guess all that they have are the clothes on their backs and a few possessions. They have whatever they can beg from people.

THERAPIST: Now, let's look at what you have. You have a nice house, a pension, a wife, two daughters, you go to restaurants, you have friends. How does that compare with what the homeless people have?

PATIENT: I guess I'm a lot better off.

THERAPIST: That's something to keep in mind when you're feeling like a failure.

A variation of this exercise is to ask patients what it would sound like to try to convince someone who is at the zero point that they (the patients) have nothing and therefore are failures. The zero-point comparison can be used for people who criticize their own intelligence, looks, social skills, accomplishments, and other personal qualities. The therapist can point out that by thinking of what they have as "greater than zero," they can imagine themselves having more positive qualities rather than having less than the ideal.

Homework

The therapist can introduce this exercise by giving patients Form 6.8 (at the end of the chapter) and explain that it is important to be creative at times in thinking about ourselves. "One way of being creative is to think of anything you have or anything that you do as being above, or better than, zero, and then focus on improvements that you could make in your present situation. Think of the things that you feel bad about in your life. Make a list of them. Then indicate how each of these is better than zero. This is an exercise in developing appreciation for what is true today."

Possible Problems

As with any exercise that fosters a larger perspective, patients may view this exercise as invalidating. It is important to point out that the intention of the exercise is not to invalidate the suffering but to put the suffering in the context of appreciating what is also true in a positive sense. Rather than focus on what is missing, patients are asked to spend a few moments focusing on what they *do* have. Some people complain that comparing themselves to the zero point is not realistic, since their comparison group, or peers, are so much more accomplished. The therapist can point out that comparing ourselves to the zero point helps us recognize and appreciate what we do have and keeps us aware of the fact that life can be much worse than it already may seem to be. This exercise can be used as an introduction to the one described below, Taking It All Away.

Cross-Reference to Other Techniques

Other relevant techniques include use of the continuum, positive tracking, depolarizing comparisons, rational role play, double standard, pie chart, and negation of problem.

Form

Form 6.6 (Zero-Point Comparisons, p. 218).

TECHNIQUE: DEPOLARIZING COMPARISONS

Description

Similar to the person who makes perfectionistic comparisons is the person who thinks entirely in terms of 0 versus 100%, all or nothing: "Either I'm extremely successful [beautiful, rich, interesting, etc.], or I'm a failure." Comparisons involve only the extreme poles. The consequence of this kind of thinking is the feeling "No matter what I do, it is never good enough." Similar to the continuum technique the exercise of depolarizing comparisons encourages patients to consider comparing themselves with people all along the range of evaluations—from 0% to 25% to 50% to 75% to 100% performance (attainment, ability, etc.).

For example, a woman believed that she was "stupid" because she was not as smart as someone else in her office who was an exceptionally brilliant lawyer. Her automatic thoughts were, "I'm an idiot. I can't do anything right. I'll never get anywhere." Her perfectionistic standards led her to compare herself with the smartest person that she could imagine and then polarize herself to the extreme.

She was introduced to the concept of the normal distribution curve, where the average IQ is 100 and 75% of the total sample population have no college education. The therapist asked her to compare herself with 5 points along the distribution: (1) the point representing the stupidest person in the world, (2) the point indicating below-average IQ (85 IQ), (3) the point indicating average IQ (100), (4) the point for above-average IQ (115), and (5) the point for genius IQ (175). By depolarizing her comparisons and including a range of points for evaluation, she was able to recognize that she was much more intelligent and educated than 90% of the population. She was surprised to realize that she is smarter than 90% of people, rather than thinking that she is an idiot because one person is smarter than she is.

Similar to the zero-point technique, this exercise required her to identify how she differed from people who would score at each of the 5 points along the scale and what it would be like to try to convince these people that she was a loser because she was not smarter than everyone. This experience dramatically diminished her self-critical thoughts about her own competence.

Not all patients place in the top 10%, needless to say. What if the patient is average or below average? We have found that most people who are average are willing to accept the norm as their achievement, especially when they can point to qualities involving integrity and kindness that may be more important than achievement. For example, a foreman in a factory criticized himself because he was not a good writer. When we examined the evidence, it was clear that he was below average in this particular area. However, what actually bothered him more was his "should" statement that he should be an excellent writer. We reframed this idea as a *preference*, not a requirement, and examined other things that he did well (see Diversifying Criteria, below).

Question to Pose/Intervention

"You seem to be comparing yourself to people at the very top—the absolutely best in the field. What if you were to compare yourself to people at different levels—say, at 20%, 50%, 75%—rather than just 95% or 100%?"

Example

In this case the patient thought that she was stupid because she did not do "well" on her chemistry exam. In fact, she received a B and had a very high cumulative grade-point average.

THERAPIST: You feel you did poorly on the exam because you got a B. How bad do you feel, from 0% to 100%?

PATIENT: I feel terrible. I'd say close to 90% bad. I expected to get an A. I guess I'm not that smart.

THERAPIST: OK, your thought is that you aren't so smart. What else does that thought lead you to conclude?

PATIENT: I guess that I'm really mediocre. Ken got an A, and I always thought I was as smart as Ken.

THERAPIST: Sometimes we focus on the person at the top when we compare ourselves to other people. I guess that Ken did better than anyone else on the test. How would you compare yourself to the rest of the class—how did they do?

PATIENT: The average grade was C.

THERAPIST: So if you compared yourself to people at the midpoint—that's the C—you did better. What percentage of people got better than a B?

PATIENT: I'd say about 10% of the people.

THERAPIST: What percentile were you in?

PATIENT: Probably the 80th percentile.

THERAPIST: How would you compare yourself to people who were at the 40th percentile?

PATIENT: I did twice as well as they did.

THERAPIST: It sounds like the only percentile that was better than yours was the 90th percentile. Why would you feel bad about doing better than 80% of the people?

PATIENT: I guess that it's not so bad as it feels. Most people didn't do as well as I did.

Homework

The therapist introduces the issue of depolarizing comparisons by suggesting that "we often compare ourselves to people at the top, but it is more realistic to compare ourselves to people performing at all different levels. Over the next week, I'd like you to consider the negative things you are saying about yourself [e.g., failure, stupid, ugly, etc.]. Using this table (Form 6.7, at the end of the chapter), make a list of these negative qualities that you think you have and then compare yourself to people at each level—those at the 25% level, the 50% level, 75%, and 100%. How do you compare to people at these levels? How does this comparison make you feel, and what does this make you think?"

Possible Problems

Many perfectionistic patients have difficulty with this technique. They complain that it does not make sense to use the full range, since they expect more from themselves. We have found several techniques to be helpful in such situations. First, consider the costs and benefits of using the entire range of comparisons. By using the entire range, patients are able to appreciate what they have accomplished. However, patients may object that they will lose their motivation (their "edge") or become mediocre if they settle for comparing themselves with people in the bottom half. Second, examine the evidence that people lose their edge when they go beyond narrow comparisons at the topmost level. In fact, some people procrastinate because they believe they cannot perform at 100%. Third, consider possible positive outcomes from performing at a less-than-perfect level—that is, do the people at the 50% or 40% level have any positives in their lives, such as less pressure?

Cross-Reference to Other Techniques

As indicated, other techniques that might be helpful include cost–benefit analysis, construction of alternatives, using the continuum technique, vertical descent, and graded task assignments.

Form

Form 6.7 (Depolarizing Comparisons, p. 219).

TECHNIQUE: LOOKING AT OTHERS' COPING

Description

As indicated above, many times we believe that people who have done worse than we have are much worse off than we are. In fact, this is often not the case. Consider income. We may believe that we need to make a certain amount of money in order to have any self-esteem, but the fact is that there are millions of people who make less than we do who feel fine about themselves and enjoy a lot of things in their lives. In using this exercise we ask patients to consider people who have done worse as a positive role model of succeeding in spite of lower performance. This technique seems counterintuitive, but it may liberate patients from the demanding standards and unfair comparisons that contribute to lowered self-esteem.

A variation of this exercise involves asking patients to consider how people who have gone through a similar loss (trauma, setback, conflict, etc.) have coped with it in a productive way. For example, if the patient has lost his or her job, he or she might consider how others have coped well with losing their jobs. What's their secret?

Question to Pose/Intervention

"You are focusing on how you did *not* measure up to your high standards. You are focusing on the negative things going on your life. Consider other people who have not done as well as you have [or who have experienced a loss like you have]. What positives do they experience in their lives? How have other people survived? What were they able to do that was positive?

Example

THERAPIST: You sound like you are down on yourself because you didn't make as much money this year as you wished you had. Are there people who make less money than you do?

PATIENT: Most people make less than I do, but I expected to make a lot more.

THERAPIST: So things didn't live up to your expectations. Do you know any people who make less?

PATIENT: Almost all the people I work with.

THERAPIST: Can you tell me about some of them? For example, are they able to experience any positive things in life?

PATIENT: Actually, Jane makes about half of what I make. She enjoys her friends. She has a simple but nice apartment, and she seems to have an upbeat attitude.

THERAPIST: How does she manage such pleasantness if she makes so much less than you do?

PATIENT: She doesn't have my expectations.

THERAPIST: Maybe there's something that Jane can teach you about life. What could that be?

PATIENT: How to have fun?

Another patient was worried about his impending divorce and suddenly seeing herself as a lonely failure.

THERAPIST: Do you have friends who are divorced?

PATIENT: Yeah. Larry is divorced, and Frank has been through it twice.

THERAPIST: How did Larry deal when he got divorced?

PATIENT: Well, he was actually fairly happy to get out of the marriage. He complained about the financial aspects of the divorce, but he got his own apartment, and he started dating on the Internet.

THERAPIST: What could you learn from Larry about how to handle this situation?

PATIENT: Well, I guess that when there's money involved, it focuses your attention (*laughs*).

THERAPIST: That's true. That might help you deal with any guilt feelings. Probably once the lawyers get involved, you'll feel less guilty and more concerned with protecting your assets. By the way, how did Larry handle this aspect?

PATIENT: He got a good lawyer.

THERAPIST: OK. What else did he do to make the divorce work out for himself.

PATIENT: He got himself a nice apartment. That's going to be expensive.

THERAPIST: Are you worth it?

PATIENT: You're right. It's *my* money!

THERAPIST: OK. What else can you learn from him?

PATIENT: Don't sit around and stew over it. Get out and meet people. Do things.

THERAPIST: So, one way of putting things in perspective is to see how other people have handled divorce.

PATIENT: That's true. It doesn't seem so bad now. If they are able to manage it, why couldn't I?

Homework

Using Form 6.8 (at the end of the chapter), the therapist can ask patients to describe the conflict, loss of job, income, relationship, rejection, or disapproval on which they are focused. Then patients should consider any other people they know (or have known in the past) who have experienced either a similar or more difficult situation and coped well in the face of the adversity. What could be learned from them?

Possible Problems

Similar to other techniques that seek to place things in perspective, this exercise can be experienced as invalidating. One patient complained, "You're trying to make this seem OK—but it hurts me a lot." The therapist should attempt to balance validation of patients' painful emotional experiences with the recognition that others have coped successfully with painful losses and that we can gain wisdom and perspective from these people.

Cross-Reference to Other Techniques

Other relevant techniques include double standard, problem solving, constructing alternatives, decatastrophizing, negation of problem, and activity scheduling.

Form

Form 6.8 (How Have Others Coped?, p. 220).

TECHNIQUE: DIVERSIFYING CRITERIA

Description

Quite often, we judge ourselves, or others, on the basis of one factor to the exclusion of many other possible factors. For example, the college student who receives a C—an average grade—on a history exam and concludes "I'm a failure, I haven't learned anything" is focusing only on the questions she got wrong and disregarding all of the other questions that she got right. Is this reasonable thinking on her part? Didn't she learn something in the course that was not on the test, in addition to those correct answers? How about her other courses?—surely she learned something in those courses as well. She also learned a lot from interacting with her friends and all the facets of college life—none of which was tested. She focused on one dimension to evaluate herself and did not consider the other areas in which she has learned many things.

Another example is the socially anxious individual who thinks "I looked like a fool at that meeting." The evidence he points to is that he hesitated when he spoke. But what would be some additional criteria or examples of competent behavior at this meeting or at all of the other meetings he has attended? The Example section provides an excerpt of a dialogue with a socially anxious businessman.

Question to Pose/Intervention

"Sometimes we think that we don't have a certain quality because we do not do well in one or two situations. For example, I worked with a man who believed he was stupid because he didn't do well on his job review interview. But he had other ways of showing his intelligence—for example, he was good at his job, per se (just not at being interviewed), and he was good at dealing with people. When you criticize yourself, you may lose awareness of your positive qualities and behaviors. Think of the quality that you believe you lack. Now think of some creative ways of observing that quality in yourself or in others."

Example

THERAPIST: You said that you looked like a fool at the meeting because you hesitated. How long did the meeting run?

PATIENT: About 90 minutes.

THERAPIST: How many times did you speak?

PATIENT: Probably about 10 times.

THERAPIST: What would be some ways that we could evaluate someone's competence at a meeting?

PATIENT: Well, I think that showing up on time, having the information you need, communicating the information, convincing the other people, getting an agreement—those would be some signs of doing a good job.

THERAPIST: Did you do any of those things?

PATIENT: Yes, I did all of them.

THERAPIST: So when you focus on your one hesitation as signifying a poor performance, you are not considering all of the other ways in which you performed well at the meeting? Perhaps you need to expand your criteria for success.

This narrowness of criteria was exemplified by a 73-year-old woman who had been married for almost 50 years. Her belief was "My husband doesn't love me because he doesn't want to have sex with me." She had held this belief for most of her marriage. We decided to expand her criteria for "love."

THERAPIST: What are some other ways in which a husband shows that he loves his wife?

PATIENT: He can be faithful, affectionate, give her things, help her when she's feeling down, do things with her.

THERAPIST: Has your husband done any of these things?

PATIENT: Yeah. And he tells me he loves me.

THERAPIST: Perhaps you're focusing on only one sign of love—sex. It sounds like you're saying that there are a lot of ways that he does love you.

As we examined her husband's past history, it surfaced that her family doctor—who also was her husband's doctor before they married—had warned her that he was not that interested in sex. As it turned out, he suffered from a lifelong depression, which reduced his sex drive, but which did not preclude him from loving his wife in other ways.

Homework

Using Form 6.9 (at the end of the chapter), patients list one quality they want more of (i.e., they believe they are lacking in this quality), indicate all the different ways of observing that quality, and identify examples of demonstrating that quality.

Possible Problems

Some individuals are "negative trackers": They only count the negatives. They discount the positives because they believe that the positives are "expected." This thinking can be challenged by asking them to list examples of people who lack some of these taken-for-granted positives. For example, if the patient believes that "knowing how to be polite" is taken for granted, then he or she should list examples of people who have shown poor manners.

Cross-Reference to Other Techniques

Other relevant interventions include the semantic technique, evidence for and against, examining insufficient information searches, double standard, and positive tracking.

Form

Form 6.9 (Developing New Ways to Evaluate a Quality, p. 221).

TECHNIQUE: Taking It All Away

Description

Much of what we experience in daily life we take for granted, assuming that it will always be there. Depression is often the consequence of discounting the positives in our lives, not appreciating the sources of rewards that are available, not noticing the good things around us. One form of therapy, used in Japan for depression, views depressed individuals as people who have lost touch with their environment—both the objects and the people. Patients are isolated, by the therapist, in a dimly lit room, where they contemplate the objects and people with whom they no longer have contact. This deprivation heightens patients' awareness of the meaning of these objects and people. The therapist then reintroduces, one by one, objects and people to each patient. Patients are asked to focus on the object or person and to describe what they appreciate about it/him/her. For example, an orange is pealed and placed in front of the patient, who comments, "I can smell the fragrance of the orange, I remember the sweetness of the juice." Similarly, patients' partners are brought in to the room, and patients describe the experiences they recall appreciatively. In this way, awareness and connection with the world is rebuilt.

I have adapted this exercise to our therapy format. I ask patients who believe they value nothing to imagine that *everything* has been taken away—their body, memory, family, job, house, car, all their possessions, their capacity to feel—everything. They must now ask a Supreme Being, who has removed all of these things, to return them one by one, not knowing how many they will get back. But he has to make a case for each one of them. And he must prove that they are worth having. If not, then he has to describe what his life will be like without them.

Question to Pose/Intervention

"Imagine that everything you have—and are—were taken away. What would you want back and why would you want it? "Imagine that there is a Supreme Being from whom you must request the restoration of each person or thing that you want back. You do not know how many of these requests will be granted. The Supreme Being has to be convinced that what you want back is really important to you—that you really appreciate it. I will play the role of the Supreme Being, and you can ask me to give you back the people and things that have been taken away from you. Keep in mind that *everything* has been taken away. You have absolutely nothing right now—no body, no mind, no memory, no friends, no family, no possessions. You have been reduced to absolutely nothing. Now begin by asking me for one thing at a time, and try to convince me that you really want it back and could really appreciate it.

Example

I used this technique with a young Wall-Streeter who believed that his life was over and not worth living because he had made a bad decision about a trade.

THERAPIST: Close your eyes and imagine that everything has been taken away—your memory, all your senses, your body, your family—your wife and child—your parents, friends, your job, house, car, all of your possessions. Now I want you to imagine that you are asking God, or some Supreme Being, to return these things. God has to be convinced that you can make a good case for valuing these things if they were restored to you.

The patient seemed uncomfortable, but he asked for his senses back first. He justified this prioritization, by saying that he could not appreciate any of the other things without the capacity to see, hear, and feel.

THERAPIST: What is it that you want to see, hear, and feel?

PATIENT: I want to see my wife, my son. I want to feel them close to me.

THERAPIST: But why do you want that? What good will it do you?

PATIENT: Because I love them.

THERAPIST: What if we limited your sensory abilities to perceiving only them? Would that be enough?

PATIENT: No. I want to be able to see the sun again. I want to hear my parents, by brother. I want to hear music.

THERAPIST: What if you never heard music again? Or saw the sun?

PATIENT: I'd miss that!

We then went through a variety of other things that he had to request be returned to him and justify his appreciation of them. What was intriguing to me was how emotionally charged this exercise was for him. Here was a "tough Wall-Streeter" who had begun to see that the most important things in his life were literally right before his eyes.

Two weeks later his depression had lifted. He told me that the exercise had impressed on him how important his life was—despite the bond deal that did not work. He recalled the following incident for me: "Our next-door neighbor came over the other day. She's a woman a few years older than my wife. To our shock, she said, 'You may have noticed that my son Jerry hasn't been coming around for the last month. I thought I should tell you that he's been upset since his father died from cancer.' I began to cry. I realized how much my family means to me and how much I mean to them."

Homework

Using Form 6.10 (at the end of the chapter), the therapist asks patients to engage their imagination in a fantasy in which they have lost everything—their body, senses, memory, family, possessions, job, friends—and are given the task of finding the meaning or importance of each of these losses and making a case for receiving them back: Describe why each is important and why each is appreciated. This is a powerful exercise that challenges the idea that nothing is worthwhile, and the state in which everything is taken for granted; Form 6.10 may be useful in eliciting some thoughts and feelings about the value of what is around us.

Possible Problems

Again, patients may consider this exercise to be invalidating, because the loss or conflict is "real" to them. Losses and conflicts *are* real, but so is everything else that we ask patients to consider. Whether patients live out these other possibilities or experiences in their lives will depend on their ability to recognize their role in patients' existence. This recognition comes from developing more mindfulness—more attuned awareness of the present reality. The therapist can say: "Consider the fact that every second you are breathing. However, you almost never notice it. Now focus on your breathing and imagine that this is taken away for 5 minutes. Obviously, you would die. It is real, but you did not notice it until you imagined it stopping."

Cross-Reference to Other Techniques

Other relevant techniques include continuum, setting a zero-point, decatastrophizing, constructing alternatives, problem solving, double standard, viewing it from the balcony, and activity scheduling (i.e., focusing on appreciating and becoming more mindful of the items in the list).

Form

Form 6.10 (Asking for Things That Are Important to Me, p. 222).

TECHNIQUE: EXAMINING OPPORTUNITIES AND NEW MEANINGS THAT COME FROM LOSS OR CONFLICT

Description

Losses and conflicts are inevitable aspects of life. While recognizing that these losses and conflicts may be painful and require significant adjustment, it is also possible to acknowledge that these losses also may provide opportunities for reconstructing meaning, opening new awareness, or responding to new challenges with personal growth. The patient who is experiencing divorce may report that she is depressed because of the loss of intimacy and continuity in her life, but the divorce also may (1) provide an opportunity for recognizing and redefining personal values of intimacy and attachment, (2) create new opportunities for new relationships with friends or a new intimate partner, and (3) catalyze growth in her work arena and in her experience of connectedness to others. Rather than looking on the dark side of the loss, the patient can be encouraged to consider the opportunities, challenges, and meanings that are possible consequences of the current situation. Victor Frankel, one of the founders of cognitive therapy, described this perspective in his provocative book *Man's Search for Meaning*, a description of life in a Nazi death camp, where finding meaning was the only way to cope.

This basic issue—finding the positive in the negative situation—became poignantly clear to me during September 2001, in New York City, where I live. I was emotionally distraught by all the images of people at the World Trade Center who had been killed in the terrorist attack. But, at the same time, I was filled with a sense of community, hope, pride, and strength by watching my fellow New Yorkers honor the firefighters and police who had lost their lives in rescuing thousands of people. It was a high price to pay—certainly—to see so many heroic people die. But it also made clear that there are heroes—something that can make us feel optimistic and connected to one another.

Question to Pose/Intervention

"Although you may be focused right now on the loss [or conflict]—and it may feel very negative to you—it is also possible to consider it in light of new meanings that you can give to your life. What good can come out of this situation? What have you learned about what you value? About what is important to you? Are there new opportunities, new behaviors, new relationships, new challenges, or new ways of seeing things that you can experience because of this loss [or conflict]?"

Example

THERAPIST: So, Jane, you are feeling down since the breakup with Bill? When you feel down, what kinds of thoughts do you have?

PATIENT: I think about how I no longer have someone I love in my life.

THERAPIST: It sounds like having a deep and meaningful relationship is important to you. that it is something you value.

PATIENT: Yes, although I know I have friends, and my work is going well. But I do feel so much better when I'm close to someone.

THERAPIST: Does that say something good about you?

PATIENT: I guess it says that I have a lot of love to give. I like the intimacy, the connection.

THERAPIST: It sounds like intimacy and connection and being able to love someone are important parts of who you are.

PATIENT: Yeah. It's hard to live without that.

THERAPIST: Yes, it's hard not to have those things right now. The pain that you experience must be telling you something about who you are. What does it tell you?

PATIENT: It tells me that I want to have love in my life.

THERAPIST: Perhaps we can look at what that says about you that is good, even if it is painful.

PATIENT: I want a meaningful relationship with someone who is special to me.

THERAPIST: So, being able to love and give and connect with someone is part of who you are. We don't want to change that.

PATIENT: No. But how will I find someone if I'm so depressed?

THERAPIST: It may not be the right time now. But since this is an important value to you, we need to keep in mind that this is something special you want to share only with a special person. Not everyone will measure up.

PATIENT: But I'll feel lonely.

THERAPIST: Perhaps, for a while, your loneliness can tell you that you have a lot to give. It's painful, but it says something good about you. Perhaps some of that love and kindness can be directed toward caring for yourself.

PATIENT: I like that sound of that.

Homework

The therapist can ask patients to focus on what the loss or conflict tells them about what they value and what is important to them: "A lot of negative experiences may help us clarify what we value and what is important to us. Does this experience teach you anything like that?" In addition, the therapist can ask patients to list some of the new opportunities for learning or growth or behavior that may develop from the current situation. Patients can use Form 6.11 (at the end of the chapter) to record their responses.

Possible Problems

For some patients, finding the meaning or significance of the event may trigger even more depression, because they believe they currently do not have what they want and may never get it. It is essential that the therapist validate the emotional distress in the current situation but also point out how the values and desires implicit in patients' responses may point to potential strengths. Each value can be a motivating force in their life. As noted in the above dialogue, the person's response to the end of a relationship, triggering feelings of loneliness and thoughts of needing intimacy, can be turned into an important value—the importance of meaningful connections with others. This value can then motivate the patient to deepen other relationships and to relate in a more honest and direct way.

Cross-Reference to Other Techniques

Other relevant techniques include constructing alternatives, positive reframing, problem solving, role playing against the negative thoughts, activity scheduling, and identifying and modifying personal schemas.

Form

Form 6.11 (Examining Opportunities and New Meanings, p. 223).

FORM 6.1. Pie Chart Exercise

Consider the different pieces in the "pie" below. Each piece represents a cause of the event; some causes may require more than one piece, because they had more influence on the event. Label each piece as a possible cause of the event. How big a piece is left for you as a cause of the event?

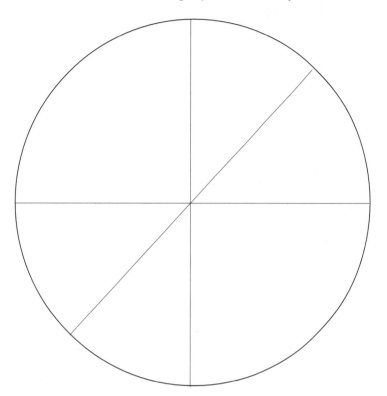

What is the negative event that bothers you: _____

List all of the possible causes of this event, including your own role in the event:

_____

_____

_____

_____

FORM 6.2. The Continuum Exercise

Using the scale below, indicate where you would place the current event that is bothering you. Now fill in events for each 10-point mark on the scale. Is it hard to fill in some points that are lower than your current event? Why is that? Would you consider rerating the current outcome or event after you have filled out this scale? What is the reason why you would—or would not—rerate the outcome or event?

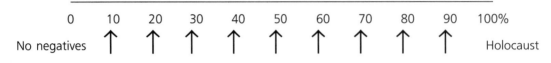

Question: Where would you place the current event?

Comments:

FORM 6.3. The Double-Standard Exercise

Consider some of the negative things that you are saying about yourself or your current experience. Now think about the advice you would give a friend. Would you be as critical of your friend as you are of yourself? Why not?

Current negative thoughts	Advice I would give a friend	Why would I be more critical of myself than of a friend?

FORM 6.4. View from the Balcony

A lot of times we experience things only from our own perspective, which is mired in the intensity of our emotions. Any interaction can be viewed from many other perspectives. Imagine that you take your current experience and try to view it as though you were observing it from a balcony. How do you see it? What are the advantages of seeing it from this new perspective?

How I currently see what is going on (negative thoughts, feelings, etc.)	How I might see it from the balcony	Advantages of seeing it from the balcony

FORM 6.5. Considering Alternatives

When we are upset, we often focus on one point of view—our own—not realizing that there are many different ways of viewing things. Consider the current situation and your point of view. Describe the situation in the left-hand column and your negative thoughts—your "interpretations"—in the middle column. Now, in the right-hand column, list different ways of seeing the current situation—different interpretations, behaviors and opportunities you might pursue, etc.

Describe the current situation that is bothering you.	What are your negative thoughts?	What are some different ways of viewing this situation? Are there new opportunities made available? Are there different possibilities that you could pursue? List these.

FORM 6.6. Zero-Point Comparisons

Think of someone who completely lacks the quality that I think that I lack—that is, the person at the zero point. What is he or she like? How do I differ? What do I have or do that represents an improvement over the zero point? What would it be like to try to convince someone at the zero point that I am a failure?

The person at the zero point has these qualities or things	I have these qualities or things

FORM 6.7. Depolarizing Comparisons

Sometimes we compare ourselves to people who perform at the top level (100%) and find ourselves lacking. Try to use a full range of comparisons when evaluating yourself, using the questions below.

Question	Answer
What quality am I criticizing in myself?	
How would I compare myself with people who have 0% on this quality?	
25%?	
50%?	
75%?	
100%?	

FORM 6.8. How Have Others Coped?

When we go through a loss or a conflict, we often focus on the worst possible outcome or meaning. It can be helpful to realize that other people have gone through similar or even worse experiences. Many of these people found ways of coping or ways of thinking that were especially helpful. What can you learn from the way they coped?

Describe current situation	Who else has experienced something like this?	How did they view this situation and how did they cope?

FORM 6.9. Developing New Ways to Evaluate a Quality

We often think that we lack a particular quality (e.g., intelligence) because we do not do well in certain situations (e.g., chemistry exams). However, there are many ways to show different aspects of intelligence or other positive qualities. Think about the quality that you want more of, and then think of examples of positive behavior that might show that you have some of that positive quality. Use positive rather than negative terms when wording the quality to be evaluated—for example, "successful experiences" rather than "failure." Focus on observable, verifiable behaviors or performances, rather than inferences about underlying qualities.

Example: Quality to be evaluated: *I have successful experiences.*

Different ways to observe it: *Performance throughout school years, scores on tests, feedback from professors.*

Indicate how you might demonstrate some of this quality in different situations.

Quality to be evaluated:
Different ways to observe it:
Do I demonstrate any examples of this quality? Specify:

FORM 6.10. Asking for Things That Are Important to Me

Imagine that you have lost everything—your senses, your body, your memory, your family, job, possessions—absolutely everything. Then list what you want back, in order of importance, and make a case for why you want each back.

What I want back	Why it's important to me

FORM 6.11. Examining Opportunities and New Meanings

Current situation (or loss)	What this tells me about my needs and values	New opportunities and challenges in my life

CHAPTER 7

~

Schema-Focused Therapy

Beck's earlier description of psychopathology proposed that each diagnostic condition was characterized by schemas, habitual patterns of thinking that were quite general, that marked vulnerability (Beck, 1976; Beck et al., 1978). Depressive schemas reflected concerns about loss, failure, rejection, and depletion; anxiety schemas reflected threat and injury; and anger schemas reflected humiliation and domination. Beck, Freeman and associates (1990) developed a model of specific schemas for the various personality disorders, relating avoidant personality to schemas of inadequacy and rejection, narcissistic personality to schemas of entitlement and special status, and so forth. Young (1990) developed a schema model focused on the specific content of personality vulnerability. Both the Beck et al. model and the Young model draw on Adler's (1926) description of how individuals are likely to either compensate for their perceived inadequacies or avoid situations that might activate these schemas (see Leahy, 2001, for a description of how schemas interfere with making progress in cognitive therapy). In this chapter we will examine how the therapist can assist the patient in identifying and modifying their individual schemas.

TECHNIQUE: IDENTIFYING SCHEMAS

Description

Underlying vulnerability to depression, anxiety and anger is the core belief that the individual holds about self or others. Beck et al. (1990) and Young and Flanagan (1998) have identified a number of core schemas that individuals endorse, and they suggest a correspondence between these schemas and personality disorders. In the present context, we do not need to diagnose personality disorder in order to evaluate schematic content. Furthermore, the specific content of personal schemas or core beliefs is not necessarily captured by the list of schemas provided in the literature on personality disorders; schemas are, by their nature, idiosyncratic and may include any consistent manner in which the individual views self or other. Thus schemas may correspond more directly with Kelly's (1955) idea of "personal construct"—that is, an idiosyncratic and biased manner in which the individual views self or other.

Examples of core beliefs from Beck et al. (1990) include beliefs about being vulnerable, socially inept, incompetent, needy, weak, helpless, self-sufficient, easily controlled by others, responsible, competent, righteous, innocent, special, unique, glamorous, and impressive. Young (1990) identifies the following as personal schemas: themes of dependence, subjugation, vulnerability to harm or illness, fear of losing self-control, emotional deprivation, abandonment, mistrust, defectiveness, social undesirability, incompetence, guilt, shame, unrelenting standards, and entitlement.

The current technique of identifying schemas involves either use of vertical descent or simply noticing consistencies in the way in which the individual views self or other. For example, with vertical descent (explained in Chapter 1) the therapist begins a sequence of questions that may lead to a fundamental or core belief. An example of this is the following: "She won't like me" → "I can't stand getting rejected" → "It means I'm unlovable." Thus the core belief may be "I am unlovable." The therapist also can tentatively identify core schemas or beliefs by noticing consistencies in patients' reports. For example, the therapist may notice that patients continue to label themselves as stupid and incompetent (i.e., schema = incompetent) or unlovable (i.e., schema = unlovable). Despite the beliefs of some therapists that identifying schemas is a long and arduous task, it may be possible to begin to identify these core beliefs in the first few sessions.

I recommend the schema form developed by Beck and his associates (Butler, Brown, Beck, & Grisham, in press), because it validly discriminates among the various personality disorders. Young (1990) also has developed a schema questionnaire that may be helpful.

Question to Pose/Intervention

Vertical Descent

"When you think that [such and such would happen], it would bother you because it would make you think . . . ?" → "And if this were true, you would feel bothered because you would think [or it would mean] . . . ?" An example is the following: "If I don't do well on the exam, then it would mean that I failed" → "What would it mean to you if you did fail?" → "That I am a failure" → "And what would that make you think?" → "I won't be able to take care of myself" → "And what would happen then?" → "I might starve to death." In this case, the core belief or schema is vulnerability to harm/loss, failure, or "biological vulnerability."

Noticing Common Patterns

The therapist might comment: "I noticed in your discussions that you keep focusing on [common pattern]. Examples of common patterns include viewing the self as ugly, undesirable, incompetent, evil, helpless, unlovable. The patient who continually refers to what she perceives as her unappealing looks is revealing her personal schema of being physically defective and possibly unlovable. Of course, the therapist might inquire further: "What would happen if you were not lovable [or if you were defective, ugly, etc.]?" In one case, the patient believed "My husband would abandon me. I can't be happy without being married." Her personal schemas involved the themes of physical defectiveness, being abandoned, feeling needy, and unable to self-reward. In this particular case it was helpful to identify these schemas, since prior to her marriage, she was much happier on her own. She was able to recognize that she did not need a man to be happy.

Example

Vertical Descent

THERAPIST: You said you are worried that your face is not exactly the way you want it to be. You are focusing a lot on some imperfections that you see. Is that right?

PATIENT: Yes. I think I'm looking older.

THERAPIST: OK. So let's see what looking older would mean to you. "If I look older it bothers me because it means what to me?"

PATIENT: It means I'm not attractive.

THERAPIST: OK. So you are equating "older" with "not attractive." And if you are not attractive, this
would bother you because it would mean . . . ?

PATIENT: My husband won't want me anymore.

THERAPIST: And if that happened, then what?

PATIENT: Then I would be alone. And then . . . I don't know . . . life would be miserable.

THERAPIST: So your thought is that you would look older, not attractive, get rejected and abandoned,
and end up alone and miserable?

PATIENT: Right. That's how I feel.

THERAPIST: Why would you be miserable if you didn't have a husband?

PATIENT: I guess I don't think I could make myself happy.

THERAPIST: So your thought is that life can't be rewarding without a husband?

PATIENT: Right.

In this particular case the patient revealed several schemas about herself—themes of being unattractive, abandoned, and unable to be happy while alone. She also discounted, in further inquiry, the
many other positive qualities she brought to her marriage, such as intelligence, common interests,
common bond, empathy, and support for her husband. Men, in her schemas, only focused on looks and
could not be trusted to value anything else.

Noticing Common Patterns

THERAPIST: You've told me that in your relationships with men, you always find yourself in this one-
down position. For example, your ex-husband, you said, treated you like a servant and never met
your needs sexually or emotionally. Your current boyfriend seemed to take advantage of you, and
you also described how your father ignored you when you were depressed. Is there a pattern
here?

PATIENT: Yeah, men treat me like shit.

THERAPIST: OK. So that is what you are seeing about the men. But is there a pattern in how you see
yourself in these relationships?

PATIENT: I guess I see myself as someone who never gets her needs met.

THERAPIST: When you think about that pattern—never getting your needs met—does that make you
think anything about yourself?

PATIENT: My needs aren't important.

THERAPIST: OK. So if you saw yourself as having needs that were not important, does that make you think anything about yourself?

PATIENT: I guess *I'm* not important.

THERAPIST: Why would you not be important?

PATIENT: Because I'm fat, and I was never as pretty as my older sister who got all the attention.

THERAPIST: So your view of yourself is that you are fat, and that is why your needs are not important?

PATIENT: I never put it in those words before. But that is how I see it, I guess. Who could love a fat ugly kid?

THERAPIST: So you see yourself, then, as not really deserving love. Perhaps that is why you find yourself in relationships with men who don't meet your needs?

PATIENT: Yeah, it just feeds on itself, doesn't it?

THERAPIST: It feeds back into your negative belief about yourself—"I am fat and ugly, I am unlovable, my needs don't count, men don't meet my needs, and that proves my point." I guess that it becomes a self-fulfilling prophecy?

PATIENT: Yeah. Always happening the same way.

THERAPIST: Your view of yourself as fat, ugly, defective, unlovable is what we call your own personal schema or self-concept. This schema is maintained by the choices you make in men. Your personal view or schema of yourself as defective and unlovable is maintained.

PATIENT: It's a never-ending pattern.

Homework

To help patients identify common schemas, the therapist can ask them to identify several automatic thoughts during the week and conduct vertical descent on each one. The core beliefs, identified by vertical descent should yield a number of common schemas. In addition, patients may complete Young's (1990) schema questionnaire (Form 7.1, at the end of the chapter). It is also useful for patients to review previous homework assignments (e.g., thought records) and determine if any schemas about self or others emerge.

Possible Problems

Some patients confuse *schemas* with *reality*, believing that their habitual patterns of viewing things are not personal constructions but simply "the facts." The therapist can help these patients realize that, at this stage, we are only trying to identify patterns in the way people view things—we are not challenging or disputing anything. It may be, for example, that the patient's view that "Others are rejecting" can be supported by the "facts"—simply because the patient consistently chooses rejecting partners.

Cross-Reference to Other Techniques

As indicated, the vertical descent procedure is very helpful in identifying schemas. Other useful exercises include identifying automatic thoughts, assumptions, conditional rules, case conceptualization, looking for variations in a belief (i.e., identifying triggers), and guessing the thought.

Form

Form 7.1 (Personal Belief Questionnaire, pp. 248–255).

TECHNIQUE: EXPLAINING SCHEMATIC PROCESSING

Description

Most people recognize that they have some common biases in the way that they view things. Schematic processing is such a bias. For example, people very concerned about failure focus on difficulty, mistakes, motivation, and achieving their goals, while typically comparing themselves to others' performances. In Chapter 5 we described "limited search" and "confirmation bias" as examples of biased information processing. Here we are explaining biased information processing by referring to the more technical concept of "schematic processing." We can define schematic processing as a bias to selectively recall or attend to information of a specific content—for example, by selectively focusing on looks and evaluating attractiveness by examining every detail of physical imperfection; or by focusing on signs of rejection from others. Schematic processing also can include selective *forgetting* of material—that is, a form of cognitive avoidance.

Question to Pose/Intervention

"We all are somewhat selective in what we focus on and what we think is important. We tend to notice and remember some things that others might not notice or recall. Let's imagine that you put on some glasses that had red lenses. You might notice that almost everything you look at is tinted red. This red lens is a metaphor for the *schema* through which you view yourself and the world. Examples of these kinds of schemas include being overly focused on achievement, rejection, abandonment, control, approval, helplessness, or attractiveness. There are many different kinds of schemas or concepts that we all use. We are going to try to see if there are certain kinds of schemas or concepts that you are using on a regular basis.

"One thing about schemas is that they make us pay attention to some things more than to others. For example, if you have a schema about rejection, you might attend to lots of things that you interpret as rejection—the way people look at you, what they say, or how they act. They might not be rejecting you, but you might have this bias to see rejection in lots of things. And if you were really focused on rejection—if that was your schema or concept—then you might remember lots of things about rejection. And you might not notice people liking you or approving of you. You might have this bias that determines how you focus on and remember things. So that is what we mean by the idea of a schema; it makes you focus your attention on, remember, and think about certain things more than others."

Example

THERAPIST: One of the things that we are interested in is whether or not you view things in certain ways—whether or not you have certain biases about things that happen to you. (*Gives the description of schematic processing described in the above section.*)

PATIENT: What do you think my schemas are?

THERAPIST: Well, we can look at that in a while. Right now, I want to see if we both understand how schemas work. Let's say that you had a schema about being special—the need to be superior. What kinds of things would you focus on?

PATIENT: I might focus on trying to do better than everyone.

THERAPIST: Right. You might. And then how would you look at your own performance?

PATIENT: I guess I might always worry that I wasn't always the best. I'd worry about failing.

THERAPIST: OK. So you might focus on "Are other people doing better than me?" or "What if I get something wrong?"

PATIENT: Yeah, I guess.

THERAPIST: Then you might really focus a lot on achievement and comparison. What do you think you might also say to yourself—something like "I could have done better, so it doesn't count"?

PATIENT: That's true. I might not take credit for what I *do* accomplish.

THERAPIST: Or you might predict that you will fail, and if you didn't do a really superb job, you might think you are a failure.

PATIENT: Yeah, perfectionism.

THERAPIST: And looking back on your life, you might recall any examples that you were not the best and dwell on them. So you would focus on being special, you would focus on anything you did that wasn't perfect, you'd take no credit for your positives, and you'd predict you wouldn't do as well as you should do. That's how schemas work.

PATIENT: I wonder what my schemas are.

Homework

Patients can be assigned the reading on schemas in Form 7.2 (at the end of the chapter).

Possible Problems

Some patients believe they do not have schemas but rather are objective observers of reality. They may not be motivated to consider their habitual patterns of thinking, and they may not be willing to consider the subjective, constructivist processes underlying these patterns. Indeed, patients may regard that this line of questioning or instruction as invalidating and as trying to "trick" them into "thinking positive thoughts." It is important to stress that discussing habitual patterns of thinking or specific patterns of focusing attention on issues does not imply incorrect perceptions. It may be true, for example, that the schema "People reject me" has empirical validity for a particular patient. The question later raised will be why this is so. Is it a consequence of poor choices, maladaptive behavior, or bad luck? Or is there a process whereby the patient does not accurately process information about positive responses from others? We discuss this process of schema maintenance later in this chapter.

Cross-Reference to Other Techniques

Related techniques include identifying automatic thoughts—especially labeling and personalizing—vertical descent, underlying assumptions, and case conceptualization,

Form

Form 7.2 (Guide to Understanding Schemas, pp. 256–258).

TECHNIQUE: IDENTIFYING SCHEMA COMPENSATION AND AVOIDANCE

Description

Alfred Adler (1964) observed that many individuals compensate for a sense of inferiority by striving for power or superior functioning. Individuals who view themselves as weak might compensate by acting in an aggressive manner. The schema-focused model stresses the importance of compensatory functioning. Examples of compensatory strategies, with the underlying negative schema in parentheses, follow: body building (weak, "unmasculine"), clinging in relationships (helplessness), obsession with accumulating money (failure, "ordinary," not special), and glamorous (unattractive, unlovable). For example, a young man who viewed himself as physically frail as a child became proficient in martial arts. His thought was, "If I can defeat people in hand-to-hand combat, then I will never be weak again."

Related to schema compensation is schema avoidance. As noted, with the avoidance pattern, individuals do not put themselves in a position where the schema can be activated. For example, the individual with a schema related to personal undesirability or defectiveness (i.e., who views herself as unlovable) might use schema avoidance by not allowing herself to enter into relationships. She may scan the environment for any sign of rejection and quickly exit the scene. The individual who believes that he is incompetent will avoid situations that are challenging.

Question to Pose/Intervention

The therapist should provide the patient with the form for understanding schemas (Form 7.2). Then the therapist can ask, "Now that you have identified your schemas, can you think of how you try to avoid situations where your schema might upset you? Are there things you do to compensate for your schema?"

Example

THERAPIST: You seem to be concerned that you are not as pretty as you were 10 years ago. [The patient is a 42-year-old woman.] What is it that concerns you about this change?

PATIENT: Well, I'm losing my looks. I'm starting to look old, and if it keeps going like this, I'll be really unattractive.

THERAPIST: What makes you think you are not looking as attractive as you thought you did?

PATIENT: I checked myself in front of the mirror, and I noticed some lines in my skin. And my hair doesn't have the shine it used to have.

THERAPIST: So, when you check carefully in front of the mirror, you see some imperfections? Is that what you mean by "unattractive" and "losing my looks"?

PATIENT: Yeah. I don't look the way I used to look.

THERAPIST: Does that make you do anything differently?

PATIENT: I spend a lot of time with my makeup in the morning. I saw a plastic surgeon last week about getting injections in my lips and skin. Maybe I can even get a face-lift.

THERAPIST: You are doing a lot of different things that you think will help you with that feeling of being unattractive. Do you avoid anything because of these feelings about not being attractive enough?

PATIENT: Yeah. I avoid sitting under a bright light because my skin doesn't look as good. And I avoid going to parties, especially if there are lots of younger women around.

THERAPIST: What do you think would happen if you went to the party?

PATIENT: Well, if I went, I would not stand in the bright light! But I guess I'd still be concerned that I looked so much older than the other women there.

THERAPIST: As long as you don't go to the party, you can avoid feeling unattractive?

PATIENT: Yeah.

THERAPIST: When did you first think you were unattractive?

PATIENT: Oh, when I was a teenager, I wore these really goofy glasses and the kids made fun of me. I was a really homely kid.

THERAPIST: Then what happened?

PATIENT: Well, I sort of changed a bit. I filled out and the boys liked that. And then I got contacts. But I always felt like I was really ugly underneath.

THERAPIST: Did that feeling of being "ugly underneath" lead you to do anything?

PATIENT: Yeah. I haven't talked about this in a long time! I was a topless dancer for a year when I was in college. It made me feel pretty, like I had power over all these men who gawked at me and wanted me.

Homework

The therapist can ask patients to identify (1) various negative labels they apply to themselves and others, and (2) the things they do to compensate for or avoid these "problems." For example, if the patient believes "I'm really ordinary," what behaviors does he engage in to make sure that his ordinariness does not manifest itself? If the patient is worried that she is really helpless and unable to take care of herself, what strategies does she use to assure herself that others will take care of her? If the patient's schema is one of incompetence, what behaviors or challenges are avoided?

Possible Problems

Because schemas are often deeply embedded in the individual's personality—and have functioned as habitual patterns for many years—some individuals have difficulty gaining any distance from them. For example, the individual who believes that she is basically unlovable may have avoided pursuing intimacy or chosen partners who reinforced her negative schema. She may not look at her behavior as one of compensation or avoidance; she may simply look at it as logical, if unfortunate. The therapist can point this out to the patient: "You may view a lot of the negative things that happened to you as just natural. But let's at least consider the possibility that some of these things may be related to your personal schema." One useful question to ask is: "If you had a different personal schema, what choices would you have made?"

Lastly, examples of schema activation, avoidance, and compensation can be elicited in session or as homework assignments. Patients can identify triggers that activate these negative schemas: "When do you think you're likely to think [I'm inadequate, inferior, helpless]?" These triggers can then be utilized as targets for trouble times, when cognitive therapy techniques can be utilized (e.g., cost–benefit analysis, examining the evidence, using the double standard, arguing back at the thought, and acting against the thought [schema]).

Cross-Reference to Other Techniques

Other relevant techniques include vertical descent (to identify the personal schemas), identifying assumptions and conditional rules, and examining the value system.

Form

Form 7.3 (Avoiding and Compensating for My Schema, pp. 259–260).

TECHNIQUE: DEVELOPING MOTIVATION TO MODIFY THE SCHEMA

Description

Schemas are, by nature, resistant to change (Beck, 1976; Beck et al., 1990; Guidano & Liotti, 1983; Leahy, 2001b; Young, 1990), and patients typically utilize a number of mechanisms to avoid change—such as cognitive and emotional avoidance, "the protective belt" (Guidano & Liotti, 1983), compensation for the schema, and schema avoidance. In the course of modifying schemas in cognitive therapy, this resistance to change may include inability to recollect important memories, dissociation, avoiding therapy, noncompliance with homework, and challenging the therapist. Schemas are self-preserving, and attempts to modify them may not be easy. Moreover, the schema has been reinforced or confirmed by selective exposure and information processing for many years. Some patients may believe that their schemas about self and others are painful but accurate and that attempts to modify these foundational beliefs will leave them exposed and without any adaptive strategies. Other patients may believe that the process of schema modification will be a painful and unending process that will accomplish nothing useful.

The approach I advocate is to demystify this process for patients. Rather than give patients the impression that we are embarking on a long journey into the dark regions of the unconscious, thereby replicating the psychoanalytic treatment patients may fear, the cognitive therapist describes a straightforward approach in which schemas are treated like all other thoughts—that is, they can be identified and tested against reality. Schemas can be temporarily replaced by alternative beliefs, which can be tried out in the real-life contexts patients encounter.

In order to engage in this work, however, patients' motivation for changing the schema must be elicited and discussed. This stage includes providing patients with an idea about what schema work entails, examining any fears or apprehensions about accessing earlier memories, dissuading patients from the view that this is a form of watered-down psychoanalysis, and emphasizing the pragmatic and commonsense approach of cognitive therapy.

Question to Pose/Intervention

"If we work on your schemas, you will likely encounter some thoughts and behaviors that might feel uncomfortable. Just like getting over a fear of elevators means getting on the elevator and feeling uncomfortable, we will work on your schemas in a way in which you might do things and think things that will involve some discomfort. But the goal is to get past that discomfort and challenge and change the schema. Let's look at the costs and benefits to you of modifying the schema. How would your life be different? How would your relationships, work, self-confidence, and other areas be different if you were no longer so negatively affected by these schemas?"

Example

THERAPIST: It sounds like you have a schema about yourself as helpless and unable to take care of yourself. Does it concern you that you have been thinking this way?

PATIENT: Yes. I think this is the way I've been thinking since I was a kid.

THERAPIST: So it's a longstanding problem? If we were to look at how this schema affects different parts of your life, what do you think we would find?

PATIENT: It affects a lot, like my relationship with my husband. He treats me like I'm a kid, and I let him do it. I haven't learned to drive—and I'm 45 years old! I'm like a baby.

THERAPIST: What other areas of your life have been affected by the schema of helplessness and incompetence?

PATIENT: Well, I lived at home for a long time, and I took a job that wasn't really challenging. I don't do much to make myself independent.

THERAPIST: What are the costs for you of this schema?

PATIENT: I don't assert myself with my husband—or anyone. I stayed in a lousy job for 12 years. I don't do things on my own. I feel lousy about myself.

THERAPIST: Any benefits to thinking you are helpless?

PATIENT: Maybe I get my husband to do things for me.

THERAPIST: Any downside to that?

PATIENT: It makes me feel like I'm stupid and powerless.

THERAPIST: Challenging and changing your schema might involve doing things that are uncomfortable. I mean, if you had a fear of elevators, you would have to get on elevators over and over. That would be uncomfortable. So challenging your schema will be uncomfortable at times. What do you think about that?

PATIENT: I won't change overnight, I know. But what do you expect me to do?

THERAPIST: Well, we can identify the different ways your schema gets activated. We can identify the thoughts and feelings you have in this area. We can try to come up with some more rational, more adaptive ways of thinking. How would that be?

PATIENT: That sounds good.

THERAPIST: Yeah, but your schema will fight back. It'll say, "This is a bunch of lies. You know you're helpless and incompetent. Who are you kidding?" Your schema is not going to give up so easily.

PATIENT: I know. It keeps coming back to me. My mother made me feel this way. She . . .

THERAPIST: We can get into that material as well. Not that this is psychoanalysis. No. This is different. We are going to actively and energetically fight these negative beliefs. We will use all of the cognitive therapy techniques at our disposal.

PATIENT: Well, I heard that this was short-term therapy.

THERAPIST: This kind of work might require a longer period. Maybe a year, at least. It depends on you, on what you want and how motivated you feel. We can both try hard, you can learn some new skills.

PATIENT: I've been like this all my life, I guess.

THERAPIST: Maybe you've suffered enough! As I said, this therapy will ask you to do things your schema doesn't want you to do. For example, if you think of yourself as helpless, maybe you will have to do some things that are independent and uncomfortable. Maybe learn to drive?

PATIENT: Oh, I'm too old.

THERAPIST: That's the schema talking, I think. Too old? How smart are the people driving on the highway?

PATIENT: Some of them are morons.

THERAPIST: Is your schema telling you that you are less than a moron?

PATIENT: Yeah.

THERAPIST: How would you argue back at that statement? How would you tell the schema that it's wrong?

PATIENT: I guess I would have to say, "Moron? I graduated from college. I read all the time. I have done well on my job. I am no moron!"

THERAPIST: So, you have started to challenge your schema. How does it feel?

PATIENT: Pretty good.

THERAPIST: That's a beginning.

Homework

The therapist can ask patients to complete Form 7.4 (at the end of the chapter), to examine the implications of modifying their personal schemas. In addition, the therapist can ask patients how their lives would be different if they had more positive schemas: "What new relationships, experiences, feelings, and thoughts would come if you had more positive schemas about yourself and other people?"

Possible Problems

One major problem for patients is confusing schema work with psychoanalysis. Schema work can be completely subsumed within cognitive therapy (Beck et al., 1990), with no references to the unconscious or any other psychoanalytic concepts. We stress to patients that (1) work on schemas will be structured, (2) the therapist will provide self-help homework assignments, (3) sessions will have agendas, and (4) the focus will remain on actively challenging, testing, and even acting against the schemas.

Another problem that commonly arises is the feeling of hopelessness about modifying the schemas. Patients may find it unrealistic that their personalities will be modified in therapy, when they have been "this way" their entire adult lives. The therapist can respond by indicating that the goal is not to change their personalities, but rather to change the impact their schemas has on them. They will remain basically the same people. However, the schemas about being incompetent or helpless, for example, may have less of a negative impact if therapy is pursued. There are no guarantees, of course, but since patients have never tried schema-focused work, it is unlikely that they have evidence against its efficacy. We encourage patients to take an experimental attitude—that is, "Let's see if some things improve." Moreover, it is important to encourage modest expectations—for example, "This is not an all-or-nothing cure."

Cross-Reference to Other Techniques

Other relevant techniques include cost–benefit analysis, looking for variations in schema-related beliefs across situations, identifying hidden assumptions, conditional rules, vertical descent, and case conceptualization.

Form

Form 7.4 (Developing Motivation to Change My Schema, p. 261).

TECHNIQUE: Activating Early Memories That Are Schema Sources

Description

In order to gain distance from a dysfunctional schema, patients can examine the origins of the schema during childhood or adolescence. For example, the patient who currently believes that she is ugly and fat can examine where she learned this negative self-attribution. Did her siblings or peers ridicule her? Did her father or mother criticize her appearance? Were there perfectionistic preoccupations about appearance in her family? Early memories can be activated by the therapist asking directly "Who taught you this?" or "Does this label of yourself as [fat, stupid, worthless, etc.] bring back any memories from your childhood?" Alternatively, the patient can focus on a negative emotion (e.g., shame) and attempt to form an image that goes with that emotion. This emotional induction can then be used to access earlier memories: "Can you recall when you first had this feeling? Are there any images from your childhood?" As the patient accesses these memories, the therapist should elicit additional details, emotions, and thoughts. (For further examples, see Beck et al., 1990; Greenberg & Paivio, 1997; Hackmann, Clark, & McManus, 2000; Young, 1990.)

Question to Pose/Intervention

"A lot of times we can trace the source of your negative beliefs and schemas to early memories—things that you experienced as a kid. Let's try to get in touch with your schema for helplessness [or whatever]. Close you eyes and focus on the thought of being really helpless. Try to get the feeling that goes with that thought. Now try to put a picture or a scene in your mind from childhood or sometime longer ago when you had that feeling and that thought."

Example

THERAPIST: You have this thought that you are helpless. That seems to be one of your core schemas. Close your eyes and try to focus on the thought "I am really helpless. I can't do anything." Keep your eyes closed and try to get the feeling that goes with that thought.

PATIENT: (*eyes closed*) I feel like my body can't move. Like I am frozen.

THERAPIST: Can you find an image up in your mind that goes with that feeling of being frozen and helpless?

PATIENT: I remember—I must have been about 5 years old—and I was walking across the living room and I stopped and I thought, "I don't know which way to go. I need my mother to tell me."

THERAPIST: So that feeling helpless and frozen. That's the image?

PATIENT: Yeah. And I asked my mother, "Where should I go?"

The following dialogue occurred with a patient who thought he could never be good enough. His schema was that others would expect perfection from him.

THERAPIST: You identified your schema that you have to do a perfect job. Now close your eyes and concentrate on that thought "I have to be perfect" and the thought "I'm not measuring up."

PATIENT: I'll try.

THERAPIST: Focus now on "I'm not measuring up." Notice any sensations or feelings in your body.

PATIENT: I noticed my heart is racing. I'm tense.

THERAPIST: Where?

PATIENT: All over.

THERAPIST: Keep focusing on "I'm not good enough." Is there a memory or image that comes to you?

PATIENT: Yeah. My mother complaining that I got a B, when I had one B and four A's. I felt my heart sink.

Homework

The homework parallels the demonstration of this technique in session. Patients are asked to identify their various schemas (from the schema questionnaire and from prior sessions). These schemas are then listed. The task is to take three 20-minute periods in which they focus on the early memories or images that accompany each schema, recording these on Form 7.5 (at the end of the chapter), along with feelings and thoughts associated with the memory.

Possible Problems

Sometimes patients find the memories to be so painful that they begin to doubt the value of the therapy. The therapist should remind these patients that some memories and experiences in schema work are painful. However, the memories may become much less painful as therapist and patient work at reconstructing the schema and establishing new and more adaptive ways of seeing self and other. The therapist can indicate that if a memory is too painful to stay with, then it should be set aside to be discussed in session.

Recollections of schema-relevant memories may, for a short period of time, "reconfirm the schema." Recalling a mother telling her that she was not attractive reinforced the defectiveness schema for one adult woman. The therapist can explain that the first step in changing something is to find out more about it. Identifying the source of the schema does not automatically modify anything. Those techniques will be utilized in subsequent sessions.

Cross-Reference to Other Techniques

Many of the emotional processing (or experiential) exercises are relevant here, including accessing the emotion, writing a story, and identifying hot spots. In addition, the recollection of the early memory also can involve identifying and categorizing automatic thoughts, vertical descent, and guessing the thoughts.

Form

Form 7.5 (Early Memories of Schemas, p. 262).

TECHNIQUE: WRITING LETTERS TO THE SOURCE

Description

One technique that has proven to be useful in modifying the effects of traumatic or difficult experiences is to have patients engage in the assertive act of writing a letter to the source of the trauma or schema. Patients need not—and almost never do—send the letter to the source of the schema. However, rather than feel dominated and controlled by the earlier experience, patients are encouraged to write a self-affirming statement that depicts what happened, the feelings and thoughts that were generated, and how the source of the schema was wrong, malicious, or unfair.

Question to Pose/Intervention

"This person who taught you to believe these negative things about yourself—who taught you your negative schemas—is still affecting you today. You have some unfinished business here. Let's go back to your memory of what happened—the time[s] you were taught to believe these negative things. I want you to compose an assertive statement to that person. You never have to send it to anyone. But you are now going to think of yourself as strong and as someone who is defending [him- or herself]. The stance is one of 'I am not going to take it any more.' In this letter describe the memory of being taught that negative schema. Tell that person why [he or she] is wrong, how you felt, and what [he or she] should have done and should have said."

Example

THERAPIST: When you recall your father telling you that you were stupid, how does it make you feel today?

PATIENT: I have mixed feelings. Part of me is angry—but then I feel afraid. I guess I still have this feeling like he could hit me. If I get angry, he will beat me.

THERAPIST: This happened when you were a child. What do you think about the likelihood that he would hit you today?

PATIENT: He would never touch me. I'm bigger than he is! I remember telling him, when I was 15, that if he ever hit me again, I'd kill him.

THERAPIST: OK, so that fear is from the past. But it sounds like you feel he kept telling you that you were stupid. But then you feel afraid, even thinking about asserting yourself with him.

PATIENT: I guess that's still true.

THERAPIST: OK. What I'd like you to do as a homework assignment is to write a letter to him. You are not to send the letter. Just write a letter to him that recalls the lousy things he did to you, the times he called you stupid. Tell him how you felt then and how you feel now. Then tell him what that made you feel about him and why he is wrong.

PATIENT: OK. It makes me nervous, though, to think about this.

THERAPIST: Why?

PATIENT: Because whenever I stood up to him when I was a kid, he would yell at me and hit me.

THERAPIST: You're not a kid anymore.

The patient wrote out his personal letter to his father and brought it to the next session.

PATIENT: (*reading letter*) "You never gave me any credit for anything that I did. All you did was tell me that I should follow your stupid rules. You were a bully. You would tell me that I was stupid, irresponsible, careless. You were the one who was stupid. You were a terrible father. A good father would make his kid feel good about himself and teach him self-confidence. You never did that. You weren't responsible either. You were drunk when you came home, and you would yell at me and Mom. That's not responsible. There are times that I hated you. I am not stupid. I went to college, but you didn't. Maybe you couldn't stand it that your son might have a mind of his own. My friends think I'm smart, and my boss thinks I am doing a good job. Is that stupid? Maybe I should forgive you, but I can't right now. I'm just really angry."

THERAPIST: How did it feel to write this out?

PATIENT: Scary. Like I was going to get punished. But I felt better after. I got something off my chest. And it made me think that he was wrong about me.

Homework

The therapist can restate the instructions given above about writing a letter to the source of the negative schema, using Form 7.6 (at the end of the chapter).

Possible Problems

As illustrated in the case example, many patients are reluctant to write a letter to the source. They fear that they will suffer retaliation, they may fear that writing the letter will only reopen old wounds, and they may feel guilty. Some patients believe that this exercise is another attempt at "positive thinking" and that the source may be correct about the negative schema. The therapist should inquire about any reluctance or fears and address them by helping patients normalize the fears (e.g., "You were taught to believe this and not to stand up for yourself—naturally you have mixed feelings now"). In addition, the therapist can elicit the negative thoughts about assertion (e.g., "I don't have any right," "Maybe she was right," "This will make things worse"). These thoughts can be addressed by using the double-standard technique (e.g., "Who would have a right to assert themselves?"), examining the evidence against the thought (e.g., "What evidence do we have now that the schema is incorrect?" or "How could we test out this negative belief?"), and taking an empirical approach to whether it would make things worse to address the source of the schema (e.g., "Let's test your prediction that you will feel worse. What would it tell you if you did not feel worse? Is this another way that the schema protects itself from changing?").

Cross-Reference to Other Techniques

Other relevant techniques include ventilation stories, accessing the emotions and images, rewriting the story, imagery rescripting, examining the evidence for and against, case conceptualization, double standard, and rational role play.

Form

Form 7.6 (Writing a Letter to the Source of Your Schemas, p. 263).

TECHNIQUE: CHALLENGING THE SCHEMA

Description

The negative schema is like any other negative thought that can be addressed using cognitive therapy techniques. Once the schema is activated and identified, the therapist can utilize the full range of cognitive therapy techniques. These techniques include the following, as discussed in earlier chapters:

1. Distinguishing thoughts from facts
2. Rating degree of emotion and degree of belief in the thought
3. Looking for variations in a specific belief
4. Categorizing the distortion in thinking
5. Vertical descent
6. Calculating probabilities in the sequence
7. Guessing the negative thought
8. Defining the terms
9. Cost–benefit analysis
10. Examining the evidence
11. Examining the quality of the evidence
12. Defense attorney
13. Role playing both sides of the thought
14. Distinguishing behaviors from persons
15. Examining variations of behavior in various situations
16. Using behavior to solve the negative thought

Question to Pose/Intervention

"Now that we have identified your negative schema, we can utilize a lot of techniques to modify it. For example, we can use all of the cognitive therapy techniques that you use for any other thought."

Example

THERAPIST: Your negative schema seems to be that you are basically stupid and incompetent. Isn't that what your father taught you?

PATIENT: Yeah. He was always labeling me as stupid.

THERAPIST: OK. Let's look at this label of "stupid." What kinds of experiences trigger this thought for you?

PATIENT: Well, whenever I have to take an exam, I worry before that I'll fail.

THERAPIST: OK. Do you have an exam coming up?

PATIENT: Next week.

THERAPIST: What automatic thoughts do you have when you think about the exam?

PATIENT: I think "I'll really screw up. I don't know all of the material. There are things I didn't read."

THERAPIST: And if you didn't know all the material, then . . .

PATIENT: I'd fail.

THERAPIST: And what would it mean to you if you failed?

PATIENT: I'm stupid. There it is again!

THERAPIST: OK. How much do you believe, from 0% to 100%, that you are stupid when you think about the exam?

PATIENT: Maybe 75%.

THERAPIST: And what feelings and emotions go with that thought "I might fail the exam. I am stupid"?

PATIENT: Anxious. Really anxious. And, humiliated.

THERAPIST: How anxious, from 0% to 100%?

PATIENT: About 90%.

THERAPIST: OK. What is the cost of thinking that you might be stupid?

PATIENT: I'm always anxious before an exam. I walk around worrying all the time. I can't sleep.

THERAPIST: And what is the benefit of these thoughts that you are stupid and might fail?

PATIENT: Maybe I'll try harder.

THERAPIST: Is there evidence that you try harder?

PATIENT: Sometimes. But a lot of the time I procrastinate. And a few times I even dropped out of courses early on because I was afraid I wouldn't do well.

THERAPIST: So those are additional costs to this idea that you are stupid. You also said that you had this thought that you don't know everything for the course. Is "not knowing everything" evidence or a reason that you will fail?

PATIENT: Sometimes I think that.

THERAPIST: Does anyone taking this course know everything?

PATIENT: No. I know that some of the people in the class haven't done most of the reading.

THERAPIST: Your assumption, though, is "If I don't know everything, then I will fail"—kind of a perfectionistic belief, don't you think?

PATIENT: Yeah. But that's how I feel a lot of the time.

THERAPIST: I can see that. But I wonder if there is any evidence that you could do well on an exam while not know everything.

PATIENT: I've done well on lots of exams, and there are a lot of things I don't know.

THERAPIST: Let's go back to the meaning of the word *stupid*. How would you define it?

PATIENT: Not knowing things. Not doing well.

THERAPIST: What is the opposite of *stupid*?

PATIENT: *Brilliant*. Someone who just knows everything.

THERAPIST: So you just thought "I don't know everything, therefore I might fail, because I might be stupid." It sounds like you have only two points on the intelligence continuum—stupid and brilliant.

PATIENT: Yeah. That's the all-or-nothing thinking you talked about.

THERAPIST: Right. What are some points along the continuum that fall between 0% and 100% and reflect some intelligence?

PATIENT: I guess points that mean "bright enough" or "smart." Or "average." Maybe "above average."

THERAPIST: Do any of those other points apply to you?

PATIENT: It depends on the task, I guess. Maybe on some tasks I'm average. But most things I'm above average. Sometimes I'm really very smart.

THERAPIST: OK. How does what you just said reconcile with the idea that you are stupid if you don't know everything?

PATIENT: It doesn't. I don't have to know everything. No one does.

THERAPIST: If your friend John were taking the exam and he said, "I haven't read everything, so I'm going to fail," what would you tell him.

PATIENT: (*laughing*) That's stupid! No. I'd tell him that he's smart, he's done well on other exams. No one knows everything. The exam is graded on a curve, anyway.

THERAPIST: Is there some reason why you would have a different standard for yourself than for your friend John?

PATIENT: I guess I was always told that I was stupid if I didn't do perfectly.

THERAPIST: And what do you think about that kind of standard?

PATIENT: It's not fair.

THERAPIST: Is it wrong? Are you stupid?

PATIENT: No.

THERAPIST: How do you know?

PATIENT: I've done well in my classes, and my SATs were pretty high. I may not be a perfect genius, but I am *not* stupid.

Homework

The therapist can list the targeted negative schemas (e.g., ugly, incompetent, helpless) on Form 7.7 (at the end of the chapter) and ask patients to use several cognitive therapy techniques to challenge the schemas. For example, a typical homework assignment might be the following:

1. Write out five negative schemas about yourself and about how you view other people.
2. Identify situations (or people) that trigger the negative schemas.
3. Rate your degree of belief in the schema of each situation. Identify your emotions for each and rate them.
4. List the evidence for and against each negative schema.
5. Write out arguments why the schemas are not realistic.
6. Rerate your negative belief in each schema and rerate your emotions.

Possible Problems

Simply challenging a negative schema in a homework assignment is not likely to induce permanent, or even dramatic temporary, change. Some patients may say, "I know it's irrational, but I still feel that it is true." The therapist can explain the following: "Beliefs that you've held most of your life take a long time to change. Just as it takes a long time of repeating exercise to get into shape physically, it takes a long time to change your schemas. Change is not an all-or-nothing undertaking. There are degrees of change. Slight modifications in the degree of belief or in the emotions triggered can count as change. Even being more aware of the schema is a change.

Another problem that arises is that the therapist may not have identified the interventions best suited to a particular patient. Some patients get more out of some exercises (e.g., double standard) than others (e.g., examining the logic). The therapist and patient can take an experimental approach: "Let's keep trying different exercises and see which ones work best for you. Then we can really concentrate on those methods."

Cross-Reference to Other Techniques

As indicated, all of the cognitive therapy techniques discussed earlier are relevant to challenging negative schemas. In addition, The therapist and patient can make up flash cards, on which the patient writes down the most common negative thoughts on one side and the best rational responses on the opposite side. These flash cards can be read daily, especially before going into situations (e.g., tests, social interactions, making phone calls) that act as triggers for the negative schema.

Form

Form 7.7 (Challenging Personal Schemas, p. 264).

TECHNIQUE: EXAMINING YOUR LIFE USING A MORE POSITIVE SCHEMA

Description

Our life stories are often experienced as if there were only one way things could go. The individual who has the schema that he or she is inferior may view his life experiences as entirely logical and reasonable. Experiences of not pursuing more challenging and independent work or procrastinating or getting rejected all will seem schema-consistent: "Of course these things happened this way. I'm inferior. This is what happens to inferior people."

In contrast, developing an alternative perspective of one's life history—and viewing choices and events as schema maintaining—can help the individual realize how his or her schema affects outcomes. With this technique we ask patients to consider how their life choices might have been different had they used a more positive schema. For example, one patient had the schema that he was incompetent and undeserving. When he imagined applying the opposite schema—one of competence and worthiness—he realized he might have made very different choices. He might have completed his homework in college, taken more challenging work, been less risk-aversive, and pursued more desirable partners. By recognizing that his life experiences—which he uses as evidence that he is incompetent—might really be more of a function of *believing* that he is incompetent, he might consider how his future choices could be affected by developing a more positive schema.

An alternative is to consider how the self would have developed under the care of more nurturant and reliable parents. For example, the man who was physically abused by his father and told that he was stupid could consider how he would have turned out differently had his father been caring, supportive, and rewarding. The value of this exercise is the realization that there might be a potential for developing a new perspective by becoming more caring and supportive toward oneself. After all, if the negative schema was learned, then a more positive schema can replace it via new learning

Question to Pose/Intervention

"We all go through life thinking about ourselves in certain ways. But if you have a negative schema—let's say, the schema that 'I am not competent'—then you might make certain choices in school, at work, in relation to friends and partners. Then you point to those choices as evidence that your schema is true. For example, if you think of yourself as incompetent, you might procrastinate in school, pursue work that is not challenging, and give up easily. However, your schema of incompetence led you to those choices. What if you had started out with a more positive schema—let's say, "I am really smart"? Then you might have made different choices, and these different choices would have supported your more positive schema. So schemas are like self-fulfilling prophecies.

"Let's go back over various aspects of your life and examine how you would have approached them if you'd had more positive schemas. What different choices would you have made about things at school? Work? Friends? Partners? [Eating, health, exercise, drinking, drugs, money, how you live, etc.]

[Alternatively] "Let's imagine that your parents were more supportive and more caring and reliable. What if they had been really terrific parents? How would that have affected your schema? Your choices?"

Example

THERAPIST: Let's imagine that you had a more positive schema about yourself as a child. Rather than viewing yourself as stupid, you would have viewed yourself as really smart and decent. Let's go back to choices and experiences in your life that might have been affected by this more positive schema.

PATIENT: You mean, go back and think about a different life?

THERAPIST: Yes. Let's see how your negative schema affected things by looking at how your life might have been different—and still could be different in the future—with a more positive schema.

PATIENT: OK. You mean, if I had started off thinking, as a kid, that I was smart, not stupid, like my father told me?

THERAPIST: Yeah.

PATIENT: I don't know. I'd probably have studied more in school, actually done the homework. In college, I would have worked harder, maybe taken some courses that I thought were too hard for me.

THERAPIST: How about work?

PATIENT: Well, I would not have stayed in that no-win job for 6 years, that's for sure! I probably would have worked harder to get more training and advance further than I did.

THERAPIST: How about your drinking? What if you'd had a more positive schema about yourself?

PATIENT: Definitely. My drinking is all tied up in that negative stuff about being stupid and a failure. I probably would have been better at work if I hadn't been drinking as much.

THERAPIST: What if you'd had parents who were really loving and supportive? What if your father—rather than hitting you and calling you stupid—had told you that you were smart and really a terrific kid?

PATIENT: I wouldn't have been so screwed up. I certainly would have been more successful in things. I would have worked harder in school to make him proud of me.

THERAPIST: If you'd had more loving and supportive parents, then you would have a more positive schema. And if you had a more positive schema—like thinking of yourself as smart and decent—you would have made different choices.

PATIENT: Yeah, but life didn't turn out that way.

THERAPIST: Well, we can start to change that. Two things can happen. First, you can start being the good parent to yourself. That is, you can start loving and supporting and caring for yourself. And, second, you can develop a new, more positive schema—and start making choices based on this new schema.

PATIENT: That would be terrific if I could. But can I?

Homework

Patients are asked to go back to childhood and through each stage in life and examine important choices, behaviors, and relationships from the perspective of the following: "How would these things have been different if you'd had a more positive schema from the beginning?" Form 7.8 (at the end of the chapter) lists 12 life areas to help patients revision their experiences.

Possible Problems

As with any retrospective report from people who may be depressed, reflecting on the past may lead to regret and self-criticism: "I could have had a better life if I hadn't been thinking so negatively. I am such an idiot!" The therapist should caution that this exercise is not meant to encourage regret but rather to help patients recognize how powerful schemas are and how their lives can be changed by developing a new, more positive schema. The focus is on developing these new positive schemas, so that whatever mistakes were made in the past can be avoided.

Cross-Reference to Other Techniques

Other relevant techniques include identify the underlying assumptions, challenging the "should" statement, identifying conditional rules, examine the value system, using case conceptualization, developing a new adaptive assumption, and activating early memories that are the source of the schema.

Form

Form 7.8 (Life through the Lens of a Different Schema, p. 265).

TECHNIQUE: CHALLENGING THE SOURCE OF THE SCHEMA THROUGH ROLE PLAY

Description

Many individuals feel trapped by their memories of someone close hurting them in the past, and they feel helpless to reverse the effect. In this exercise patients engage in an empty-chair role play in which they challenge and argue against the source of the negative schema. The purpose here is to engage patients in dominating and defeating the credibility of the person who demoralized them at an earlier time.

Question to Pose/Intervention

"I'd like you to imagine the person who treated you so badly sitting here, in this empty chair. Imagine this person is right here, and you are going to tell [him or her] how wrong [he or she] is.

Example

THERAPIST: Remember when your mother told you that you were being selfish because you were crying and upset?

PATIENT: Yeah. She made me feel like my needs didn't matter, like I was selfish just to be alive.

THERAPIST: OK. Let's imagine that she is sitting here in this chair, and I have given you truth serum so you have to tell her exactly what you think. You can't hold anything back. Tell her why she is wrong.

PATIENT: (*Talking to empty chair*) You were being selfish, not me. A good mother should make her kid feel like she's loved. You failed me. You were too wrapped up with your own problems to pay any attention.

THERAPIST: Tell her why you are not selfish.

PATIENT: I'm not selfish at all. First of all, I took care of *you*. And I helped at home all the time. I took care of Billy [younger brother]. And then when I got married, I took care of my husband and my children. If anything, I should be more selfish.

THERAPIST: Tell her how you feel toward her.

PATIENT: I feel angry and hurt. You let me down. You hurt me.

THERAPIST: Tell her about the future—what she can't do to you.

PATIENT: You can't hurt me anymore. You can't tell me I'm selfish. I won't take it.

Homework

This in-session technique should be used in conjunction with the exercise of writing a letter to the source (see Form 7.6 at the end of the chapter).

Possible Problems

Assertive role plays in session sometimes evoke feelings of fear, defeat, and humiliation. Many individuals who have been taught their negative schemas through psychological humiliation or abuse experience considerable fear, shame, and guilt when engaged in the role play. The therapist can help patients examine how these were the very feelings experienced in learning the schema, and these are the feelings that come from the schema. Thus, to challenge and defeat the source of the schema will involve challenging any thoughts related to shame (e.g., "This happened to me because I am worthless") or fear (e.g., "I'll get punished").

Cross-Reference to Other Techniques

Other techniques that can be used include writing a letter to the source, activating memories of the source of the schema, activating the emotion, examining how life would have been different with a different schema, and examining compensation and avoidance of schema.

Form

Form 7.6 (Writing a Letter to the Source of Your Schemas, p. 263).

TECHNIQUE: DEVELOPING A MORE POSITIVE SCHEMA

Description

The goal of schema therapy is to reduce the impact of the negative schema on current functioning. This goal is ultimately accomplished by conceptualizing a new, more positive and adaptive schema. Because most individuals have more than one schema, this new adaptive schema needs to be multifaceted. The therapist can assist patients in identifying a new balanced schema and examining how this new schema might affect their choices and experiences. One tip: To make the new schema more flexible, encourage patients to use qualifiers—for example, "*Sometimes* I am really smart," "*Often* I am appealing to people."

Question to Pose/Intervention

"Let's imagine that you feel a lot better about yourself because you have a new schema. Rather than thinking of yourself as incompetent [or any other negative schema], you think of yourself as being *fairly competent*. What would be the consequence of thinking of yourself in this new way? What cognitive therapy techniques might you use to support your new schema?"

Example

THERAPIST: You think of yourself as being really stupid and irresponsible because of how your father treated you. What could be a new, more positive schema about yourself?

PATIENT: That I am smart and a really decent guy.

THERAPIST: OK. What would be the evidence that you are smart?

PATIENT: I finished college, got a master's degree, and am doing reasonably well at work. I have a high IQ.

THERAPIST: If you think of yourself as being smart, what kinds of thoughts would you have when you meet people?

PATIENT: I'd think about how they'd see that I'm on the ball.

THERAPIST: And how about work—would anything change in that context if you see yourself in these positive terms?

PATIENT: I would take on more challenging work, maybe try to advance further.

THERAPIST: How about getting your finances straightened out?

PATIENT: Yeah. I should get my credit cards paid down and start saving some money—that would definitely be smart!

Homework

Patients can examine all of their negative schemas and how they can be rephrased into positive and more adaptive schemas. For each new schema patients should use Form 7.9 (at the end of the chapter) to list all of the different decisions, opportunities, thoughts, and experiences that should be made more probable as a result of the new schema.

Possible Problems

Some patients view this as just "feel-good talk"—that it is not real and does not feel real. The therapist can explain that "trying on" a new schema requires time to feel comfortable with it. Reviewing the costs and benefits of the new schema, the evidence in support of it, and using the double-standard technique and rational role plays, when needed, to support the new schema on an ongoing basis are important. Simply repeating, "I am competent," for example, will not be sufficient. Continued practice with cognitive techniques to challenge the negative schema and the old negative thoughts will be essential.

Cross-Reference to Other Techniques

Patients can utilize many of the cognitive therapy techniques to support the new, more positive schema. For example, what positive automatic thoughts, assumptions, and behaviors follow from the positive schema? What new positive vertical descent could be utilized? How could patients act as if they believed the positive schema and engage in problem solving and planning based on it?

Form

Form 7.9 (Effects of My Positive Schema, p. 266).

FORM 7.1. Personal Belief Questionnaire

Name: _____ Date: _____

Please read the statements below and rate *how much you believe each one*. Try to judge how you feel about each statement *most of the time*.

4	3	2	1	0
I believe it totally	I believe it very much	I believe it moderately	I believe it slightly	I don't believe it at all

Example	How much do you believe it?				
1. The world is a dangerous place. (Please circle)	4 Totally	3 Very much	2 Moderately	1 Slightly	0 Not at all
1. I am socially inept and socially undesirable in work or social situations.	4	3	2	1	0
2. Other people are potentially critical, indifferent, demeaning, or rejecting.	4	3	2	1	0
3. I cannot tolerate unpleasant feelings.	4	3	2	1	0
4. If people get close to me, they will discover the "real" me and reject me.	4	3	2	1	0
5. Being exposed as inferior or inadequate will be intolerable.	4	3	2	1	0
6. I should avoid unpleasant situations at all cost.	4	3	2	1	0
7. If I feel or think something unpleasant, I should try to wipe it out or distract myself (for example, think of something else, have a drink, take a drug, or watch television).	4	3	2	1	0
8. I should avoid situations in which I attract attention, or be as inconspicuous as possible.	4	3	2	1	0
9. Unpleasant feelings will escalate and get out of control.	4	3	2	1	0
10. If others criticize me, they must be right.	4	3	2	1	0
11. It is better not to do anything than to try something that might fail.	4	3	2	1	0
12. If I don't think about a problem, I don't have to do anything about it.	4	3	2	1	0

(continued)

Personal Belief Questionnaire *(page 2 of 8)*

		Totally	Very much	Mod- erately	Slightly	Not at all
13.	Any signs of tension in a relationship indicate the relationship has gone bad; therefore, I should cut it off.	4	3	2	1	0
14.	If I ignore a problem, it will go away.	4	3	2	1	0
15.	I am needy and weak.	4	3	2	1	0
16.	I need somebody around at all times to help me to carry out what I need to do or in case something bad happens.	4	3	2	1	0
17.	My helper can be nurturant, supportive, and confident—if he or she wants to be.	4	3	2	1	0
18.	I am helpless when I'm left on my own.	4	3	2	1	0
19.	I am basically alone—unless I can attach myself to a stronger person.	4	3	2	1	0
20.	The worst possible thing would be to be abandoned.	4	3	2	1	0
21.	If I am not loved, I will always be unhappy.	4	3	2	1	0
22.	I must do nothing to offend my supporter or helper.	4	3	2	1	0
23.	I must be subservient in order to maintain his or her good will.	4	3	2	1	0
24.	I must maintain access to him or her at all times.	4	3	2	1	0
25.	I should cultivate as intimate a relationship as possible.	4	3	2	1	0
26.	I can't make decisions on my own.	4	3	2	1	0
27.	I can't cope as other people can.	4	3	2	1	0
28.	I need others to help me make decisions or tell me what to do.	4	3	2	1	0
29.	I am self-sufficient, but I do need others to help me reach my goals.	4	3	2	1	0
30.	The only way I can preserve my self-respect is by asserting myself indirectly; for example, by not carrying out instructions exactly.	4	3	2	1	0

(continued)

		Totally	Very much	Mod-erately	Slightly	Not at all
31.	I like to be attached to people but I am unwilling to pay the price of being dominated.	4	3	2	1	0
32.	Authority figures tend to be intrusive, demanding, interfering, and controlling.	4	3	2	1	0
33.	I have to resist the domination of authorities but at the same time maintain their approval and acceptance.	4	3	2	1	0
34.	Being controlled or dominated by others is intolerable.	4	3	2	1	0
35.	I have to do things my own way.	4	3	2	1	0
36.	Making deadlines, complying with demands, and conforming are direct blows to my pride and self-sufficiency.	4	3	2	1	0
37.	If I follow the rules the way people expect, it will inhibit my freedom of action.	4	3	2	1	0
38.	It is best not to express my anger directly but to show my displeasure by not conforming.	4	3	2	1	0
39.	I know what's best for me, and other people shouldn't tell me what to do.	4	3	2	1	0
40.	Rules are arbitrary and stifle me.	4	3	2	1	0
41.	Other people are often too demanding.	4	3	2	1	0
42.	If I regard people as too bossy, I have a right to disregard their demands.	4	3	2	1	0
43.	I am fully responsible for myself and others.	4	3	2	1	0
44.	I have to depend on myself to see that things get done.	4	3	2	1	0
45.	Others tend to be too casual, often irresponsible, self-indulgent, or incompetent.	4	3	2	1	0
46.	It is important to do a perfect job on everything.	4	3	2	1	0
47.	I need order, systems, and rules in order to get the job done properly.	4	3	2	1	0
48.	If I don't have systems, everything will fall apart.	4	3	2	1	0

(continued)

		Totally	Very much	Mod- erately	Slightly	Not at all
49.	Any flaw or defect of performance may lead to a catastrophe.	4	3	2	1	0
50.	It is necessary to stick to the highest standards at all times, or things will fall apart.	4	3	2	1	0
51.	I need to be in complete control of my emotions.	4	3	2	1	0
52.	People should do things my way.	4	3	2	1	0
53.	If I don't perform at the highest level, I will fail.	4	3	2	1	0
54.	Flaws, defects, or mistakes are intolerable.	4	3	2	1	0
55.	Details are extremely important.	4	3	2	1	0
56.	My way of doing things is generally the best way.	4	3	2	1	0
57.	I have to look out for myself.	4	3	2	1	0
58.	Force or cunning is the best way to get things done.	4	3	2	1	0
59.	We live in a jungle, and the strong person is the one who survives.	4	3	2	1	0
60.	People will get at me if I don't get them first.	4	3	2	1	0
61.	It is not important to keep promises or honor debts.	4	3	2	1	0
62.	Lying and cheating are OK as long as you don't get caught.	4	3	2	1	0
63.	I have been unfairly treated and am entitled to get my fair share by whatever means I can.	4	3	2	1	0
64.	Other people are weak and deserve to be taken.	4	3	2	1	0
65.	If I don't push other people, I will get pushed around.	4	3	2	1	0
66.	I should do whatever I can get away with.	4	3	2	1	0
67.	What others think of me doesn't really matter.	4	3	2	1	0
68.	If I want something, I should do whatever is necessary to get it.	4	3	2	1	0

(continued)

		Totally	Very much	Mod-erately	Slightly	Not at all
69.	I can get away with things, so I don't need to worry about bad consequences.	4	3	2	1	0
70.	If people can't take care of themselves, that's their problem.	4	3	2	1	0
71.	I am a very special person.	4	3	2	1	0
72.	Since I am so superior, I am entitled to special treatment and privileges.	4	3	2	1	0
73.	I don't have to be bound by the rules that apply to other people.	4	3	2	1	0
74.	It is very important to get recognition, praise, and admiration.	4	3	2	1	0
75.	If others don't respect my status, they should be punished.	4	3	2	1	0
76.	Other people should satisfy my needs.	4	3	2	1	0
77.	Other people should recognize how special I am.	4	3	2	1	0
78.	It's intolerable if I'm not accorded my due respect or don't get what I'm entitled to.	4	3	2	1	0
79.	Other people don't deserve the admiration or riches they get.	4	3	2	1	0
80.	People have no right to criticize me.	4	3	2	1	0
81.	No one's needs should interfere with my own.	4	3	2	1	0
82.	Since I am so talented, people should go out of their way to promote my career.	4	3	2	1	0
83.	Only people as brilliant as I am understand me.	4	3	2	1	0
84.	I have every reason to expect grand things.	4	3	2	1	0
85.	I am an interesting, exciting person.	4	3	2	1	0
86.	In order to be happy, I need other people to pay attention to me.	4	3	2	1	0
87.	Unless I entertain or impress people, I am nothing.	4	3	2	1	0
88.	If I don't keep others engaged with me, they won't like me.	4	3	2	1	0

(continued)

		Totally	Very much	Mod-erately	Slightly	Not at all
89.	The way to get what I want is to dazzle or amuse people.	4	3	2	1	0
90.	If people don't respond very positively to me, they are rotten.	4	3	2	1	0
91.	It is awful if people ignore me.	4	3	2	1	0
92.	I should be the center of attention.	4	3	2	1	0
93.	I don't have to bother to think things through—I can go by my "gut" feeling.	4	3	2	1	0
94.	If I entertain people, they will not notice my weaknesses.	4	3	2	1	0
95.	I cannot tolerate boredom.	4	3	2	1	0
96.	If I feel like doing something, I should go ahead and do it.	4	3	2	1	0
97.	People will pay attention only if I act in extreme ways.	4	3	2	1	0
98.	Feelings and intuition are much more important than rational thinking and planning.	4	3	2	1	0
99.	It doesn't matter what other people think of me.	4	3	2	1	0
100.	It is important for me to be free and independent of others.	4	3	2	1	0
101.	I enjoy doing things more by myself than with other people.	4	3	2	1	0
102.	In many situations, I am better off to be left alone.	4	3	2	1	0
103.	I am not influenced by others in what I decide to do.	4	3	2	1	0
104.	Intimate relations with other people are not important to me.	4	3	2	1	0
105.	I set my own standards and goals for myself.	4	3	2	1	0
106.	My privacy is much more important to me than closeness to people.	4	3	2	1	0
107.	What other people think doesn't matter to me.	4	3	2	1	0

(continued)

	Totally	Very much	Mod-erately	Slightly	Not at all
108. I can manage things on my own without anybody's help.	4	3	2	1	0
109. It's better to be alone than to feel "stuck" with other people.	4	3	2	1	0
110. I shouldn't confide in others.	4	3	2	1	0
111. I can use other people for my own purposes as long as I don't get involved.	4	3	2	1	0
112. Relationships are messy and interfere with freedom.	4	3	2	1	0
113. I cannot trust other people.	4	3	2	1	0
114. Other people have hidden motives.	4	3	2	1	0
115. Others will try to use me or manipulate me if I don't watch out.	4	3	2	1	0
116. I have to be on guard at all times.	4	3	2	1	0
117. Oftentimes people deliberately want to annoy me.	4	3	2	1	0
123. I will be in serious trouble if I let other people think they can get away with mistreating me.	4	3	2	1	0
124. If other people find out things about me, they will use them against me.	4	3	2	1	0
125. People often say one thing and mean something else.	4	3	2	1	0
126. A person whom I am close to could be disloyal or unfaithful.	4	3	2	1	0

(continued)

Personal Belief Questionnaire *(page 8 of 8)*

Patient Name: _____   Date on PBQ: _____

Scored by: _____   Date of scoring: _____

PBQ Scale		Raw score		Z-score	Z-scores of comparison groups	
					Patients with corresponding personality disorder	Patients with no personality disorder
Avoidant	Sum of items 1–14	= ____	(Raw score – 18.8)/10.9	= ____	.62	–.69
Dependent	Sum of items 15–28	= ____	(Raw score – 18.0)/11.8	= ____	.83	–.49
Passive–Aggressive	Sum of items 29–42	= ____	(Raw score – 19.3)/10.5	= ____	No Data	–.38
Obsessive–Compulsive	Sum of items 43–56	= ____	(Raw score – 22.7)/11.5	= ____	.31	–.51
Antisocial	Sum of items 57–70	= ____	(Raw score – 9.3)/6.8	= ____	.31	–.18
Narcissistic	Sum of items 71–84	= ____	(Raw score – 10.0)/7.6	= ____	1.10	–.38
Histrionic	Sum of items 85–98	= ____	(Raw score – 14.0)/9.3	= ____	No Data	–.29
Schizoid	Sum of items 99–112	= ____	(Raw score – 16.3)/8.6	= ____	No Data	–.14
Paranoid	Sum of items 113–126	= ____	(Raw score – 14.6)/11.3	= ____	.51	–.55

Note. Z-scores are based on a sample of 756 psychiatric outpatients with mixed diagnoses.

FORM 7.2. Guide to Understanding Schemas

What are schemas?

We have found that people differ in what gets them depressed, anxious, or angry. We refer to these differences as *schemas*. Schemas are the habitual ways in which you see things. For example, depression is characterized by schemas about loss, deprivation, and failure; anxiety is characterized by schemas about threat or fear of failure; and anger is characterized by schemas about insult, humiliation, or violation of rules. Research on personality indicates that people differ in the themes that underlie their depression, anxiety, or anger.

Each of us looks at our experiences in terms of certain habitual patterns of thinking. One person might focus a lot on issues of achievement, another on issues around rejection, and someone else on fears of being abandoned. Let's say that your schema—your particular issue or vulnerability—is related to achievement. Things can be going well for you at work, but then you have a setback that activates your schema about achievement—your issue about needing to be very successful so that you will not see yourself as a failure. The setback at work might lead to the schema about being a failure (or being "average," which is equated with failure), and then you get anxious or depressed.

Or let's say that your schema is related to issues about abandonment. You might be very vulnerable to any signs of being rejected and left alone. As long as a relationship is going well, you are not worried. But because of this schema, you might worry about being left or being rejected. If the relationship breaks up, it leads you to feel depressed because you can't stand being alone.

How We Compensate For Our Schemas

If you have a schema about a specific issue, you might try to compensate for this vulnerability. For example, if you have a schema about failure or that being average is bad, you might work excessively hard—you are trying to compensate for your perception that you might turn out to be inferior or not live up to your standards of perfection. You might compensate by checking your work over and over again. As a consequence, people might see you as *too* absorbed in your work. You might have a hard time relaxing, because you are worried that you are not working enough, that something is left undone, or that you are losing your motivation.

If your schema is about being abandoned, you might compensate for it by giving in to your partner all the time. You might be afraid of asserting yourself, because you fear being abandoned. Or you might constantly seek reassurance from your partner so that you can feel secure, but the reassurance doesn't work for very long. You keep seeing signs of your partner pulling away. Another way that you might compensate for your schema about abandonment is to form relationships with people who do not meet your needs but with whom you are willing to connect because you don't want to be alone. Or you stay in relationships far beyond a point that seems reasonable to you, because you think you can't stand being on your own.

As you can see, trying to compensate for your underlying schemas can create problems of its own. The "compensation" may lead you to sacrifice your needs, work compulsively, pursue no-win relationships, worry, demand reassurance, and other behaviors that are problematic for you. And the most important thing about these compensations is that you never really address your underlying schema. For example, you might not ever question your belief that you have to be special, superior, avoid being average, avoid being alone, etc. Therefore, you never really change your schema. It's still there—ready to be activated by certain events. It is your continual vulnerability.

(continued)

How We Avoid Facing Our Schemas

Another process that creates problems is "schema avoidance," which means that you try to avoid facing any issues that tap into your schema. Let's say that you have a schema about being a failure; your view is that deep down inside, you might really be incompetent. One way you might avoid testing out this schema is to never take on challenging tasks or to quit early on tasks. Or let's say you have a schema about being unlovable or unattractive. How do you avoid facing the schema? You might avoid socializing with people you think won't accept you. You might avoid dating. You might avoid calling friends because you already assume that people think you have nothing to offer. Or let's say that you are afraid of being abandoned. You could avoid this schema by not allowing yourself to get close to anyone, or you could break off with the person early in the relationship so that you don't get rejected later.

Another way that people avoid their schemas—whatever those schemas are—is by emotional escape through substance use or extreme behaviors such as drinking too much, using drugs to dull your feelings, binge eating, or even acting out sexually. You may feel that dealing with your thoughts and feelings is so painful that you have to avoid or escape them by these addictive behaviors. These behaviors "hide" your underlying fears from you, at least while you are bingeing or drinking or using drugs. Of course, the bad feelings come back again, because you are not really examining and challenging your underlying schemas. And, ironically, these addictive behaviors feed into your negative schemas, making you feel even worse about yourself.

Where Do Schemas Come From?

We learn these negative schemas from our parents, siblings, peers, and partners. Parents might contribute to these negative schemas by making you feel that you are not good enough unless you are superior to everyone, telling you that you are too fat or not attractive, comparing you to other children who are "doing better," telling you that you are selfish because you have needs, or intruding on you and ordering you around, or threatening to kill themselves or abandon you. There are many different ways that parents teach children these negative schemas about themselves and others.

For example, think about the following actual experiences that some people recalled about how their parents "taught" them their negative schemas:

1. "You could do better—why did you get that B?": schema about the need to be perfect or avoid inferiority.
2. "Your thighs are too fat and your nose is ugly": schema about fatness and ugliness.
3. "Your cousin went to Harvard—why can't you be more like him?": schema about inferiority and incompetence.
4. "Why are you always complaining? Can't you see that I have problems taking care of you kids?": schema about the selfishness of needs.
5. "Maybe I should just leave and let you kids take care of yourself": schema about burden and abandonment.

Another source of schemas, as we indicated, might be people other than your parents. Perhaps your brother or sister mistreated you, leading you to form schemas of being abused, unlovable, rejected, or controlled. Or perhaps your partner has told you that you are not good enough, leading to schemas of being unattractive, unworthy, and unlovable. We even internalize schemas from popular culture, such images of being thin and beautiful, having a perfect body, "what real men should be like," perfect sex, lots of money, and enormous success. These unrealistic images reinforce schemas about perfection, superiority, inadequacy, and defectiveness.

(continued)

Guide to Understanding Schemas *(page 3 of 3)*

How Will Therapy Be Helpful?

Cognitive therapy can help you in a number of important ways:

- Learn what your specific schemas are.
- Learn how you are compensating and avoiding your schemas.
- Learn how your schemas are maintained or reinforced by the choices you've made or the experiences you've had.
- Examine how your schemas were learned.
- Challenge and modify these negative schemas.
- Develop new, more adaptive, and more positive schemas.

FORM 7.3. Avoiding and Compensating for My Schema

In the form below are a number of ways people may view themselves or others. Examine the list in the left-hand column to see which of these thoughts look familiar to you. If any strike you as one of your schema, list what you did to avoid or compensate for the problem in the right-hand column. For example, a man who thought he was basically "not masculine" worked out excessively with weights and learned karate (i.e., compensation). A woman who thought she was really not that smart (i.e., incompetent) worked excessively hard in school (i.e., compensation). Another woman who thought people could not be trusted avoided dating (i.e., avoidance). Try to examine how you have handled your own personal schemas. You can even add some other examples of personal schemas in the left-hand column.

Personal schemas	Things I do to compensate or avoid
Incompetent or inept	
Helpless	
Weak	
Physically vulnerable (to sickness or injury)	
Cannot trust others	
Responsible/irresponsible	
Immoral or evil	
Cannot be controlled by others	
Tough	
Special/unique	
Need to be outstanding	
Glamorous	
Impressive	

(continued)

Avoiding and Compensating for My Schema *(page 2 of 2)*

Personal schemas	Things I do to compensate or avoid
Unconnected to others	
Unlovable	
Uninteresting	
Disorganized	
Undeserving	
Selfish	
Others are judgmental of me	
Other schemas . . .	

FORM 7.4. Developing Motivation to Change My Schema

Changing your schema will involve hard work and some discomfort at times—for example, doing things that your schema says you can't do. What are the advantages and disadvantages to you of changing your negative schemas?

Personal schemas	Advantages	Disadvantages

Form 7.5. Early Memories of Schemas

We are interested in identifying the early memories that are related to your personal schemas. In a quiet room, with no distractions, close your eyes and focus on the schema most troubling to you. Repeat your schema in your mind—for example "I am unlovable" or "I am incompetent.

to get in touch with the feelings behind that schema. Make the feelings more intense. Now, once you have the feelings and thoughts in your mind, try to recall experiences from childhood, or other times in your life, when you had these feelings and thoughts. Let yourself see the scene in detail. What was happening, what did the people look like, what were they doing? Focus on your physical sensations (e.g., tense, heart pounding, sweating, feeling cold), your emotions (e.g., angry, helpless, afraid, sad, etc.) and your thoughts in this image. When you feel "done," open your eyes and record your experience below.

Personal schema	Memory of first thinking and feeling this way	Sensations, feelings, and thoughts that go with this memory

FORM 7.6. Writing a Letter to the Source of Your Schemas

Write a letter or statement to the person (or people) who are the source of your negative beliefs about yourself and others. Be assertive and strong. Tell them why they are wrong and how you are different from the way they viewed you. Tell them that you are standing up for yourself. Tell them how they failed. In the bottom part of the form, write out any thoughts and feelings that you had while doing this exercise.

Your assertive letter or statement to the source of your negative schemas:

The thoughts and feelings I have about writing this letter:

FORM 7.7. Challenging Personal Schemas

Technique	Response
Identify personal schema	
Define your schema	
Degree of belief in schema (0%–100%)	
Emotions triggered by schema	
What situations trigger your schema?	
Cost and benefit of schema	Cost Benefit
Evidence for and against	For Against
Use the double standard technique Would you apply this to someone else?	
Why is this schema unrealistic?	
View yourself on a continuum—not in all-or-nothing terms [e.g., Rate yourself and others on a scale from 0% to 100%)	
Act against your schema (What can you do that opposes your schema?)	
Rerate belief in schema	

FORM 7.8. Life through the Lens of a Different Schema

Consider how your choices and behaviors in each of the areas listed below would have been different if you'd had a more positive schema.

Areas, choices, and behaviors	How things would have been different with a more positive schema
School	
Choice of jobs	
Performance on jobs	
Procrastination	
Friendship	
Partner/intimate relationships	
Health	
Smoking	
Drinking	
Money	
Leisure	
Where I live	
Other	

FORM 7.9. Effects of My Positive Schema

My new positive schema is that I am _____

Areas, choices, and behaviors	How it will be different in the future for me
School	
Choice of jobs	
Performance on jobs	
Procrastination	
Friendship	
Partner/intimate relationships	
Health	
Smoking	
Drinking	
Money	
Leisure	
Where I live	
Other	

CHAPTER 8

~

Emotional Processing Techniques

Although cognitive-behavioral therapy stresses the importance of cognition or thought in activating or maintaining negative moods or anxiety, there has been increasing emphasis on considering the role of emotional processing (Caspar et al., 2000; Greenberg & Paivio, 1997; Greenberg & Safran, 1987; Greenberg, Watson, & Goldman, 1998; Leahy, 2002). In this chapter we review techniques related to activation of emotion through experiential or emotion-focused therapy exercises, such as those developed by Greenberg and his colleagues. In addition, we examine how cognitive-behavioral techniques can be utilized to explore and understand how patients process and conceptualize emotion. We review the work on mindfulness (Kabat-Zinn & University of Massachusetts Medical Center/Worcester Stress Reduction Clinic, 1991; Segal et al., 2002) and on conceptualization and strategy of emotional processing (Leahy, 2002).

Greenberg's emotionally focused therapy is often viewed as an experiential approach that is somewhat different from the traditional cognitive therapy model. However, in the current context of attempting to identify and modify thoughts, I view Greenberg's work as extremely valuable. It can be used to assist patients in (1) identifying specific emotions, (2) experiencing the thoughts that are contained with the "emotional scheme" (as Greenberg uses this term), (3) identifying what they need, and (4) gaining direction in getting their needs met. Moreover, part of Greenberg's (2001) emotionally focused approach is the concept of "metaemotion"—that is, how patients view their emotions. In my own work, I borrowed from, and attempt to complement, Greenberg's important insights. In this chapter we examine various techniques that assist patients in accessing emotion, thoughts associated with emotion, and the metacognitive or metaemotional beliefs, and modifying the emotional impact through rescripting.

TECHNIQUE: ACCESSING THE EMOTION

Description

In contrast to cognitive therapy, which stresses the central role of thoughts and beliefs in the activation and maintenance of depression and anxiety, the emotionally focused approach views emotions as primary. Indeed, emotions are viewed as comprising an emotional schema that "contains" the important cognitive content examined by cognitive therapists (Greenberg, 2002a; Greenberg & Safran, 1987). Greenberg distinguishes between primary and secondary emotions, wherein the primary emotion is the basic feeling, and the secondary emotion may be the individual's more overt emotion—one that covers or defends against the primary emotion. For example, the individual may overtly express or experience anger (i.e., the secondary emotion), but the primary emotion behind the anger may be feeling hurt. It may be "easier" for a particular person to experience anger, because feeling hurt may convey a sense of weakness or failure that is intolerable. In addition, Greenberg and Safran (1987) propose that some individuals express "instrumental emotions"—that is, their emotional expression is "aimed" at evoking responses in others. For example, a patient may cry in order to make others feel guilty, but her underlying, more primary emotion is fear. In any case, the therapist should assist patients in identifying these different layers of emotions. Greenberg (2002a) suggests a number of experiential techniques that may prove useful. These include asking patients to name the emotion, notice feelings in the body, focus on, and stay with, the emotion, identify thoughts that go with the emotion, identify what information contained in the emotion, keep an "emotion log," notice interruptions or interferences with feeling the emotion, state what the emotion is saying, and state what patients need for themselves.

In the current context, emotion-focused techniques and conceptualization can be very helpful to cognitive-behavioral therapists, because activating and accessing emotional experiences assist patients in recognizing the cognitive elements that are contained in each emotional scheme. These techniques also can be useful in accessing fundamental personal schemas, which are often associated with intense emotion.

Question to Pose/Intervention

"I notice that when you talk about [identify problem area], you seem to feel something very deeply. Certain issues seem to bring up emotions for you. Let's stay with this issue. Try to focus on a situation that represents or symbolizes this issue. Close your eyes and try to feel the emotion that comes with this memory [or image]. As you focus on this emotion, try to notice any feelings in your body. Notice your breathing. Notice your physical sensations. Are you noticing any feelings? Any thoughts? Images? Does this emotion make you feel like saying something, asking for something, doing something?

"Are there any ways in which you notice yourself interrupting or interfering with the experience of this emotion? Are you finding that you drift away, try to keep yourself from having the emotion, or tell yourself you can't handle it? Focus on your internal sensations and describe them."

Example

The patient had recently gone through a break-up with a woman he had been involved with for two years.

THERAPIST: You said that you were feeling sad. Do you notice any other emotion or feeling?

PATIENT: I don't know. It's hard for me to put my finger on it.

THERAPIST: Do you notice any sensations or feelings in your body?

PATIENT: It's a feeling in my chest, like I want to cry. And my stomach—some kind of tension. And then a feeling like my heart is beginning to race.

THERAPIST: Let's stay with that feeling in your chest. Close your eyes and try to concentrate on it. What do you notice?

PATIENT: It's a feeling in my chest . . . a feeling of heaviness, and then I can feel my heart racing, and then I feel like I am going to cry. But I stop myself.

THERAPIST: So, you notice this crying might come out, and you stop it, and then what does that feel like?

PATIENT: My heart is racing.

THERAPIST: OK. If you *did* cry, what would that feel like, do you think?

PATIENT: I don't know. Like getting something out. Like letting go. But then I would feel, maybe I would lose control. I would look like I lost control.

THERAPIST: And then what would happen?

PATIENT: You might think less of me.

THERAPIST: So, if you cried, I would think less of you. That's how you feel. And if you cried, what would happen to that racing heartbeat?

PATIENT: I don't know. I try not to think about it.

THERAPIST: OK. Let's go back to the feeling in your chest and this feeling that you are going to cry. Can you focus on this feeling now? Can you let that feeling happen?

PATIENT: (*beginning to cry*) I just don't know. I feel so terrible. Excuse me.

THERAPIST: OK. That's the way you are feeling at this moment. And can you tell me, with this feeling, are there any thoughts that go with the crying?

PATIENT: I feel like saying, "I can't stand being alone." It's always going to be this way.

THERAPIST: In that feeling is the fear that you will always be alone. And when you are crying, if you were to ask for something, what would it be?

PATIENT: "Please come back."

THERAPIST: So you want her to come back?

PATIENT: Yes. I know it wasn't good, but I can't stand this loneliness.

THERAPIST: And your racing heartbeat?

PATIENT: I feel ashamed. I want to hide.

THERAPIST: Why do you want to hide?

PATIENT: Because I seem so pathetic.

THERAPIST: So you are feeling that it is pathetic to be sad and to cry?

PATIENT: Yes.

THERAPIST: Let's go back to this sadness, this feeling in your chest, and the feeling of wanting to cry. Close you eyes and concentrate on that feeling of sadness. Let's imagine a blank screen, and now a picture drifts onto that screen. Your sadness puts that picture on the screen. What image comes up on the screen?

PATIENT: I see myself in my room, bent over. It's dark. I'm alone (*crying*).

THERAPIST: And what are you feeling in that room all alone?

PATIENT: I'll always be alone—like my heart is breaking.

Homework

Greenberg (2002a) suggests that patients use an emotion log (see Form 8.1 at the end of the chapter) to record any feelings during the coming week. The therapist can explain the following: "It's important for both of us to find out about the feelings you are having. These are the emotions that are so important to you. They can be emotions of any kind—sad, happy, afraid, curious—anything. I'd like you to try to notice these emotions during the week and record them in your emotion log. We can use this log later to see the range of feelings you are experiencing. I also would like you to write down any examples during the week when you begin to notice an emotion but then try to block it from happening. Maybe you might notice that you are feeling anxious, and you try to make it go away or maybe you distract yourself. Perhaps you notice some sadness or you feel like crying and you try to block it. Try to notice if you are trying to block some of these feelings. Write down any examples."

Possible Problems

Some patients who pursue cognitive therapy have the misconception that this therapy is antiemotional. They think the goal is to feel and behave in entirely rational ways. The therapist can explain that the role of rationality is only to help patients handle emotions more productively. The goal is not to eliminate emotions. Furthermore, the therapist can stress that emotions are like hunger and pain—they teach us what we need. Emotions contain thoughts, and focusing on the emotion is like opening up a file cabinet with a wealth of important information. Other patients may fear that gaining access to their emotions will lead to a flood of negative feelings that will engulf them. These beliefs about accessing emotions can be important when we discuss emotional schemas—that is, how individuals conceptualize their emotions and respond to their emotions once they are accessed.

Cross-Reference to Other Techniques

Other relevant techniques include explaining how thoughts create feelings, distinguishing thoughts from facts, rating degree of emotion and belief in the thought, identifying hot spots, identifying emotional schemas, and enhancing emotional processing.

Form

Form 8.1 (Emotion Log, p. 281).

TECHNIQUE: WRITTEN VENTILATION

Description

Pennebaker and his colleagues proposed that expressing emotion by freely writing down recollections of traumatic or troubling events may have a palliative effect on anxiety, depression, and physical well-being (Pennebaker, 1993; Pennebaker & Beall, 1986). In the free expression of emotion—that is, *ventilation*—patients recall a troubling event and write down a detailed description of it, paying close attention to the emotions that surface and the meaning of the event. Although the immediate effect may be an increase in negative feelings as the negative event and the memories become more salient, there is often a decrease in negativity and a reduction in stress within days or weeks.

Question to Pose/Intervention

"I'd like you to think back about this event that bothered you so much. Try to get a very clear recollection of the event and the experience you had. I'd like you to take about 20 minutes and write down all of your thoughts and feelings about that event. What was it like for you? It would be helpful to give as many details as possible. Try to make your recollection feel as real as possible."

Example

The patient was a woman in her thirties who recalled being sexually abused as a child by a friend of her brother.

THERAPIST: You described how this older kid sexually abused you when you were a kid. It might be hard to go back and describe that experience, but let's try to find out more together about what that was like for you. I know it must have been very hard and will be very hard now thinking about it.

PATIENT: It was terrible.

THERAPIST: OK. What we will do is look back at that experience. Get the details and your feelings about it. You can write this down as your memory comes back; describe all of the details and feelings. Write out any thoughts that you remember having then.

The patient returned to the next session with the homework assignment completed.

THERAPIST: Let's look at what you wrote and see what it felt like and what you thought. Could you read to me the story that you wrote?

PATIENT: (*reading*) He was my brother's friend. I was 13 and he was 17. His name was Ken and he was bigger than me and my brother looked up to him. My parents were away for the day. My brother had gone downstairs to the den to be with his girlfriend, and Ken was upstairs with me, joking around. He told me he had a knife, then he showed me the knife, and I felt afraid. He took me into the bedroom and told me that we were going to play a game. I was afraid to say anything because I thought he was crazy. Then he began kissing me. I told him to stop, but he said that he was going to play the game whether I liked it or not. Then he showed me the knife again and said I'd better do what he said. Then he said, "You'll like it anyway." I was terrified. But I did what he told me to do. He made me suck him. I felt like throwing up. But I was completely aware of what was happening. When it was over, I put my clothes on, and he told me that if I told anyone, he would kill me. I never told my brother or my parents. I felt afraid and then I felt ashamed.

THERAPIST: Which part of this memory bothers you the most in reading it?

PATIENT: The part where I thought he threatened to kill me if I told.

THERAPIST: You read it to me and you are sitting here in my office how do you feel about it now?

PATIENT: I guess I feel nervous. But I also feel safer. I told the story, and nothing is going to happen to me now. It was a long time ago.

THERAPIST: Have you ever told the whole story before?

PATIENT: No. I just wanted to forget it, and I didn't think it would do any good—just make me more anxious. And I felt ashamed, anyway.

THERAPIST: How do you feel now?

PATIENT: Well, I don't really feel ashamed telling you. You're a professional. But I wonder how my husband would feel. He might judge me. So I feel that part of me needs to keep this to myself, because someone else might not understand.

Homework

The therapist can say the following:

"It's important to be able to recall some memories that were painful and hurt you, because they may still linger on for you. Getting that memory out by writing it down and then telling the story can help us understand what the experience meant to you and what it felt like. We can also use the memory in some new ways in therapy—ways in which you will feel more in control later and that can help you understand things and move beyond the past. Right now, though, it may be painful to recall some of these things, but that pain may be the beginning of a much better process for you.

"I'd like you to think back about this event that bothered you so much. Try to get a very clear recollection of the event and the experience you had. Now I'd like you to take about 20 minutes to write down all of your thoughts and feelings about that event. What was it like for you? Please provide as many details as possible. Try to make the recollection feel as real as possible."

Possible Problems

The therapist should be cautious to avoid retraumatizing patients by having them recall traumatic memories without guidance. It is recommended that patients describe the event in session prior to writing down the longer story. If the recollection during the session is too upsetting—for example, the patient seems overwhelmed by the story—the therapist can help him or her gain some distance by using relaxation techniques prior to telling the story. The therapist also can interrupt the storytelling to initiate anxiety management through deep breathing, muscle relaxation, attentional distraction, etc. Moreover, the therapist can remind the overwhelmed patient that the office is safe and the therapist is the patient's ally; the therapist can even ask the patient to identify all the reasons why he or she is safe today in this office, telling the story, how the abusive individual or terrible experience is not going to appear or happen today.

Some patients believe accessing their emotions and reliving the trauma will set them back even further. This is a meta-emotional belief: "If I have a bad feeling, it will never go away." The therapist can identify this belief and examine how it operates to inhibit full emotional processing. For example, the belief that a negative emotion must be avoided, at all costs, contributes to the inability to fully reexperience the memory, discover that it can be tolerated, and learn that reality is different from the original traumatizing experience. Attempts to block the memory (as indicated in the upcoming discussion of "hot spots") include racing through the story, leaving out details at crucial moments, not reporting feelings associated with an apparently traumatic event, dissociating in the session, or displaying inappropriate affect (e.g., laughing or responding in a rote or bland fashion).

Cross-Reference to Other Techniques

As indicated above, the therapist can provide reassurance, have patients identify evidence of current safety, utilize breathing and muscle relaxation techniques, and elicit elements of the story in session prior to the written ventilation assignment. Other techniques that suitably follow the ventilation assignment include vertical descent, identifying schemas, safety behaviors, writing letters to the source of the schema, and imagery rescripting.

Form

Form 8.2 (Writing a Story, p. 282).

TECHNIQUE: IDENTIFYING "HOT SPOTS"

Description

The patient may get "stuck" in certain parts of the image or memory. These "hot spots" may elicit either strong emotions (e.g., tearfulness, anxiety, fear) or inhibition of emotion (e.g., dissociation, mechanical responses). As patients recalls the image or story, the therapist should attend to any strong shifts in emotion and ask patients to repeat that specific image or part of the story. These hot spots often entail the emotional schemas that contain the most problematic automatic thoughts (see Cason, Resick, & Weaver, 2002; Grey, Holmes, & Brewin, 2001).

Question to Pose/Intervention

"As you recall the story [or form the image], try to notice if any specific details or parts of the story are especially difficult for you. Notice if there is any change in your emotion or feeling; you might become more upset with a specific image or detail. Or you might find yourself "spacing out" at a specific detail, perhaps because it is too difficult to pay attention to it. As you repeat that detail or image, ask yourself what about it is especially upsetting. What thoughts does this detail generate? What feelings?"

Example

THERAPIST: I noticed that as you read the story about your mother hitting you that you sort of spaced out. You seemed to have no emotion at the part where she began to yell at you.

PATIENT: Really? I didn't even notice that.

THERAPIST: OK. Let's go back. Read that part again, the part where she is yelling at you.

PATIENT: (*reading from her story*) "Then she began to yell at me, 'You're stupid. I never should have had you'" (*visibly nervous now*).

THERAPIST: What feelings did you have then?

PATIENT: I felt afraid . . . and ashamed.

THERAPIST: Tell me about the feelings of being afraid and ashamed.

PATIENT: I felt that I was nothing, and she was going to stomp me into the ground. And I felt like I was pretty worthless, worth nothing, actually.

THERAPIST: That part was hard to take, so you spaced out rather than feel what was happening.

PATIENT: Right. It's hard to recall it even now.

Homework

The therapist can ask patients to write down a memory of a traumatic or upsetting event with as much detail as possible. Then patients should read the story aloud several times, noting specific parts are most upsetting. They go back over these more upsetting parts and write down any feelings and thoughts that go with these hot spots. Form 8.3 (at the end of the chapter) can be used.

Possible Problems

Hot spots are, by their very nature, difficult to handle. Patients may become so upset that they refuse to do the homework. In these cases, it may be more useful to have patients schedule longer (double) sessions, in which these more difficult memories can be accessed and the hot spots identified. Furthermore, because dissociation is, by its nature, difficult for the dissociater to notice, the therapist should have patients repeat the story in the session, while the therapist looks for any signs of emotional avoidance (e.g., mechanical/rote reading of the story, reading certain parts very rapidly, or spacing out and drifting).

Cross-Reference to Other Techniques

Other techniques that can be useful include written ventilation, identifying emotional schemas, imagery rescripting, identifying automatic thoughts, and looking at the trauma from the balcony.

Form

Form 8.3 (Identifying Hot Spots, p. 283).

TECHNIQUE: IDENTIFYING EMOTIONAL SCHEMAS

Description

Individuals differ as to their conceptualizations of, and strategies for dealing with, emotions (Leahy, 2002). Once an "unpleasant" emotion (e.g., sadness, anger, or anxiety) has been activated, the individual may respond with a variety of thoughts or behaviors. For example, some individuals, noticing that they feel anxious, may respond with the following problematic ideas about their anxiety: It will have a long duration, they have no control over this emotion, others would not have the same feelings (low consensus), they feel ashamed or guilty about feeling the anxiety, and they do not accept the emotion. Moreover, these individuals may then believe that they cannot allow themselves to experience this emotion, cannot express it because others would not understand or validate them; they should be entirely rational and certainly not have mixed feelings. I have developed the Leahy Emotional Schemas Scale (LESS; Leahy, 2002) that can be used to identify these various emotional schemas. Many of these dimensions are related to depression, anxiety, and different personality disorders (Leahy 2000; 2002).

Question to Pose/Intervention

"When we feel anxious, sad, angry, or confused, we may have different thoughts about experiencing these feelings. For example, some people may believe that these feelings will last a long time, whereas others believe they are temporary. Some people believe that they should not have certain feelings, whereas others accept these feelings. We can find out how you think, react, and feel about your emotions and feelings by having you complete this form [LESS]."

Example

THERAPIST: I noticed that you get upset about being anxious. When you notice that you are breathing rapidly and your heart is pounding, you seem to get upset about these sensations.

PATIENT: Yes. I think that I'm losing control.

THERAPIST: OK. So you are thinking "When I have these feelings, I will lose control." What do you do to avoid losing control?

PATIENT: I try to hold my breath, and then I try to take deep breaths.

THERAPIST: Is it possible that holding your breath and then taking deep breaths can make you hyperventilate? Can it make you short of breath?

PATIENT: I don't know. Can it?

THERAPIST: Well, we can test it out later. But let's go back to your emotions. You said that it upsets you to feel anxious. What else is going through your mind about these feelings?

PATIENT: Well, I don't think I should feel this way. I'm intelligent and rational, and I have a lot going for me.

THERAPIST: Do you believe you should be rational and logical and not emotional?

PATIENT: Yeah, I guess so—not like a robot, though but not this emotional.

THERAPIST: And when you feel this way, what other thoughts do you have?

PATIENT: It doesn't make sense. There's nothing really bad happening. I mean, I'm in a relationship, and I am doing well at work. I shouldn't be so emotional.

THERAPIST: So these emotions don't make sense to you. And how do you feel talking about them?

PATIENT: I don't think anyone could understand. People see me as always on top of things. They'd be surprised. I guess they might think I am really screwed up.

THERAPIST: So your thoughts about these feelings are that you have to get rid of them immediately, and then you either hold your breath or take really deep breaths. Then you think that you should be rational and logical, that people see you this way, and that your emotions don't make sense, since nothing really bad is happening. It sounds like you feel that people would think less of you, so you are sort of ashamed and you think no one could understand.

Homework

The therapist should have *patients* complete the Leahy Emotional Schemas Scale (Form 8.4, at the end of the chapter). See the section above (Questions to Pose) for instructions regarding this homework assignment. The LESS has fourteen dimensions regarding thoughts and feelings about emotion (see Form 8.5). The patient's responses to the LESS can be the focus of further inquiry.

Possible Problems

Some patients may have difficulty reflecting on how they think about and handle their emotions. This difficulty is often evident in patients who utilize emotional avoidance as a coping strategy. Patients who are actively alcoholic, using cocaine, marijuana, or binge eating on a regular basis may be so out of touch with their emotions that they cannot identify thoughts about, and responses to, these emotions. The LESS scale can be used with these patients in the session. For example, the therapist might say, "When you come home to your apartment and first walk in the door, what feeling do you have?" For one patient, who binged and abused alcohol, her first thoughts were "This is so empty, my life is so empty." The therapist could then go through some of the items on the LESS scale to identify her beliefs that she had to get rid of her feelings, that these feelings would overwhelm her, and that no one could ever understand her.

Furthermore, patients may have different emotional schemas for different kinds of emotions. The same individual may have different emotional schemas for anxiety than for sexual feelings. For example, one patient believed that her anxiety about taking a test would not last forever, that other people might have the same kinds of feelings, and they would understand hers. In contrast, her belief about her sexual fantasies was that she should be in control of her feelings, that these feelings could go out of control, they were shameful, and people would think less of her if she shared them. She then blamed others for these feelings. Thus the therapist can explore if the patient has different "theories" or "strategies" for dealing with different emotions.

Cross-Reference to Other Techniques

As we will see in the section below on enhancing emotional processing, the cognitive therapist can utilize a wide range of techniques to examine each dimension of the emotional schemas. This range can include eliciting or accessing the emotion, examining the costs and benefits of certain strategies, evidence for and against these beliefs, the double-standard technique, carrying out experiments (e.g., to see if others will reject them for their emotions), vertical descent, examining the relationship between emotional schemas and personal schemas, identifying the source of beliefs about emotions, role playing, etc.

Forms

Form 8.4 (Leahy Emotional Schemas Scale, pp. 284–285); Form 8.5 (Fourteen Dimensions of the Leahy Emotional Schemas Scale, pp. 286–287).

TECHNIQUE: ENHANCING EMOTIONAL PROCESSING

Description

As indicated above, each dimension of the emotional schemas model is relevant to how emotions are processed. The metaemotional or metacognitive model of emotional processing proposes that conceptualizations of, and strategies for responding to, activated emotions will affect the maintenance of depression, anxiety, or anger (Leahy, 2000). In this section, I provide suggestions on how these emotional dimensions can be utilized. Specific examples for each of these are provided in Form 8.6 (at the end of the chapter). For example, the individual who believes that he or she cannot accept his or her emotions can examine what would happen if he or she did "accept" these emotions (e.g., "If I accept my emotions, I will never get rid of them"). Negative attitudes toward accepting emotions may reflect beliefs that emotions are shameful, out of control, intolerable, or will escalate if allowed. Beliefs about the necessity of suppressing emotion may add further strength to the intrusive nature of these emotions (Purdon, 1999; Purdon & Clark, 1993).

Question to Pose/Intervention

Utilizing some of the questions outlined in Form 8.6, the therapist can ask patients the following kinds of questions:

"Are there some people who accept and understand your feelings?" (Validation)
"Do the emotions make sense to you? What could be some good reasons why you are sad, anxious, and angry" (Comprehensibility)

"What are the reasons that you think your emotions are not legitimate?" (Comprehensibility)
"Why shouldn't you have the feelings that you have?" (Shame, Guilt)

Other questions can be based on the different emotional schemas.

Example

THERAPIST: You said that you felt ashamed of your sexual feelings for Mike. What makes you feel ashamed of these feelings?

PATIENT: I'm married to Larry. A good wife doesn't have these kinds of feelings.

THERAPIST: Your thought is "I can't be a good wife and have fantasies about other men"? When you have these feelings for Mike, what do you do with them?

PATIENT: I try to tell myself that I shouldn't have these feelings—I shouldn't think about them. But then it just makes me nervous, and I can't get him out of my mind. I know he wouldn't be right for me anyway. I'm afraid if I let myself go with this fantasy, I would just act on it. But, I don't know—I probably would never do that.

THERAPIST: OK. So you feel guilty and ashamed and then you try to stop having these feelings, but they get stronger. What would happen if you just simply acknowledged that you had these feelings and didn't try to suppress them?

PATIENT: Maybe they'd get stronger?

THERAPIST: Do you think that married people fantasize about other people? Or do you think of yourself as the only one?

PATIENT: Oh, I'm sure almost everyone fantasizes.

THERAPIST: Is there a difference between having a fantasy and acting on it? Aren't your thoughts different from your behavior?

PATIENT: Of course. Right. I would never do anything. It's just a fantasy.

THERAPIST: It sounds like you think you should have only one set of feelings—feelings of fidelity, 100% of the time. What would it mean if you had doubts or fantasies?

PATIENT: Part of me thinks it means I'm a bad person, but another part makes me think—well, it's human.

THERAPIST: If you thought of these feelings as another way of being human, what would happen?

PATIENT: I might feel a lot less guilty—and maybe I wouldn't fantasize as much.

Homework

Utilizing Form 8.6, the therapist can have patients examine some of the dimensions of emotional processing and respond, in writing, to each of the questions provided.

Possible Problems

As indicated, some patients enter cognitive therapy expecting to emphasize rationality as a solution to all problems, and discussing their emotions may seem counterproductive to them, simply another version of dynamic therapy. The therapist can explain that the purpose in examining their emotions is to help them manage those emotions by thinking about them differently—indeed, that this *is* a cognitive approach to emotion. Making sense of emotion, allowing emotion, decatastrophizing emotion, and feeling less guilty about an emotion are all part of a cognitive approach to emotional processing.

Cross-Reference to Other Techniques

Many of the techniques used to challenge automatic thoughts and modify dysfunctional assumptions are relevant in evaluating emotional schemas. These include examining the costs and benefits, evidence, double standard, vertical descent, role play, and behavioral experiments.

Form

Form 8.6 (Emotional Schemas: Dimensions and Interventions, pp. 288–290).

TECHNIQUE: IMAGERY RESCRIPTING

Description

Traumatic experiences may persist in memory for years, resulting in posttraumatic stress disorder (PTSD). Attempts to modify traumatic images by relying solely on verbal disputation may not adequately activate the fear structure and may not provide the patient with a powerful enough counter to the thoughts and feelings contained in the image. Imagery rescripting allows patients to recreate their story, in dramatic detail, in a way that changes the nature of the original traumatic event. For example, the patient who recalls being beaten by his father as a child can rescript the image so that the father is small, weak, and foolish, and the patient is strong, aggressive, and hostile toward the father. The imagery rescripting activates a stronger, more competent emotional component of the self that counters the defeated and victimized weaker self. Valuable descriptions of this technique, and variations on it, can be found in the work of Resick, Smucker and Dancu (Resick, 2001; Smucker & Dancu, 1999). Imagery rescripting is especially helpful for individuals who have been abused.

Question to Pose/Intervention

"When you have these terrible images and memories, you feel defeated and attacked. Let's go back and change the image and the story. This time I want you to imagine that you are strong, tall, aggressive, and angry. Your [abuser] is weak, small, and stupid. I want you to imagine yourself dominating and criticizing and punishing your [abuser]. Tell him [or her] how stupid and awful he [or she] is. Tell him [or her] that you are a much better person."

Example

THERAPIST: You said that your father used to beat you and lock you in the basement. What did that feel like for you?

PATIENT: I felt like I was a piece of shit. I felt weak, like no one cared about me, and I couldn't do anything. I was just beaten.

THERAPIST: I wonder how you feel right now, as we are talking about this?

PATIENT: Scared. Like it could happen again.

THERAPIST: OK. So as you described it [earlier], he would come home drunk, and start screaming, and then he'd hit you, over and over.

PATIENT: Yes, there was no escaping him.

THERAPIST: OK. Let's imagine that he is really really small, about 2 feet high, and that he has this little tiny high-pitched voice. And let's imagine that you are really big and strong and ferocious. I'd like you to clench your fists, as if you were going to punch someone. Let's imagine you are towering over him.

PATIENT: (*clenching her fists*) I can see him as this little midget with this squeaky voice, screaming at me that I am not doing what I'm supposed to be doing.

THERAPIST: OK. Now let me hear you tell him off. Tell him you're in charge.

PATIENT: (*talking loudly down to the imaginary father*) You can't tell me what to do, you little piece of crap! You are *nothing* compared to me.

THERAPIST: Tell him why he's nothing compared to you.

PATIENT: You're just a drunk and a failure and a lousy father. I went to college—no thanks to you—and I raised a kid and I earn a living and I'm a decent person. And you are nobody!

THERAPIST: Tell him what you will do if he hits you again.

PATIENT: I'll kill you. I'll stomp on you until you are nothing. I'll throw you out of the goddamn window!

Homework

The therapist can ask patients to recall a former experience of abuse or humiliation and to write down the details of the traumatic experience. This reality-based recounting is followed by a new fantasy script. In this rescripted story, patients are instructed to describe themselves as strong, confident, aggressive, and confrontational. The patients dominate the scene, reducing their abuser or humiliator to a piddling annoyance. Afterward, patients can write down their thoughts and feelings about doing this exercise.

Possible Problems

Some patients become even more anxious when they confront their feared abuser in the rescripted version. Magical thoughts such as "The abuser will come back and hurt me" or "If I am assertive, I'll be punished" are not uncommon. The therapist should be aware of patients' hesitancy in utilizing this rescripting technique. Any signs of increased anxiety, dissociation, responding in a rote and mechanical way, or the sudden desire to terminate therapy should be addressed. The therapist can ask about the automatic thoughts, perhaps supplying the sentence stem: "If I stand up to the abuser in this image, I become afraid because I think . . . " This kind of automatic thoughts and assumptions often reflect the sense of powerlessness, shame, and humiliation that accompanied the abuse. Standard cognitive therapy techniques can be utilized to challenge these negative thoughts about self-esteem or assertion. For example, one patient noticed that she had thoughts "I deserved the abuse," "If I stand up to them, they will kill me," and "Passivity will protect me." These fearful thoughts were then examined through cost–benefit analysis, rational role play, double standard, and empty-chair techniques.

Cross-Reference to Other Techniques

Imagery induction, schema work (identifying core schemas, schema avoidance, schema maintenance), case conceptualization, feared fantasy, assertion, writing letters to the source, and double-standard techniques are helpful.

Form

Form 8.7 (Rescripting the Story, p. 291).

FORM 8.1. Emotion Log

Type of Emotion	Monday	Tuesday	Wednesday	Thursday	Friday	Saturday	Sunday
Happy							
Interested							
Excited							
Caring							
Affection							
Love							
Loved							
Compassion							
Grateful							
Proud							
Confident							
Hurt							
Sad							
Regret							
Irritated							
Angry							
Resentful							
Disgust							
Contempt							
Ashamed							
Guilty							
Envious							
Jealous							
Anxious							
Afraid							
Other							

FORM 8.2. Writing a Story

Describe your memory of your story in as much detail as you can:

What feelings or emotions did you experience in this story?

What thoughts do you have looking back at this story?

What parts of this story—what memories—were the most painful? Why?

How do you feel after writing down this story?

FORM 8.3. Identifying Hot Spots

Describe the story or image in as much detail as you can.	Which specific parts of this story are most upsetting? These are the hot spots.	What feelings and thoughts do you have at these hot spots?

FORM 8.4. Leahy Emotional Schemas Scale

We are interested in how you deal with your feelings or emotions—for example, how you deal with feelings of anger, sadness, anxiety, or sexual feelings. We all differ in how we deal with these feelings, so there are no right or wrong answers. Please read each sentence carefully and rate it, using the scale below, as to how you've dealt with your feelings during the past month. Put the number of your response next to the sentence.

Scale:
1 = very untrue of me
2 = somewhat untrue of me
3 = slightly untrue of me
4 = slightly true of me
5 = somewhat true of me
6 = very true of me

1. ____ When I feel down, I try to think about a different way to view things.
2. ____ When I have a feeling that bothers me, I try to think of why it is not important.
3. ____ I often think that I respond with feelings that others would not have.
4. ____ Some feelings are wrong to have.
5. ____ There are things about myself that I just don't understand.
6. ____ I believe that it is important to let myself cry in order to get my feelings "out."
7. ____ If I let myself have some of these feelings, I fear I will lose control.
8. ____ Others understand and accept my feelings.
9. ____ You can't allow yourself to have certain kinds of feelings—like feelings about sex or violence.
10. ____ My feelings don't make sense to me.
11. ____ If other people changed, I would feel a lot better.
12. ____ I think I have feelings that I am not really aware of.
13. ____ I sometimes fear that if I allowed myself to have a strong feeling, it would not go away.
14. ____ I feel ashamed of my feelings.
15. ____ Things that bother other people don't bother me.
16. ____ No one really cares about my feelings.
17. ____ It is important for me to be reasonable and practical rather than sensitive and open to my feelings.
18. ____ I can't stand it when I have contradictory feelings—like liking and disliking the same person.
19. ____ I am much more sensitive than other people.
20. ____ I try to get rid of an unpleasant feeling immediately.
21. ____ When I feel down, I try to think of the more important things in life—what I value.
22. ____ When I feel down or sad, I question my values.
23. ____ I feel that I can express my feelings openly.

(continued)

24. _____ I often say to myself, "What's wrong with me?"

25. _____ I think of myself as a shallow person.

26. _____ I want people to believe that I am different from the way I truly feel.

27. _____ I worry that I won't be able to control my feelings.

28. _____ You have to guard against having certain feelings.

29. _____ Strong feelings only last a short period of time.

30. _____ You can't rely on your feelings to tell you what is good for you.

31. _____ I shouldn't have some of the feelings I have.

32. _____ I often feel numb emotionally, like I have no feelings.

33. _____ I think that my feelings are strange or weird.

34. _____ Other people cause me to have unpleasant feelings.

35. _____ When I have conflicting feelings about someone, I get upset or confused.

36. _____ When I have a feeling that bothers me, I try to think of something else to think about or do.

37. _____ When I feel down, I sit by myself and think a lot about how bad I feel.

38. _____ I like being absolutely definite about the way I feel about *someone else*.

39. _____ Everyone has feelings like mine.

40. _____ I accept my feelings.

41. _____ I think that I have the same feelings other people have.

42. _____ I aspire to higher values.

43. _____ I think that my feelings now have *nothing* to do with how I was brought up.

44. _____ I worry that if I have certain feelings, I might go crazy.

45. _____ My feelings seem to come from out of nowhere.

46. _____ I think it is important to be rational and logical in almost everything.

47. _____ I like being absolutely definite about the way I feel about *myself*.

48. _____ I focus a lot on my feelings or my physical sensations.

49. _____ I don't want anyone to know about some of my feelings.

50. _____ I don't want to admit to having certain feelings, but I know that I have them.

FORM 8.5. Fourteen Dimensions of the Leahy Emotional Schemas Scale

Validation

Item 8.	Others understand and accept my feelings.
(Item 16.)	No one really cares about my feelings.
(Item 49.)	I don't want anyone to know about some of my feelings.

Comprehensibility

(Item 5.)	There are things about myself that I just don't understand.
(Item 10.)	My feelings don't make sense to me.
(Item 33.)	I think my feelings are strange or weird.
(Item 45.)	My feelings seem to come from out of nowhere.

Guilt

Item 4.	Some feelings are wrong to have.
Item 14.	I feel ashamed of my feelings.
Item 26.	I want people to believe that I am different from the way I truly feel.
Item 31.	I shouldn't have some of the feelings I have.

Simplistic View of Emotion

Item 18.	I can't stand it when I have contradictory feelings—like liking and disliking the same person.
Item 35.	When I have conflicting feelings about someone, I get upset or confused.
Item 38.	I like being absolutely definite about the way I feel about *someone else*.
Item 47.	I like being absolutely definite about the way I feel about *myself*.

Higher Values

Item 21.	When I feel down, I try to think of the more important things in life—what I value.
(Item 25.)	I think of myself as a shallow person.
Item 42.	I aspire to higher values.

Control

(Item 7.)	If I let myself have some of these feelings, I fear I will lose control.
(Item 27.)	I worry that I won't be able to control my feelings.
(Item 44.)	I worry that if I have certain feelings, I might go crazy.

Numbness

Item 15.	Things that bother other people don't bother me.
Item 32.	I often feel numb emotionally, like I have no feelings.

(continued)

Rational

Item 17.	It is important for me to be reasonable and practical rather than sensitive and open to my feelings.
Item 46.	I think it is important to be rational and logical in almost everything.
Item 30.	You can't rely on your feelings to tell you what is good for you.

Duration

Item 13.	I sometimes fear that if I allowed myself to have a strong feeling, it would not go away.
(Item 29.)	Strong feelings only last a short period of time.

Consensus

(Item 3.)	I often think that I respond with feelings that others would not have.
(Item 19.)	I am much more sensitive than other people.
Item 39.	Everyone has feelings like mine.
Item 41.	I think that I have the same feelings other people have.

Acceptance of Feelings

(Item 2.)	When I have a feeling that bothers me, I try to think of why it is not important.
(Item 12.)	I think I have feelings that I am not really aware of.
(Item 20.)	I try to get rid of an unpleasant feeling immediately.
Item 40.	I accept my feelings.
(Item 50.)	I don't want to admit to having certain feelings, but I know that I have them.
(Item 9.)	You can't allow yourself to have certain kinds of feelings—like feelings about sex or violence.
(Item 28.)	You have to guard against having certain feelings.

Rumination

(Item 1.)	When I feel down, I try to think about a different way to view things.
(Item 36.)	When I have a feeling that bothers me, I try to think of something else to think about or do.
Item 37.	When I feel down, I sit by myself and think a lot about how bad I feel.
Item 24.	I often say to myself, "What's wrong with me?"
Item 48.	I focus a lot on my feelings or my physical sensations.

Expression

Item 6.	I believe that it is important to let myself cry in order to get my feelings "out."
Item 23.	I feel that I can express my feelings openly.

Blame

Item 11.	If other people changed, I would feel a lot better.
Item 34.	Other people cause me to have unpleasant feelings.

FORM 8.6. Emotional Schemas: Dimensions and Interventions

Validation

Are there some people who accept and understand your feelings? Do you have arbitrary rules for validation? Do people have to agree with everything you say? Are you sharing your emotions with people who are critical? Do you accept and support other people who have these emotions? Do you have a double standard? Why?

Comprehensibility

Do the emotions make sense to you? What could be some good reasons why you are sad, anxious, and angry, etc? What are you thinking (what images do you have) when you are sad, etc. What situations trigger these feelings? If someone else experienced this event, what kinds of different feelings might they have? If you think your feelings don't make sense right now, what does this make you think? Are you afraid that you are going crazy, losing control? Are there things that happened to you as a child that might account for why you feel this way?

Guilt and Shame

Why do you think your emotions are not legitimate? Why shouldn't you have the feelings that you have? What are some reasons that your feelings make sense? Is it possible that others could have the same feelings in this situation? Can you see that having a feeling (e.g., anger) is not the same as acting on it (e.g., being hostile)? Why are certain emotions good and others bad? If someone else had this feeling, would you think less of him? How do you know if an emotion is bad? What if you looked at feelings and emotions as signs telling you that something is bothering you—like a caution sign, a stop sign, or a flashing red light? Is anyone harmed by your emotions?

Simplicity versus Complexity

Do you think that having mixed feelings is normal or abnormal? What does it mean to have mixed feelings about someone? People are complicated, so why wouldn't you have different, even conflicting, feelings? What is the disadvantage of demanding that you have only one feeling?

Relationship to Higher Values

Sometimes we feel sad, anxious, or angry because we are missing something that is important to us. Let's say you feel sad about a relationship breakup. Doesn't this mean that you have a higher value that's important to you—for example, a value of closeness and intimacy? Doesn't this value say something good about you? If you aspire to higher values, doesn't this mean that you will have to be disappointed at times? Would you want to be a cynic who values nothing? Are there other people who share your higher values? What advice would you give them, if they were going through what you are going through?

Controllable

Do you think that you have to control your feelings and get rid of the "negative" ones? What do you think would happen if you couldn't get rid of that feeling entirely? Is it possible that trying to get rid of a feeling completely makes that feeling too important to you? Are you afraid that having a strong feeling is a sign of something worse? Going crazy? Losing complete control? Isn't there a difference between controlling your actions and controlling your feelings?

(continued)

Numbness

Are there situations that trigger "spacing out"? No feelings? Are there situations that bother most people but don't bother you? Do people think that you are blunted in your feeling? Unfeeling? What kinds of strong feelings do you have? Do you ever notice having a strong feeling and then try not to have it? Do you ever have the feeling that you are going to cry, but you stop it? What do you fear would happen if you let go and let yourself have those feelings? What kinds of thoughts do you have when you experience strong feelings? Do you ever drink or use drugs or binge on food to get rid of those strong feelings?

Rationality, Antiemotional

Do you think you should always be logical and rational? What would you be concerned about if you were not rational/logical? Do you think that people who are rational or logical are "better" people? What happened in the past when you weren't logical/rational? Is it possible that some experiences are not logical/rational but simply emotional? Is there such a thing as a rational painting? A rational song? Can your emotions tell you about what hurts you? What needs to be changed? Are emotions an important source of information about our needs, desires, and even our rights as human beings? Do you know other people who are less rational than you, but who have a happier or fuller life?

Duration of Strong Feelings

Do you have fears that a strong feeling will last too long? Have you had strong feelings before? What happened? Did they end? Why did they end? Do strong feelings go up and down? If you had a strong feeling in our session, what do you think would happen? If you cried or felt really bad for few minutes, what do you think would happen? What would you gain by finding out that your strong feelings can be expressed and then go away?

Consensus with Others

Exactly what feelings do you have that you think other people don't have? If someone else had these feelings, what would you think of them? Why do you think very emotional plays or movies, novels, or stories appeal to people? Do you think that people like to find out that other people have the same feelings? Are there other people who are sad, angry, or anxious? Is it normal to be upset, have fantasies, etc? If you are ashamed of your feelings and don't tell people, might this keep you from finding out that others have the same feelings?

Acceptance or Inhibition

What will happen if you allow yourself to accept an emotion? Will you act on it? Do you fear that if you accept an emotion, it won't go away? Or do you think that *not* accepting your emotions will motivate you to change? What are the negative consequences of inhibiting a feeling? Excessive use of attention and energy? Rebound effect? Does the emotion conflict with a belief about good versus bad feelings? If you deny that something bothers you, how can you fix the problem?

Rumination versus Instrumental Style

What are the advantages and disadvantages to focusing on how bad you feel? When you are focusing on how bad you feel, what kinds of things are you thinking and feeling? Do you sit and think "What's wrong with me?" or "Why is this happening to me?" Do you focus on sadness, replaying in your mind the same things over and over? Do you sometimes think that if you keep thinking about it, you will come up with a solution? Does your worrying make you feel that you can't control your stressful thoughts? Try setting aside 30 minutes each day, during which time you will worry intensely. You have

(continued)

to set aside all your worries until that time. Rephrase your worries into behaviors that you can carry out, problems that you can solve. Distract yourself by taking action or calling a friend and talking about something other than your worries. Exactly what do you predict will happen? Have your predictions ever proved to be false? When you are ruminating, you are chewing things over. Is there some "truth" or "reality" that you just refuse to accept?

Expression

If you expressed a feeling, do you think you would lose control? Feel worse? How long would you feel worse? Can expressing a feeling help you clarify your thoughts and other feelings? Conversely, if you only focus on expressing a feeling, will you overfocus on it? Will you become self-absorbed? Are there things that you could do to distract yourself or solve your problems?

Blaming Others

What did other people say or do that made you feel the way you do? What thoughts did you have that made you feel sad, angry, anxious, etc? If you thought about this situation differently, what would you feel or think? Are your feelings dependent on what others think of you? Are you focused on getting approval, respect, appreciation, or fairness? What would be the advantage and disadvantage of not needing approval, etc? What rewards does the other person currently control? Can you have rewarding experiences despite what that person said, did, etc.? Is it possible that your feelings are a combination of what is happening to you and what you are thinking? What would you like to feel—angry, sad, curious, indifferent, accepting, challenged? What are the costs and benefits of these different feelings? Given the situation, what would you need to think in order to have each of these feelings? What would you like to have happen? How can you be more assertive? Solve problems? What thoughts would you have to change?

FORM 8.7. Rescripting the Story

When you initially experienced a trauma or stressful event, you may have viewed the other person as superior or more powerful. In the left-hand column, write down a detailed description of what happened: what the other person looked like, sounded like, said, did, etc. In the right-hand column rewrite, or rescript, this entire story. This time you are more powerful, and the other person is weak and scared. You are bigger, the other person is smaller. You are loud, he or she is quiet. You are active, aggressive, and hostile, and the other person is afraid of you. Rewrite this story in a way that is going to make you the more powerful and dominant one. Then write down your thoughts and feelings about doing this exercise.

Description of original traumatic or stressful event	Rescripting the story: describing the event from a new perspective
What thoughts and feelings did you have about the other person and yourself when this happened?	What thoughts and feelings do you have now?

CHAPTER 9

——

Examining and Challenging
Cognitive Distortions

A key view of cognitive therapy is that depression, anxiety, and anger are often the result of recurring patterns of cognitive distortions. In this chapter, I provide a brief checklist of the most common cognitive distortions and some useful interventions or questions that can be utilized to examine and challenge these distorted beliefs. Of course, many of the other techniques discussed in this book can be used for cognitive distortions. This chapter is intended to serve as a convenient reference source for techniques, questions, or interventions that can be quickly applied to modify negative beliefs. (*Note*: Technique lists that follow are worded as if the therapist were addressing the patient.)

1. *Mind reading: You assume that you know what people think without having sufficient evidence of their thoughts—for example, "He thinks I'm a loser."*

Techniques
   1. Rate the degree of your belief and identify and rate your emotions.
   2. Identify exactly what your prediction is—for example, "He doesn't like me, so he won't talk to me."
   3. Let's conduct a cost–benefit analysis:
       a. Do you think that mind reading gives you valuable information?
       b. Will mind reading help you prevent being taken by surprise or will it prevent something bad from happening?
       c. How would your thoughts, feelings, and behavior change if you did less mind reading?
   4. Examine evidence for and against your mind reading.
   5. What is the quality of the evidence that supports your mind reading?
   6. What cognitive distortions are you using to support your belief? Are you personalizing, fortune telling, labeling, discounting positives, using a negative filter?

7. How could you prove that your thought is wrong? Is it testable?

8. Let's do a vertical descent exercise: What if your thought were true—why would it bother you? If people are thinking what you think that are thinking, does this mean something about you (e.g., "I'm undesirable" or "I'm foolish") or something about them (e.g., "They're mean")?

9. Let's challenge your need for approval: What if someone doesn't like you? Exactly what will happen? What things will remain the same?

   a. What does it make you think if someone doesn't agree with you or approve of you? Does this disagreement or disapproval mean that you are less worthwhile? Is the other person less worthwhile? Why or why not?

   b. List all of the things you can still do even if the person doesn't like you.

   c. No one gets approval from everyone. Why should disapproval bother you?

   d. What would happen if you accepted the fact that someone might not approve of you? What would be the costs and benefits to you?

10. Practice repeating the following statement 20 minutes each day: "No matter what I do, some people won't like me." What happens to the thought? Does it become boring?

11. Act against your thought. Do something positive toward the person you think doesn't like you.

2. *Fortune telling: You predict the future in negative terms involving failure or danger—for example, "I'll fail that exam" or "I won't get the job."*

Techniques

1. Rate the degree of your belief and identify and rate your emotions.

2. Identify exactly what your prediction is—exactly what will happen and when and where it will happen.

3. Let's conduct a cost–benefit analysis:

   a. Do you think that worry protects and prepares you?

   b. Do you fear that you can't control your worries?

4. Examine evidence for and against your fortune telling.

5. What is the quality of the evidence that supports your fortune telling?

6. What cognitive distortions are you using to support your belief?

7. How could you prove that your thought is wrong? Is it testable?

8. Let's do a vertical descent exercise: What if your thought were true—why would it bother you?

9. Practice repeating the following statement 20 minutes each day: "No matter what I do, it's always possible something bad could happen to me."

10. How many times have you made incorrect predictions?

11. What is your worst feared outcome—your feared fantasy?

    a. What is the worst, best, and most likely outcome?

    b. Write down a detailed description of your worst feared outcome.

    c. List all the things that would have to go wrong for this outcome to happen.

    d. List all the things that might prevent this outcome from happening.

    e. Practice repeating the image and story of the worst outcome for 20 minutes each day.

12. Describe in detail three positive outcomes. Write down detailed stories about how these positive outcomes could occur.

3. *Catastrophizing: You believe that what has happened, or will happen, will be so awful and unbearable that you won't be able to stand it—for example, "It would be terrible if I failed."*

Techniques
1. Rate the degree of your belief and identify and rate your emotions.
2. Identify exactly what your prediction is—exactly what will happen and when and where will it happen?
3. Let's conduct a cost–benefit analysis:
   a. Do you think that worry protects and prepares you?
   b. Do you fear that you can't control your worries?
4. Examine evidence for and against your catastrophizing thinking.
5. What is the quality of the evidence that supports your catastrophizing thinking?
6. What cognitive distortions are you using to support your belief? Are you fortune telling, discounting positives, using "should" statements, using negative filters?
7. How could you prove that your thought is wrong? Is it testable?
8. Let's do a vertical descent exercise: What if your thought were true—why would it bother you? Exactly what would happen?
9. Practice repeating the following statement 20 minutes each day: "No matter what I do, it's always possible that something absolutely terrible could happen to me."
10. How many times have you made incorrect predictions?
11. Exactly what would make this event terrible and awful?
12. How would you feel about this event a month later, a year later, 2 years later?
13. Are there people to whom this catastrophe has happened but who have gone on to experience positive things in their lives? How did they manage to go beyond the negative event to positive experiences?
14. Even if this catastrophe happened to you, what positive things could you still experience?
15. Would other people think that what is happening or has happened is terrible and awful? Why would they see it differently from the way you see it?
16. Even if this "terrible" thing happened, could something positive come out of it? Could it lead you to learn something? Open up new opportunities? Motivate you to reexamine your values?

4. *Labeling: You assign global negative traits to yourself and others—for example, "I'm undesirable" or "He's a rotten person."*

Techniques
1. Rate the degree of your belief and identify and rate your emotions.
2. Identify exactly what you predict about your own (or another person's) behavior.
3. How would you define [the label]? For example, how would you define *worthless* or *stupid*? What is the opposite of [the label]? For example, what is the opposite of "worthless person"? How would you define the opposite? How would we know it if we saw it?
4. Let's conduct a cost–benefit analysis:
   a. Do you think that labeling yourself will motivate you?
   b. Do you think that labeling yourself is being realistic?
   c. If you didn't label yourself, how would your thoughts, feelings, and behavior change?
5. Examine evidence for and against your negative label.

6. What is the quality of the evidence that supports this belief that you are [rotten, undesirable, etc.]?

7. What cognitive distortions are you using to support your belief? Are you thinking in all-or-nothing terms, discounting positives, using "should" statements, using a judgment focus, applying negative filters?

8. How could you prove that your thought is wrong? Is it testable?

9. Rather than focus on labeling the whole person, think about some different behaviors—positive, negative, and neutral—that you see in this person.

10. Describe the situations in which this person displays a positive and a negative behavior. Is there any pattern?

11. How was this person seeing the situation? Did he or she have a different point of view, a different need, different information?

12. Using the double-standard question, ask yourself, "Would everyone label this person in such a negative way? Why not?"

5. *Discounting positives: You claim that the positive things you or others do are trivial—for example, "That's what wives are supposed to do, so it doesn't count when she's nice to me" or "Those successes were easy, so they don't matter."*

Techniques

1. Rate the degree of your belief and identify and rate your emotions.

2. Identify exactly what you are discounting.

3. Let's conduct a cost–benefit analysis:
   a. Do you think that being strict and demanding will motivate you or others?
   b. Do you think you're being "moral" or "standing up for what's right"? Where did you get this rule?
   c. If you didn't discount the positives, how would your thinking, feeling, and behavior change?

4. Examine evidence for and against discounting positives.

5. What is the quality of the evidence that supports discounting positives?

6. What cognitive distortions are you using to support your belief? Are you using dichotomous thinking, negative filters, labeling, "should" statements, a judgment focus?

7. Are you using all of the information available or limiting your search to information that supports your belief? What is the consequence of this way of thinking?

8. Let's try a double-standard exercise: Would everyone see it this way? Why not?

9. What is your underlying assumption? Complete this sentence: "These things don't count because . . . "

10. What if we made your view that these things don't count a universal one for everyone? What would be the consequence?

11. Let's try another double-standard exercise: If you really loved someone or cared about him or her, would you count these positives? Why? What would be a reason not to count them here?

12. Try positive tracking: Keep track of your positives (or the other person's positives) every day for a week. What does this record tell you?

13. Try to reward positives: Every time you or someone else does something positive, praise yourself or the person. Will this praise increase or decrease the positive behavior?

6. Negative filtering: You focus almost exclusively on the negatives and seldom notice the positives—for example, "Look at all of the people who don't like me."

Techniques

1. List all of your negative filter statements.
2. What are the costs and benefits of filtering everything through negatives?
3. Are you not looking at all of the information? Is there some information that you are ignoring? Why?
4. Exactly what would happen, or what would it mean to you, if you did count this positive information?
5. Apply the double-standard technique: Would everyone see things this negatively? Why not?
6. What is your underlying assumption? Complete this sentence: "These things don't count because . . . "?
7. What if we made your view that these things don't count a universal one for everyone? What would be the consequence?
8. Apply another double standard: If you really loved someone or cared about him or her, would you count these positives? Why? What would be a reason not to count them here?
9. Try positive tracking: Keep track of your positives (or the other person's positives) every day for a week. What does this record tell you?
10. Try to reward positives: Every time you or someone else does something positive, praise yourself or the person. Will this praise increase or decrease the positive behavior?

7. Overgeneralizing: You perceive a global pattern of negatives on the basis of a single incident—for example, "This generally happens to me. I seem to fail at a lot of things."

Techniques

1. Rate the degree of your belief and identify and rate your emotions.
2. Identify exactly what you predict about your own (or another person's) behavior.
3. Let's conduct a cost–benefit analysis:
   a. Do you think that overgeneralizing will motivate you?
   b. Do you think that overgeneralizing is being realistic?
   c. How would your thoughts, behavior, and feelings change if you didn't overgeneralize?
4. Examine evidence for and against your overgeneralizing.
5. What is the quality of the evidence that supports your belief of "This is always happening"?
6. What cognitive distortions are you using to support your belief? Are you using negative filters, labeling, discounting positives?
7. How could you prove that your thought is wrong? Is it testable?
8. Are there situations when this [behavior, outcome, emotion, etc.] is not happening? How would you describe these situations?
9. Apply the double-standard exercise: Would everyone see things this way? Why not?
10. Try positive tracking: Keep track of your positives (or the other person's positives) every day for a week. What does this record tell you?
11. Try to reward positives: Every time you or someone else does a positive, praise yourself or the person. Will this praise increase or decrease the positive behavior?
12. Try mindfulness rather than judging. Focus only on describing what has happened without using any words of judgments. Avoid using words such as *always* and *never*—for example, "He's always like that" or "I'm never going to succeed." Focus only on behavior that you can

observe—for example, "He was driving fast"—and on how you felt—"I felt nervous." Stay in the present moment. How does this feel?

13. Imagine you are looking down from a balcony on what is happening, and you must describe what you see to a stranger. Exactly what would you say is being said and done?

8. *Dichotomous thinking: You view events or people in all-or-nothing terms—for example, "I get rejected by everyone" or "It was a complete waste of time."*

Techniques

1. Rate the degree of your belief and identify and rate your emotions.
2. Identify exactly what you predict about your own (or another person's) behavior.
3. Let's conduct a cost–benefit analysis:
   a. Do you think that viewing yourself in all-or-nothing terms will motivate you?
   b. Do you think that dichotomous thinking is being realistic?
   c. How would your thinking, behavior, and feelings change if you were less dichotomous in your thinking?
4. Examine evidence for and against your dichotomous thinking. Are there exceptions to your all-or-nothing thinking?
5. What is the quality of the evidence that supports your belief that things are "all-or-nothing"?
6. What cognitive distortions are you using to support your belief? Are you discounting positives, using negative filters, labeling?
7. How could you prove that your thought is wrong? Is it testable?
8. What if you looked at things along a *continuum* from 0% to 100%? Fill in each 10-point increment with a behavior.
9. What are some behaviors that are worse, better, or the same as this behavior?
10. Are there situations or times when this is not happening? How would you describe these situations or times?
11. Apply the double-standard technique: Would everyone see it this way? Why not?
12. Try the positive tracking: Keep track of your positives (or the other person's positives) every day for a week. What does this record tell you?
13. Try to reward positives: Every time you or someone else does a positive, praise yourself or the person. Will this praise increase or decrease the positive behavior?

9. *"Shoulds": You interpret events in terms of how things should be, rather than simply focusing on what is—for example, "I should do well. If I don't, then I'm a failure."*

Techniques

1. Rate the degree of your belief and identify and rate your emotions.
2. Identify exactly what your "should" rule is—for example, "I should be perfect" or "I should get everyone's approval."
3. Let's conduct a cost–benefit analysis:
   a. Do you think that being strict and demanding will motivate you or others?
   b. Do you think you're being "moral" or "standing up for what's right"?
   c. How would your thinking, behavior, and feelings change if you were less "should" oriented?

4. Examine evidence for and against your "should" rule. Are there people who do not have this "should" rule? What do you think of them?

5. What cognitive distortions are you using to support your belief? Are you using labeling, discounting positives, dichotomous thinking, overgeneralizing?

6. Do you label yourself in all-or-nothing terms when you don't live up to your rigid rules? What is the consequence of this labeling?

7. Double-standard technique: Would everyone see it this way? Why not? If people are not using your "should" rules, how are they looking at these things?

8. What if we made it a universal rule that everyone follow your "should" rule? What would be the consequence?

9. Morality should advance human dignity. Do your "should" rules treat people in a humane and dignified way? Or are they aimed at condemning and criticizing people?

10. Does your "should" rule come from any religious, moral, or legal beliefs? Specify exactly where you learned this "should" rule. Is this current version perhaps a misperception of what was originally taught or written?

11. Apply another double-standard: If you really loved someone or cared about him or her, would you apply this "should" rule to him or her? Why? Is there some reason why you would use this rule for some people but not for others?

12. What if you replaced your "should" rule with the statement that you might *prefer* something to be true? What if you were less extreme in your statement? For example, rather than saying "I should be perfect," you were to say "I'd prefer doing well"? Try restating all of your "should" rules in terms of less extreme preferences. How does this feel?

13. What are the costs and benefits of this new preference that is less extreme?

14. List a range of preferences (in relation to your "should" rule) from 0% to 100%. What do most people think is sufficient or adequate?

15. Try mindfulness rather than judging: Focus only on describing what has happened, without using any words of judgments and without using any "shoulds." Avoid using words such as *always* and *never*—for example, "He's always like that" or "I'm never going to succeed." Focus only on behavior that you can observe—for example, "He was driving fast"—and on how you felt—"I felt nervous." Stay in the present moment. How does this feel?

16. How will staying in the present moment change this moment? What will happen an hour from now, a day from now, a week from now?

17. Imagine you are looking down from a balcony on what is happening, and you must describe what you see to a stranger. Exactly what would you say is being said and done?

10. ***Personalizing: You attribute a disproportionate amount of the blame for negative events to yourself, and you fail to see that certain events are also caused by others—for example, "The marriage ended because I failed."***

Techniques

1. Rate the degree of your belief and identify and rate your emotions.

2. Identify exactly what your statement or thought is—for example, "This is entirely my fault."

3. Let's conduct a cost–benefit analysis:

    a. Do you think that taking it personally motivates you to try harder, or does it protect you in some way?

    b. Do you think that personalizing this event/situation is "realistic"?

    c. What thoughts, feelings, and behaviors would change if you personalized your experience less?

4. Examine evidence for and against your personalizing statement.

5. What is the quality of the evidence that supports your belief?

6. What cognitive distortions are you using to support your belief? Are you overgeneralizing, mind reading, discounting positives, using negative filters, labeling, catastrophizing, or using "should" statements?

7. How could you prove that your thought is wrong? Is it testable?

8. Use the pie-chart technique. Distribute the possible causes for this event, using a pie metaphor. To what degree was the outcome due to causes other than yourself or the other person?

9. What variations do you see in this behavior? Are you (or they) always this way? What would you conclude if there is variation?

10. What were your intentions? The other person's intentions? Are you certain your belief about their intentions is correct? How could you know?

11. Distinguish between self-*criticism* and self-*correction*. What behavior could you improve? What could you learn? What could you do differently in the future?

12. Rather than personalizing and blaming, what if you were to ask what problems needed to be solved? For example, if you are going through a breakup in a relationship, rather than blame yourself or the other person, why not ask yourself what practical problems you need to solve right now? What would be the consequences of this new way of thinking?

11. Blaming: You focus on the other person as the source of your negative feelings, and you refuse to take responsibility for changing yourself—for example, "She's to blame for the way I feel now" or "My parents caused all my problems."

Techniques

1. Rate the degree of your belief and identify and rate your emotions.

2. Identify exactly what your statement or thought is—for example, "This is entirely [his or her] fault."

3. Let's conduct a cost–benefit analysis:
    a. Do you think that blaming others will motivate them to try harder?
    b. Does blaming them protect you in some way?
    c. Do you think that blaming others is "realistic"?
    d. What thoughts, feelings, and behaviors would change if you blamed others less?

4. Examine evidence for and against your blaming statement.

5. What is the quality of the evidence that supports your belief that others are at fault?

6. What cognitive distortions are you using to support your belief? Are you overgeneralizing, mind reading, personalizing, discounting positives, using negative filters, labeling, catastrophizing, or using "should" statements?

7. If you look at their behavior along a continuum, is it really as bad as it seems to you?

8. Even if this person did this negative thing, what are some rewarding behaviors that you can still experience?

9. How could you prove that your thought (i.e., "They are entirely to blame") is wrong? Is it testable?

10. Use the pie-chart technique. Distribute the possible causes for this event, using a pie meta-

phor. To what degree are the causes of the event due to things about you, others, or the situation?

11. What variations do you see in their behavior? Do they always behave this way?

12. What were your intentions? Are you sure about your belief regarding their intentions? How could you know their intentions?

13. What information were they using? What information did you have?

14. Distinguish between criticizing others and requesting a change in their behavior. What behavior could they improve? What could you all learn? What could you and they do differently in the future?

15. Do you label people in all-or-nothing terms when they don't live up to your rigid rules? What is the consequence of this labeling?

16. Apply the double-standard exercise: Would everyone see it this way? Why not?

17. What if we made your belief a universal rule for everyone: that is, everyone should be blamed severely for this behavior. What would be the consequence?

18. Morality should advance human dignity. Does your "should" rule treat people in a humane and dignified way? Or are they aimed at condemning and criticizing people?

19. Does your "should" rule come from any religious, moral, or legal beliefs? Specify exactly where you learned this rule. Is this rule possibly a misperception of what was taught or written?

20. Apply another double-standard exercise: If you really loved someone or cared about him or her, would you apply this "should" rule to them? Why? Is there some reason why you would use this rule for some people but not for others?

21. What if you replaced your "should" rule with the statement that you might *prefer* something to be true? What if you were less extreme in your statement? For example, what if, rather than saying "I should be perfect," you were to say "I'd prefer doing well"? Try restating all of your "should" rules in terms of less extreme preferences.

22. What are the costs and benefits of this new preference that is less extreme?

23. List a range of preferences, from 0% to 100%. What do most people think is sufficient or adequate in regard to the behavior we are discussing?

12. *Unfair comparisons: You interpret events in terms of unrealistic standards—you focus primarily on others who do better than you and find yourself inferior in the comparison—for example, "She's more successful than I am" or "I'm a complete failure because others did better than I did on the test."*

Techniques

1. Rate the degree of your belief and identify and rate your emotions.

2. Identify exactly what standard you use for your own (or another person's) behavior.

3. Let's conduct a cost–benefit analysis:

   a. Do you think that viewing yourself in extreme terms will motivate you?

   b. Do you think that using extreme standards is being realistic?

   c. Do you fear "compromising" your standards? What would that mean? What would happen if you did compromise?

   d. Are you "proud" of your high standards—even if you criticize yourself when you don't live up to them?

   e. What thoughts, feelings, and behaviors would change if you used less extreme standards?

4. Examine evidence for and against your use of extreme standards. Do these standards really motivate you? Do you avoid certain things because of these standards? Are they really realistic?

5. What is the quality of the evidence that things should be viewed in such extreme ways? Are these extreme standards common in our society?

6. What cognitive distortions are you using to support your belief? Are you discounting positives, using negative filters, labeling, or using perfectionistic "should" statements?

7. What if you looked at things along a continuum, from 0% to 100%? Fill in each 10-point increment with a behavior. How would you describe these behaviors that come between 0% and 100%?

8. Where does the average person place on this continuum? Are you using the full range of human behavior? For example, the average IQ is 100, the average family income is $40,000. Is there some reason why you would not use the average as a baseline for your standards?

9. What are some behaviors that are worse, better, or the same as this behavior?

10. Specifically, what does it mean if someone does not "live up to the standard"? Exactly what will happen?

11. Are there some people who have not lived up to the standard at times? Exactly what has happened to them?

12. Apply the double-standard technique: Would everyone see things this way? Would everyone use these standards? Why not?

13. Try positive tracking: Keep track of your positives (or the other person's positives) every day for a week. What does this record tell you?

14. Try to reward positives: Every time you or someone else does something positive, praise yourself or the other person. Will this praise increase or decrease their positive behavior?

13. *Regret orientation: You focus on the idea that you could have done better in the past—for example, "I could have had a better job if I had tried" or "I shouldn't have said that"—rather than paying attention to what you could do better now. You believe that you should have known something in the past that would have prevented a bad outcome, but you really were not in a position to know for sure—for example, "I should have known that the stock market was going to collapse" or "I should have known that [he or she] would not be trustworthy."*

Techniques

1. Rate the degree of your belief and identify and rate your emotions.

2. Identify exactly what your regret is. For example, complete the following sentence: "I should have known that [X] was true."

3. Let's conduct a cost–benefit analysis:
   a. Do you think that regretting the past motivates you to be more careful in the future?
   b. Do you think that regretting things is realistic?
   c. What thoughts, behaviors, and feelings would change if you regretted things less?

4. Examine evidence for and against your regrets.

5. What is the quality of the evidence in support of your regrets?

6. Why should you have known before [X] happened? Should you know everything? Should you be able to read people's minds? Foretell the future? Never make mistakes? What is the consequence of this way of thinking?

7. What evidence was available to you? What seemed to be the most important thing at the time?
8. Is it possible you made a good decision, given the information available at the time?
9. What cognitive distortions are you using to support your belief? Are you personalizing, discounting positives, mind reading, labeling?
10. How could you prove your thought is wrong? Is it testable?
11. Apply vertical descent: What if your thought were true? Why would it bother you? Do you think this means that you can't make good decisions, that you should be overly cautious, never take risks, blame yourself if things don't work out, never trust anyone?
12. Do you conclude that since you didn't make the best decision, you are stupid, incompetent, or bad at making decisions?
13. Have you made there other good decisions? What do you conclude from these successes in decision making?
14. Apply the double-standard exercise: How would most people see this situation? Would they think you should regret it? Take all the blame?
15. Rather than criticize yourself, try self-correction. What could you learn from this experience? What could you do differently in the future?
16. Even though this decision did not work out, what are some positives that came from it? What are some positive things that you could do now or in the future?

14. *What if?*: You keep asking a series of questions about "what if" something happens, and you fail to be satisfied with any of the answers—for example, "Yeah, but what if I get anxious?" or "What if I can't catch my breath?"

Techniques
1. Rate the degree of your belief and identify and rate your emotions.
2. Identify exactly what your prediction is.
3. Let's conduct a cost–benefit analysis:
   a. Do you think that worry protects and prepares you?
   b. Do you fear that you can't control your worries?
   c. Do you think that you need a solution for every possible problem?
   d. How would your thoughts, feelings, and behaviors change if you were not using "what if" thoughts as much?
4. What cognitive distortions are you using to support your what if thinking? (Fortune-telling, mind-reading, emotional reasoning, etc.)
5. Are you trying to make things absolutely certain? Is it possible to have certainty in an uncertain world?
6. Apply vertical descent: What if your thought were true? Why would it bother you?
7. Do you think that things are dangerous unless you can make sure they are completely safe? What are the costs and benefits of this belief?
8. Do you think that coming up with ideas based on "what if something goes wrong" helps you solve problems that need to be solved?
9. Focus on current problems and behaviors. Rather than try to solve every possible problem in the future, focus right now on some short-term problems—that is, problems that need to be addressed today or this week. Do you feel more competent with this time-limited perspective?

10. Does reassurance really work for more than a few minutes? Do you find that no matter how many times you get reassurance, it doesn't last? Is this because there is no complete certainty about the future?

11. Practice repeating the following sentence 20 minutes each day: "No matter what I do, it's always possible something bad could happen to me." Does the thought become more or less powerful?

12. How many times have you made incorrect negative predictions? Could making negative predictions be a bad habit?

13. What is your worst feared outcome, your feared fantasy?
    a. What is the worst, best, and most likely outcome?
    b. Write out a detailed description of your worst feared outcome.
    c. List all the things that would have to go wrong for this fear to happen.
    d. List all the things that would prevent this fear from happening.
    e. Practice repeating the image and story of the worst outcome for 20 minutes each day. How do you feel?

15. Describe in detail three positive outcomes and write stories about how these positive outcomes could occur

16. Are you afraid of making positive predictions? Do you have a superstition that you should never "tempt fate" by making positive predictions? Test this belief out by making five positive predictions for this week and repeat each one 50 times.

15. Emotional reasoning: You let your feelings guide your interpretation of reality—for example, "I feel depressed; therefore, my marriage is not working out."

Techniques
1. Rate the degree of your belief and identify and rate your emotions.
2. Identify exactly what your emotional reasoning thought is—for example, "I feel anxious, so something bad is going to happen."
3. Distinguish between an emotion and a fact. Describe the facts—things that you can see or hear—rather than your emotional response to them.
4. Let's conduct a cost–benefit analysis:
   a. Does relying on your emotions make you feel like you are on a roller coaster?
   b. Do you think that your emotions protect you from, and prepare you for, the worst?
   c. How would your thoughts, feelings, and behavior change if you relied less on your emotions to make predictions or judgments?
5. Examine evidence for and against your use of emotional reasoning. Does the evidence support your thought that your emotions have generally been a good or bad guide to reality?
6. What cognitive distortions are you using to support your belief? Are you discounting positives, personalizing, mind reading, fortune telling, catastrophizing, negative filters?
7. How could you prove your thought is wrong? Is it testable? How could you test out the belief that your emotions predict reality?
8. Apply vertical descent: What if your thought were true? Why would it bother you?
9. Apply the double-standard exercise: What advice would you give a friend who relied primarily on his or her emotions to judge reality?

16. *Inability to disconfirm: You reject any evidence or arguments that might contradict your negative thoughts. For example, when you have the thought "I'm unlovable," you reject as irrelevant any evidence that people like you—for example, "That's not the real issue, there are deeper problems and other factors." Consequently, your thought cannot be refuted.*

Techniques

1. Rate the degree of your belief and identify and rate your emotions.
2. Identify exactly what your thought is.
3. Let's conduct a cost–benefit analysis:
   a. What is the consequence of thinking in this vague and indefinable way?
   b. What is the consequence of thinking in terms that no one else can quite understand?
   c. Are you assuming that because your thinking is vague and difficult to pin down, you are a deep thinker? Is it possible you are just confused right now?
4. Examine evidence for and against your position: Is it possible to collect evidence that goes against your thought?
5. What is the quality of the evidence that supports your thought or goes against your thought?
6. What cognitive distortions are you using to support your belief? Are you relying on emotional reasoning, discounting positives, or negative filters?
7. How could you prove that your thought is wrong? Is it testable? If your thought can't be tested—if there is no way we could possibly prove that you are wrong, then isn't your thought really "meaningless"?
8. Apply the double-standard exercise: If someone else thought this way, what advice would you give him or her?
9. If your thinking is so vague that it can't be tested, does this make you feel helpless about changing things?
10. What actions could you take that would "act against" your thought?
11. Imagine having to set up an experiment to test your thought. How would you go about collecting information? How would you describe this experiment to a stranger?

17. *Judgment focus: You view yourself, others, and events in terms of evaluations as good–bad or superior–inferior, rather than simply describing, accepting, or understanding. You are continually measuring yourself and others according to arbitrary standards, and finding that you and others fall short. You are focused on the judgments of others as well as your own judgments of yourself—for example, "I didn't perform well in college" or "If I take up tennis, I won't do well" or "Look how successful she is. I'm not successful."*

Techniques

1. Rate the degree of your belief and identify and rate your emotions.
2. Identify exactly the nature of your judgment—for example, "I should be perfect" or "I should get everyone's approval" or "They should do what I want them to do."
3. Let's conduct a cost–benefit analysis:
   a. Do you think that being strict and demanding will motivate you or others?
   b. Do you think you're being "moral" or "standing up for what's right"?
   c. Where did you get this rule?
4. Examine evidence for and against your judgments. Do other people make these judgments as severely and as often as you do?

5. What cognitive distortions are you using to support your belief? Are you using labeling, discounting positives, dichotomous thinking, or overgeneralizing?

6. Do you label yourself and others in all-or-nothing terms when you or they don't live up to your rigid rules? What is the consequence of this labeling?

7. Apply the double-standard technique: Would everyone see it this way? Why not?

8. What if we made this good–bad standard universal rule for everyone?

9. Morality should advance human dignity. Do your judgments treat people in a humane and dignified way? Or are they aimed at condemning and criticizing people?

10. Apply another double-standard exercise: If you really loved someone or cared about him or her, would you judge him or her this way? Why? Is there some reason why you would judge yourself in this way but not others?

11. What if you replaced your judgments with the statement that you might *prefer* something to be true? What if you were less extreme in your statement? For example, what if you were to say "I'd prefer doing well" rather than "I should be perfect"? Try restating all of your "should" rules in terms of less extreme preferences.

12. Try mindfulness rather than judging. Focus only on describing what has happened, without using any judgmental words. Avoid using temporal words such as *always* and *never*—for example, "He's always like that" or "I never measure up." Focus simply on behavior that you can observe—for example, "He was driving fast"—and on how you felt—for example, "I felt nervous." Stay in the present moment.

13. If you stay in the present moment, how will this moment change? What will happen an hour from now, a day from now, a week from now?

14. Try seeing this situation from the vantage point of a balcony. Imagine you are looking down from a balcony on what is happening, and you are asked to describe what you see to a stranger. Exactly what would you say is being said and done?

CHAPTER 10

—

Modifying Need for Approval

Beck and others have suggested that individuals vary along the dimensions of sociotropic and autonomous functioning, such that *sociotropic* individuals are concerned with interpersonal conflicts or relationship losses, whereas *autonomous* individuals focus more on personal standards of performance and are prone to self-criticism (Alden & Bieling, 1998; Bieling, Beck, & Brown, 2000; Blatt, 1974; Blatt & Zuroff, 1992; Clark, Steer, Beck, & Ross, 1995). In this chapter we use a case summary to review techniques that might be useful for modifying excessive need for approval—that is, one of the central concerns for individuals characterized by sociotropy.

Sara is 32 years old and employed in a public relations firm. Her work has been going well recently, but she is concerned that some of her coworkers do not like her. She joined this firm 2 months prior to our meeting for cognitive therapy. At her previous job, she'd had conflicts with an authoritarian supervisor who never thought that Sara's work was quite good enough. Sara describes her previous boss as erratic—sometimes quite friendly, sometimes isolating herself in her office, only to come out in angry tirades on occasion. After some discussion, it became somewhat clear that Sara's previous boss was worried about losing her own job, since there was a demand for downsizing. Sara sought the current job after some time of dissatisfaction with her prior position.

Sara's new position was somewhat higher in rank, salary, and responsibility than those of two women coworkers who had been there for some time. In addition, Sara had known her new boss in the context of a previous friendship and enjoyed a level of familiarity with him.

Sara's presenting complaint was her perception that her coworkers did not like her, which made her think that she was not doing a good job, failing to get the approval of her colleagues, and that her boss would fire her. She also focused more now on her divorce, which had occurred 4 years ago. The divorce was precipitated by her then husband's preoccupation with pornography on the Internet, his unwillingness to get a job to help support the two of them, and his continual criticism of Sara for gaining weight. Since the divorce, Sara has been in three relationships, none of which developed into a permanent relationship. (Techniques are indicated in brackets.)

FIRST SESSION AFTER INTAKE

THERAPIST: What kinds of events seem to trigger these bad feelings at work?

PATIENT: When I go into the office in the morning, Lisa is sort of cold toward me. She just gives me a perfunctory "Hello."

THERAPIST: What kinds of thoughts does that bland greeting trigger for you?

PATIENT: Oh, I just feel lousy.

THERAPIST: OK. *Lousy* is the feeling or emotion you have in response to the underlying thoughts. Complete the following sentence: "I feel lousy because I think . . . "

PATIENT: . . . she doesn't like me.

THERAPIST: And if that were true, it would mean what? [VERTICAL DESCENT]

PATIENT: It makes me think that I must be screwing up on the job.

THERAPIST: OK. So when you think that someone doesn't like you, you conclude it must be because you're doing a bad job? And then you feel really lousy? [EXPLAINING HOW THOUGHTS CREATE FEELINGS]

PATIENT: Yeah.

THERAPIST: What other thoughts do you have when you're feeling down at work?

PATIENT: I think that Lisa and Carol will tell my boss, Dave, that I'm doing a lousy job.

THERAPIST: OK. So your thoughts are, "If they don't like me, they will spread the word"?

PATIENT: Right. And then maybe Dave will regret hiring me. And then—I don't know—maybe I'll lose my job.

THERAPIST: I can see that these thoughts are connected to a lot of bad feelings and other really negative thoughts. When you think that Lisa and Carol don't like you, does that conclusion make you do anything differently in the office? [EXAMINING VARIATIONS OF BEHAVIOR IN DIFFERENT SITUATIONS]

PATIENT: I try to stay to myself. I go into my office and close the door. Pretty much the only person I talk to is Dave.

THERAPIST: So you isolate yourself from Carol and Lisa? What do you think that makes them think?

PATIENT: I never thought of that. They don't like me anyway.

THERAPIST: Your thought is that they think you're doing a lousy job. But is it possible that they might think that you aren't that friendly toward them? Maybe they think that you prefer Dave to them. Could they feel rejected? [EXAMINING THE EVIDENCE]

PATIENT: I never considered that possibility. I always thought they didn't like me.

THERAPIST: Well, it seems that you might be doing a number of things that contribute to your current problem. In cognitive therapy we look at the way you are thinking and try to see if you have any biases in the way you look at things. We call these biases "cognitive distortions." Here's a list of some typical cognitive distortions (Shows Form 1.5 of Automatic Cognitive Distortions). Can you see if there is anything you are doing on this list? [CATEGORIZING THE DISTORTION]

PATIENT: Let's see. Well I'm doing mind reading, saying that they don't like me. But it could be true!

THERAPIST: That's an excellent point. Your thoughts could end up being true. We don't know yet, because we haven't looked at the evidence. But it's possible. Do you spot any other automatic thought distortions? [DISTINGUISHING THOUGHTS FROM FACTS]

PATIENT: Yeah, I'm personalizing and labeling. I'm sort of taking the behavior personally—as if it says something about me. And I'm labeling myself. I guess I'm thinking that I'm a failure or I'm screwing up.

THERAPIST: Right. Those are some of the thoughts you are having. So now that we have begun to categorize these thoughts, let's weigh their costs and benefits. Is there any advantage in thinking that they don't like you? [COST–BENEFIT ANALYSIS]

PATIENT: Well, maybe I can figure out what I'm doing wrong and how to avoid offending them. Maybe I can try to stay out of their way.

THERAPIST: OK. Is there any disadvantage in focusing on your assumption that they don't like you?

PATIENT: It makes me nervous and self-critical. I feel very awkward talking to them. I just can't be myself.

THERAPIST: So, if you had to weigh out the advantages and disadvantages of focusing on figuring out whether people like you, would it be 50/50, 60/40, 40/60 or what?

PATIENT: I'd say that the disadvantages are driving me crazy. I'm always worrying about people not liking me.

THERAPIST: So how does that worry weigh out?

PATIENT: I'd say 90% for the disadvantages.

THERAPIST: OK. If you were a lot less concerned about how they felt about you, what would change in your behavior or your thoughts or your feelings?

PATIENT: I would be more relaxed. Oddly, I might even be friendlier.

THERAPIST: Now that's interesting. You are thinking that they don't like you, but then you isolate yourself. What is your reason for isolating yourself?

PATIENT: As I said, it makes me feel that I won't have any conflicts. I won't be bothering them.

THERAPIST: Yeah. And we considered the possibility that this isolating yourself—something that you do to make yourself feel safer—what we call a "safety behavior"—may actually backfire. It may make them think that you're a snob. [IDENTIFYING SAFETY BEHAVIORS]

PATIENT: A snob?

THERAPIST: Right. That you are too busy with your own thing to bother being friendly.

PATIENT: That never occurred to me. You know, when I was in high school I was sort of shy—but I was pretty and really smart. And one of my friends once told me that the other girls thought I was a snob. It really blew me away.

THERAPIST: Interesting. You were probably thinking you were awkward, and they were probably thinking that you thought you were too good for them.

PATIENT: That's incredible! But it does make sense. I'm *not* trying to look down on them. They do a good job.

THERAPIST: Right. But just as you might be doing some mind reading, so might they. Let's look at these safety behaviors. You said that you just go into your office and close the door. Do you do anything else that helps you feel safer?

PATIENT: Well, I don't look at them directly. I'm kind of soft-spoken, and I look down when I say hello, and then I go into my office.

THERAPIST: Hmm. What might that behavior make them think?

PATIENT: That I'm not friendly.

THERAPIST: OK. What if you were to do the following for the next week: Walk in, stop and say hello to Lisa and Carol, ask them how their evening was and how they're doing. Tell them that you've been feeling sort of swamped with the new job—which is why you've been isolating yourself in your office. And then, when you go into your office, leave the door open. [USING BEHAVIOR TO CHALLENGE THE THOUGHT]

PATIENT: Wow. They'll think I'm really crazy.

THERAPIST: Or friendly?

PATIENT: OK. It's worth a try.

THERAPIST: Alright. What I'd like you to do is act against your thought that they don't like you by being friendly. Let's see what happens. What do you predict? [ACTING AGAINST THE WAY YOU FEEL]

PATIENT: I guess the neurotic side of me thinks that they'll just snub me.

THERAPIST: OK. So we'll test out that thought. Another thing I'd like you to do is take the list of automatic thought distortions and write down examples of any negative thoughts you have and then categorize them. So if you have the thought, "She thinks I'm a loser," write that down in the left-hand column, and then write down "mind reading" in the right-hand column. Let's see if you can catch those thoughts and record them on this form. [SETTING UP PREDICTIONS]

NEXT SESSION

THERAPIST: How did you feel about the last session?

PATIENT: I thought it was helpful. I had never thought that people might think I'm a snob.

THERAPIST: OK. Well, let's look at your self-help homework. You were going to go into the office and give up your safety behaviors. What happened?

PATIENT: It's interesting. Lisa and Carol were both there. I came in and stopped at their desks and told them all the things that we had talked about—about my being overwhelmed and isolating myself—and then I asked them about how they were doing. Lisa was actually kind of friendly. She said, "Yeah, I was wondering why you were so unfriendly." And then we talked about her new apartment. But Carol was a bit more aloof. She didn't say much. [EXAMINING THE EVIDENCE]

THERAPIST: How did it go the rest of the week?

PATIENT: Very much the same. Carol was a bit more friendly but still a little stand-offish. I left my door open and Lisa came by for a visit. I also stopped by in Lisa's office.

THERAPIST: Did you write down and categorize your distorted thoughts? [CATEGORIZING THE DISTORTION]

PATIENT: Yeah. I had thoughts like "Carol doesn't like me" and "She thinks I'm a snob."

THERAPIST: OK. And I can see that you labeled these thoughts as "mind reading." That's correct. It can also be personalizing, too, since Carol may be acting that way for other reasons. [CATEGORIZING THE DISTORTION]

PATIENT: I guess. But it really bothered me. I kept thinking about it all week. I mean, things with Lisa are better, but now I worry a lot about Carol.

THERAPIST: OK. This is a good place for us to start, isn't it? Let's see. "If Carol doesn't like me, it would bother me because it makes me think . . . " [VERTICAL DESCENT]

PATIENT: I screwed up. There it is again.

THERAPIST: OK. If you screwed up, it would means . . . ?

PATIENT: I must be a failure. People aren't going to like me.

THERAPIST: And then what would happen?

PATIENT: I'd end up all alone.

THERAPIST: Hmm. So, if you ended up all alone, what would that mean?

PATIENT: I'd be miserable. Life would not be worth living. [IDENTIFYING UNDERLYING ASSUMPTION]

THERAPIST: It sounds like a lot could be riding on Carol not liking you. Of course, we don't know how she feels, but let's take a look at these thoughts. Let's start with the first thought, "If Carol doesn't like me, then I screwed up." Could there be other reasons why Carol doesn't like you—if that is, indeed, the case? [EXAMINING EVIDENCE; CONSIDERING ALTERNATIVE INTERPRETATIONS]

PATIENT: Well, part of it could be that I acted like a snob for the first 2 months; which means I screwed up.

THERAPIST: Any other reasons?

PATIENT: Well, Carol could resent the fact that I was brought in over her head and that Dave and I were friends. She might be jealous. I don't know.

THERAPIST: Any of that sound plausible?

PATIENT: All of it. But it's hard for me to think that someone is jealous of me.

THERAPIST: Well, it might be surprising to you, but it could also be true. So one set of thoughts is that she might be jealous of you. She might think that Dave favors you. Maybe he does.

PATIENT: He probably does.

THERAPIST: OK. Now another thought that you had is "If I screwed up, then I am a failure." We call this all-or-nothing thinking and labeling. What did you screw up? [IDENTIFYING DISTORTIONS; EXAMINING EVIDENCE]

PATIENT: Getting Carol to like me.

THERAPIST: Of course, we really don't know what Carol thinks, but even if she didn't like you, is getting her to like you part of your job description?

PATIENT: No. I'm hired to do public relations. But I'd like to get along with people.

THERAPIST: Yes, that's what we're also aiming at. But you seem to think that if you did screw up on one thing, then you would be a failure. Doesn't everyone make mistakes?

PATIENT: Yeah. [EXAMINING ALL-OR-NOTHING THINKING; DOUBLE-STANDARD TECHNIQUE]

THERAPIST: Is everyone a failure? [EXAMINING LOGICAL ERRORS]

PATIENT: No. But that's how I think.

THERAPIST: Could we distinguish between a behavior and an entire person? Let's say that one of your behaviors—going in and closing the door—was not that productive. Let's even go so far as to say, you screwed up. Aren't there some things that you are doing well on the job? [DISTINGUISHING BEHAVIORS FROM PERSONS]

PATIENT: Yeah. I think Dave thinks my work is good. One of our biggest clients wants to work exclusively with me.

THERAPIST: OK. So perhaps you might make a mistake once in a while, but you are jumping to conclusions in labeling yourself as a failure. [CHALLENGING LABELING AND ALL-OR-NOTHING THINKING]

PATIENT: My last boss was constantly telling me that I was screwing up.

THERAPIST: What was she like as a boss?

PATIENT: Terrible. Her entire staff turned over in 2 years. My friend Phyllis told me that she heard that my former boss might get fired.

THERAPIST: She sounds like a terrible boss. Why did everyone leave?

PATIENT: They couldn't stand her.

THERAPIST: So how successful was she as a boss?

PATIENT: She did a lousy job.

THERAPIST: It seems that you are really concerned with what other people are thinking about you. Let's see if we can come up with a general rule that you might be using. Let's start with "If my co-workers don't like me, then it means . . . " [IDENTIFYING UNDERLYING ASSUMPTION]

PATIENT: I screwed up.

THERAPIST: "If my boss is critical of me, it means . . . " [VERTICAL DESCENT]

PATIENT: I'm incompetent.

THERAPIST: Is the general rule "My worth depends on what other people think?" [IDENTIFYING UNDERLYING ASSUMPTION]

PATIENT: I guess. I can be going along OK for a while, but if someone doesn't like me, I just feel like crumbling.

THERAPIST: OK. So you really seem to feel that you need other people to like you. Let's call that a basic assumption on your part. [IDENTIFYING BASIC ASSUMPTIONS]

PATIENT: OK.

THERAPIST: If you have the assumption that you must get the approval of others to feel worthwhile, then you might develop some strategies to make sure that you don't get rejected or don't get judged by others. For example, one of the strategies that you seemed to use in the office was to try to show a low profile—sort of just slink in and not say much and not make waves. Part of this low-profile strategy was to look down, talk softly, and not say much. Right? [IDENTIFYING CONDITIONAL RULES]

PATIENT: Yeah. But it may have backfired. They might have thought I was a snob.

THERAPIST: That's possible. But you might have other strategies that you use to keep yourself from being judged badly.

PATIENT: Well, let's see. I think one of them is that I try to do a perfect job. And I try to always do what the boss wants me to do.

THERAPIST: OK. So these are some new rules that you might be using. They include, "Maintain a low profile, don't make waves, talk softly, try to do a perfect job, and always please the boss." Is that about right? [IDENTIFYING CONDITIONAL RULES]

PATIENT: Yeah. It's a lot of pressure on me.

THERAPIST: Right. These are what we call your "conditional rules." It's like you're saying to yourself, "If I do a perfect job, then the boss won't criticize me. And if the boss doesn't criticize me, then I'm not incompetent." [IDENTIFYING CONDITIONAL RULES]

PATIENT: That's the way I think. It's the way I feel about it.

THERAPIST: OK. So we have three different levels here. The first level is that your value depends on what others think. The second level is that you have to do a perfect job to make sure they don't judge you. And the third—the deepest level of your thinking—is that maybe you really are incompetent. [IDENTIFYING UNDERLYING SCHEMA; DEVELOPING CASE CONCEPTUALIZATION]

PATIENT: Well, I don't necessarily think I'm incompetent . . . but sometimes I guess I do think that!

THERAPIST: When is that?

PATIENT: When someone criticizes me.

THERAPIST: OK. So as long as you are doing a perfect job, you are above suspicion, and you can think you're competent. But when criticism comes along, then . . . well, that just shows that you are incompetent.

PATIENT: Yeah. I can be feeling terrific—as long as people like me and I'm not getting criticized. Then, wham! I'm totally undermined. I make a mistake . . . or someone doesn't like me . . . and then I think I'm a loser.

THERAPIST: OK. So now we are developing what we call a "case conceptualization" of your problem. We can start with the deepest level: "I'm incompetent." Then we add your strategies of laying low, not making waves, doing a perfect job. Then we come to your underlying assumption "If someone doesn't like me, then it means I'm defective or incompetent." [DEVELOPING CASE CONCEPTUALIZATION]

PATIENT: OK. Yeah, that makes sense. I always go around with this idea that someone is going to find out that I'm incompetent.

THERAPIST: Now let's see about this idea, "I'm incompetent." How would you define *competent*? [IDENTIFYING SCHEMA; SEMANTIC TECHNIQUE]

PATIENT: I'd say, "Someone who can get things done."

THERAPIST: OK. Let's imagine that you are reading your résumé to me. You are your own defense attorney, and you have to make your best case to support the defense's plea that you are competent. What's the argument, Counselor, that you are competent? [DEFENSE ATTORNEY: EXAMINING EVIDENCE]

PATIENT: Well, I graduated from college. I did really well, too. I even supported my ex-husband financially for some time. And I've done a lot of good work for my clients, got them a lot of PR. I make a decent salary.

THERAPIST: How are you doing now in your work compared to 5 years ago?

PATIENT: A hell of a lot better.

THERAPIST: So you're arguing that you are competent and getting better all the time?

PATIENT: Yeah, I guess that's true.

THERAPIST: Let's take your conditional rule—"If I do a perfect job, I can prove I'm competent and I won't get criticized." What are the disadvantages of having to do a perfect job? [COST–BENEFIT ANALYSIS OF ASSUMPTION AND RULES]

PATIENT: A lot of pressure. It's impossible.

THERAPIST: Is there any way of knowing if a job is perfect in your business? [APPLYING SEMANTIC TECHNIQUE; IDENTIFYING UNVERIFIABLE TERMS]

PATIENT: No. That's a good point. You can't really know. It's a matter of judgment. You don't know all the variables. No. You can't know what constitutes a perfect job.

THERAPIST: So trying to do a perfect job is kind of meaningless?

PATIENT: Right.

THERAPIST: If your self-esteem depends on being perfect—and that standard of perfection is meaning-less—where does that leave you? [IDENTIFYING LOGICAL ERRORS]

PATIENT: Nowhere.

THERAPIST: Not a good place to be, is it?

PATIENT: Not for me.

THERAPIST: We have to base your self-esteem on something different, something other than being per-fect, something other than what some critical boss or envious colleague might think.

PATIENT: What would that be?

THERAPIST: How about the facts?

PATIENT: What do you mean?

THERAPIST: Rather than use how others might evaluate you, we might use the actual facts about your qualities and your performance. For example, what if we took your intelligence and education. How do you compare with the average person? [USING THE NORMAL COMPARSION]

PATIENT: I'm above average.

THERAPIST: How much above average?

PATIENT: I don't know—a lot, I guess.

THERAPIST: You don't seem to take too much credit for that.

PATIENT: I don't want to sound conceited.

THERAPIST: Do you believe that you will sound conceited if you think positive things about yourself? [COST–BENEFIT ANALYSIS OF THOUGHT]

PATIENT: I guess I do. I don't want people to think that I'm conceited and a snob.

THERAPIST: Let's look at what you just said: If you think or say positive things about yourself, people won't like you. What's the consequence of that viewpoint?

PATIENT: I guess I don't think well of myself. In fact, I'm often really kind of self-effacing.

THERAPIST: What do you hope to get from being self-effacing?

PATIENT: I know it sounds irrational. I expect that people will like me. [IDENTIFYING CONDITIONAL RULES]

THERAPIST: Interesting. So you're thinking, at times, that if you put yourself down, you'll get approval. How does that kind of thinking affect your self-esteem?

PATIENT: I feel lousy about myself. And, you know, people might think less of me if I'm putting myself down.

THERAPIST: Do you ever think or say, "Gee, I did a really good job on that project—I feel good about the way I did that"?

PATIENT: No. I guess I'm afraid that I'll begin to think I'm superior and get conceited, and then people won't like me.

THERAPIST: OK. So now it makes sense, doesn't it, that you have a hard time building your self-esteem, because you sort of equate self-esteem with alienating other people? [IDENTIFYING CON-DITIONAL RULES]

PATIENT: Yeah. I guess that's the sort of thing I felt when I was growing up. My mother would tell me, "You're getting full of yourself. You think you're so much better than everyone." [EXAMINING ORI-GIN OF SCHEMAS AND RULES]

THERAPIST: What led her to say that?

PATIENT: Sometimes I felt good about how well I did in school. I remember telling my mother, "My teacher told me I did better than everyone on the essay." And then Mom told me, "You're getting too big for your britches."

THERAPIST: What lesson was Mom teaching you?

PATIENT: Don't brag about your work.

THERAPIST: And, if you do, people will think you're conceited.

PATIENT: Yeah.

THERAPIST: Tell me about Mom. What was her background?

PATIENT: Well, she came from a very strict family, and poor. She had two brothers, and her father vowed that whatever it took, they would make sure that the boys got to go to college. So both her brothers went to college, but my mother had to work. She worked in an office. She was good. But I think that she always resented her brothers. She always felt bitter about not going to college. It was a different generation then. [APPLYING ALTERNATIVE INTERPRETATION]

THERAPIST: So this is where you learned that you shouldn't take credit, you shouldn't tell anyone how well you do, and that you'll get criticized if you do.

PATIENT: I never felt that what I was doing was ever good enough for her.

THERAPIST: Is it possible that she was kind of envious of you? Here you were—smart, doing well— probably like she was doing when she was a kid. But you got to go off to college. It exemplified for her what she was never able to do.

PATIENT: That's right. It's funny. She never said anything to me about my doing well in college, but then I found out that she would tell other people—she'd brag about me, like she was taking credit for my achievements. But she never gave *me* any credit.

THERAPIST: How did that make you feel?

PATIENT: Lousy, but I kept trying, even though it never seemed to work.

THERAPIST: Do you see any parallel between trying to please your critical mother and trying to please your boss? [IDENTIFYING GENERALITY OF SCHEMA]

PATIENT: Yeah. Nothing was ever good enough. Then I blamed myself.

THERAPIST: Right. But it might be that Mom had her own problems dealing with your success. Maybe you got criticized not because you were inferior, but because you were doing so well.

PATIENT: I never thought of that—doing well! That makes sense.

THERAPIST: Right. Especially when someone is envious of you. That's the blind spot for you. When your coworkers feel envious, or your boss has her own problems and is worried about her own job, you experience withholding behavior and then you think "I must be incompetent." You can't win, playing that game, can you?

PATIENT: It always comes up like that. I'm doing well, someone doesn't approve, or withholds, and I think I'm a loser.

THERAPIST: OK, that's the origin of this pattern. Let's imagine now that you are going to confront Mom, tell her what you really think—especially based on what you and I have been talking about. Let's imagine that Mom is sitting here, in this empty chair, and that I've given you a truth serum. You've got to really let it all out. Tell her what you really think. Don't be concerned about her approval. Let her know. [ROLE PLAYING AGAINST THOUGHT; ROLE PLAYING AGAINST SCHEMA]

PATIENT: OK. (*Hesitating, talking to Mom*) I was never good enough for you. It's not my fault that your parents were so sexist. I know it was terrible for you, not being able to fulfill your potential. You're smart. But I'm smart, too. I never got any credit from you. I never heard a compliment. I needed that.

THERAPIST: Tell her how bad you felt.

PATIENT: I felt awful, growing up and not feeling that my own mother was on my side. It hurt me. It *still* hurts me.

THERAPIST: Good. Now tell her what you need her to say to you.

PATIENT: I need you to say that you really respect me, you really appreciate everything that I do. I need you to see me as a success.

THERAPIST: Excellent. And now tell her why you are a success.

PATIENT: Damn it! I did great on the SATs and I graduated with honors from college. Even when I had to work part-time, I wrote papers that my professors thought were terrific. I'm really doing well in my work. I'm a success, whether you want to admit it or not!

THERAPIST: How does saying all these things feel?

PATIENT: Terrific.

THERAPIST: Let's see how we can carry the work we've done here today forward. Here's a homework assignment for you. I'd like you to write down statements to your current boss and your prior boss about why you are competent and deserve respect. I want you to really let them have it—just as you did here. But don't show them these statements. These are for you to think about. [ASSERTION AGAINST NEGATIVE CRITICS]

PATIENT: OK. I'll do it. It's about time for me to stand up for myself.

NEXT SESSION

THERAPIST: In the last session we talked about your feeling about your mother and your boss.

PATIENT: Yeah. I wrote down some of the statements to my bosses. It felt good. It felt like I was standing up for myself.

THERAPIST: What did you say?

PATIENT: (*to previous boss, reading*) "I think you were really unfair criticizing me all the time. I did the best job I could. I'm not perfect, but you just focused on things you didn't like. You weren't a perfect boss. A good boss motivates and rewards and teaches, but you didn't do any of those things. You were so critical and difficult to deal with that everyone left. I know that I did a good job because clients told me that I did." [ASSERTION AGAINST NEGATIVE CRITICS]

THERAPIST: How did that feel?

PATIENT: Good. It's about time that I stood up for myself.

THERAPIST: Let's look at this underlying belief you have that you aren't good enough. It sounds like this is something you believed when you were a kid.

PATIENT: Yeah. No matter what I did, it wasn't good enough for my mother. She just picked on my faults, so I came to believe only in my faults.

THERAPIST: Quite early in your life you were thinking that you weren't good enough. Not good enough in what? [IDENTIFYING ORIGIN OF SCHEMA]

PATIENT: Not pretty enough. She always compared me to my cousin, who was really pretty. I was OK looking, but she was really gorgeous. So it was a difficult comparison for me.

THERAPIST: What else weren't you good enough in?

PATIENT: I thought I wasn't smart enough—I mean, I *was* smart, but not the smartest, not perfect. I didn't take credit for my achievements.

THERAPIST: You mean, you weren't given credit?

PATIENT: Right.

THERAPIST: So your mother was telling you, "You're not as pretty as your cousin and you're not the smartest." Let's take the pretty part. If you thought you weren't pretty enough, what did that belief make you do or make you avoid? [EXAMINING EFFECT OF SCHEMA; SCHEMA MAINTENANCE; SCHEMA AVOIDANCE]

PATIENT: I *avoided* more than anything else. I was always shy with guys. When Roger [her ex-husband] showed an interest in me, I grabbed it. I didn't think anyone would want me.

THERAPIST: How did this idea that you had—"I'm not pretty enough"—play itself out in the marriage?

PATIENT: He would criticize me, and he wasn't interested in sex a lot of the time. So I thought "I must be too fat" or "I'm not pretty enough."

THERAPIST: It sounds like Roger reinforced your negative view of yourself—that must have been hard. Did you do anything else because of this negative view of yourself as not pretty enough.

PATIENT: I had an affair. It wasn't really a serious affair, more of an attempt to get someone to tell me I was attractive. I broke it off because I couldn't handle it.

THERAPIST: So this idea that you weren't pretty enough led you to put up with Roger's criticism and lack of interest and then to have an affair? Interesting. What if you had started out, as a child, with the idea that you *were* pretty and you *were* intelligent. What if you'd had really positive ideas about yourself from a very young age? Would you have made different choices? [EXAMINING ALTERNATIVE POSITIVE SCHEMA]

PATIENT: Absolutely. I never thought about this before. I absolutely would make different choices. The first thing is, I wouldn't have been so shy. There was this guy Paul who was really nice, really seemed like my type—he was smart—but I always felt awkward around him. He was a little shy, too. He never asked me out. Funny, but he called me a few months ago—he and his wife are having problems. He wanted to have dinner with me. I guess I would have made more of an effort as an adolescent to get Paul interested. And I wouldn't have stayed with Roger. He was OK for the first couple of months, but he was sort of full of himself. I wouldn't have stayed with Roger.

THERAPIST: How about this idea that you aren't smart enough? What choices would you have made if you'd believed you were really smart?

PATIENT: I would have gone on for a PhD. I just assumed "I'm not bright enough to do that." But, you know, I am.

THERAPIST: Anything else?

PATIENT: Well, I would have pushed harder for a raise on my last job. I was so intimidated by my boss!

THERAPIST: OK. So those are really different ways of thinking and acting. If only your mother would have been more compassionate, more loving. It sounded like she felt bitter about her own shortcomings. She didn't get to where she wanted to be, so she took it out on you. [APPLYING ALTERNATIVE INTERPRETATION]

PATIENT: Right.

THERAPIST: Well, I wonder if you could do some self-help work on this area. I'd like you to write down some of the decisions you've made in your life, since you were a girl—decisions that reflect the ways you thought about yourself and other people. I'd like you to think about how these decisions were affected by your mother's behavior—that is, how her lack of support of you, how her own feelings of inadequacy, rubbed off on you. Then I'd like you to write down how you might have thought, decided, or felt if your mother had been more supportive, more loving, more protective of you. You can use this form [7.8, Life through the Lens of a Different Schema] and this other form [7.9, Effects of My Positive Schema]. Doing this homework might help you understand how you might have felt differently. Maybe you might think about how you could feel differently now.

PATIENT: OK.

THERAPIST: One of the things we might do is think of someone in your life who was really loving, really caring toward you. Can you close your eyes? Try to relax. Try to think about who that person was. [APPLYING COMPASSIONATE MIND]

PATIENT: OK. I've got a picture of my Aunt Beth.

THERAPIST: Tell me about Aunt Beth.

PATIENT: She was really loving. She always seemed to kiss me and hug me and tell me how wonderful—how pretty—I was. I always felt great seeing her.

THERAPIST: Hold her face in your mind and try to see what she looked like.

PATIENT: She had sort of curly brown hair. She always wore makeup, but sort of more formal, more like a lady.

THERAPIST: Imagine that you are feeling really bad about work. Your coworkers snub you and your boss is critical. What would Aunt Beth tell you? [APPLYING COMPASSIONATE MIND]

PATIENT: She'd say, "Don't worry, you're terrific. They're just jealous. You know you do a good job. You know that you're smarter than they are. You're so pretty, and I love you so much."

THERAPIST: What are your feelings right now?

PATIENT: I feel really warm. I feel like crying.

THERAPIST: Why?

PATIENT: Because she is no longer alive. She died of cancer 4 years ago.

THERAPIST: She was someone who loved you, and it's sad to lose her. She mattered so much. But we can bring her back *inside you*. Think about Aunt Beth inside you. She is the compassionate, loving voice. She is your guardian angel.

PATIENT: She was always on my side.

THERAPIST: Right. What would Aunt Beth say to you that would be soothing when your ex-husband is critical.

PATIENT: She'd say, "Don't worry about him. He doesn't count. You are smarter, a more decent, person. You are a winner. You don't need him. He would just bring you down. You're better off without him."

THERAPIST: Now we have these two parts of your mind. The critical voice that tells you that you are always wrong and never good enough, and the compassionate voice, the compassionate mind, that tells you that you are loved. The compassionate mind stands up for you and takes care of you.

PATIENT: That's what I need, someone who will take care of me, and understand me.

THERAPIST: That someone has to be *inside* of you. That someone is the compassionate mind that cares.

PATIENT: But I don't seem to be that compassionate myself.

THERAPIST: Didn't you tell me in our intake interview about how you took care of your sick dog? What did you do for her?

PATIENT: I took care of her all the time. I took her to the vet, got her the best care. I loved her.

THERAPIST: And how about your friend Paula, when she was going through a rough time—what did you do?

PATIENT: I listened. I told her that she was terrific—and she is. She was having a hard time.

THERAPIST: We need to find a way whereby you direct that compassionate mind toward yourself. That's what we are going to do.

PATIENT: That would be great.

THERAPIST: Let's look at this form—the critical and compassionate mind. The critical mind is the part of you that says you're a failure and not attractive enough. That's the part you write down in the left-hand column. The compassionate mind—well, that's going to be Aunt Beth. She's your guardian angel. She is going to soothe, nurture, love, and accept you. When you hear that critical voice, you write down what Aunt Beth would say in this column.

PATIENT: OK, I understand. She would always be on my side. She would love me.

THERAPIST: And part of her lives in you, doesn't it? Part of her and part of you took care of that sick puppy. Part of both of you took care of that sick friend.

PATIENT: I guess that's true.

THERAPIST: How do you feel now?

PATIENT: Like a burden has been lifted. Thanks for listening to me.

SUMMARY

There are numerous cognitive and behavioral techniques we could have utilized to challenge Sara's need for approval. In this chapter, I have highlighted an example of a highly competent woman who feels undermined by what appears to her to be rejection or coldness from her coworkers. This particular example allows us to see how the surface issues—fear of negative evaluation and need for approval—may be linked to a broader case conceptualization. This case conceptualization also links the patient's current situation to her earlier maladaptive schemas as defective, not good enough, and incompetent—schemas that arose in response to her envious and competitive mother's negative views of the young girl's success. Moreover, we can see how the use of Gilbert's (2002) model of the compassionate mind can assist her in utilizing a resource from her past—her memory of her loving aunt—to give credibility and force to the "rational responses" that can be used to challenge her self-critical voice.

As indicated by this example, individuals who have high needs for approval may seem quite adaptive and symptom-free, until they find themselves in an environment of rejection and criticism. The interested reader might consider how this patient's treatment could be expanded to include homework assignments involving assertiveness, collecting rejections to decatastrophize them, rational role plays, and flash cards that remind her of her rational voice that will defend her against the critical voice.

—

CHAPTER 11

Challenging Self-Criticism

One of the central issues in depression and anxiety is low-self esteem, a condition often characterized by self-criticism, unrealistically high standards for the self, and excessive focus on perceived "flaws" while discounting positives (see Harter, 1999). In this chapter I use another case example to illustrate how to modify self-critical thinking through the use of cognitive therapy techniques. The reader may also consult the excellent suggestions offered by David Burns in *The Feeling Good Handbook* (1989)and *Ten Days to Higher Self Esteem* (1999). In addition, *Self-Esteem: A Proven Program of Cognitive Techniques for Assessing, Improving, and Maintaining Your Self-Esteem* by McKay and Fanning (2000) is a useful self-help book for patients.

The patient, John, is a 26-year-old single male employed in the advertising business. He recently experienced a breakup with his girlfriend Rita, with whom he'd had an up-and-down 3-month relationship. During the past 3 weeks since the breakup, he has been ruminating about his defectiveness and thinking that he will never find another relationship. He has avoided seeing his friends and generally goes directly home to his apartment, eats fast-food dinners, watches television, and broods on the idea that he has nothing to offer. He is currently depressed and anxious about the future.

FIRST SESSION AFTER INTAKE

THERAPIST: So, John, you've been feeling pretty bad since you and Rita broke up. Tell me a little bit about the relationship.

PATIENT: It was up and down. We often argued. I guess we didn't have a lot in common. She was more interested in hanging out and drinking, and I don't drink that much. I don't think she had many interests outside of clothes and talk shows.

THERAPIST: So it was problematic?

PATIENT: Yeah.

THERAPIST: Now, when you are feeling down, can you tell me the kind of thoughts that you have?

PATIENT: I feel sad.

THERAPIST: OK. That's a feeling. I'd be interested in the kinds of things that you are thinking when you are sad. For example, when you are sitting at home alone feeling sad, what's going through your head? Complete this sentence: "I feel sad because I think … " [DISTINGUISHING THOUGHTS FROM FEELINGS; ELICITING AUTOMATIC THOUGHTS]

PATIENT: I'm alone.

THERAPIST: OK. And the thing about being alone that bothers you most is that you think … ?

PATIENT: I'll always be alone.

THERAPIST: And the reason you'll always be alone is because … [VERTICAL DESCENT]

PATIENT: I'm a loser. I have nothing to offer.

THERAPIST: And if you have nothing to offer, and you're alone, then what would happen … ?

PATIENT: Life would have no meaning.

THERAPIST: OK. So the breakup seems to signify some important things to you. It means to you that you are a loser, you have nothing to offer, you'll always be alone, and life has no meaning.

PATIENT: Right. It feels really bad to me.

THERAPIST: You know, in cognitive therapy we talk about "automatic thoughts." These are thoughts that come to us spontaneously and they seem true to us. They are often associated with feeling sad, anxious, or angry. [EXPLAINING HOW THOUGHTS CREATE FEELINGS] Examples of your automatic thoughts are "I'm a loser" or "I'll always be alone." [CATEGORIZING DISTORTIONS]

PATIENT: When I'm home alone, I think a lot of those kinds of thoughts.

THERAPIST: OK. So being alone seems to be something that triggers these thoughts?

PATIENT: Right, or thinking about not having a girlfriend.

THERAPIST: Here's a list of the kinds of automatic thoughts people have. We call them *distortions*. (Gives patient list of automatic thought distortions.) Can you see yourself on this list? Do you do some labeling—for example, "I'm a loser"—and some fortune telling—for example, "I'll always be alone"?

PATIENT: Yeah. I think I do a lot of these things.

THERAPIST: OK. We will look at your way of thinking and test it out. Let's see if these thoughts about yourself really hold up to our examination. [DISTINGUISHING THOUGHTS FROM FACTS] Let's take the thought "I'm a loser." How would you define *loser*? [APPLYING SEMANTIC TECHNIQUE]

PATIENT: Someone who can't get anything done. Someone who has nothing to offer.

THERAPIST: OK. Let's write down "I'm a loser." (*Patient complies.*) When you're alone and feeling really down, how much do you believe this belief on a scale from 0% to 100%, with 100% meaning that you believe it with absolute certainty. [RATING DEGREE OF BELIEF]

PATIENT: I'd say about 95%.

THERAPIST: And how sad do you feel, from 0% to 100%, when you have this thought? [RATING DEGREE OF EMOTION]

PATIENT: About 99%.

THERAPIST: OK. Now let's look at the evidence. Put a line down the center of the page under "I'm a loser" and put "For" at the top of the left-hand column and "Against" at the top of the right-hand column. Let's list the evidence for and against the idea that you are a loser. [EXAMINING EVIDENCE]

PATIENT: The evidence that I'm a loser? Rita and I broke up. I'm depressed. I don't have a girlfriend. That's about it.

THERAPIST: OK. What's the evidence that you are *not* a loser?

PATIENT: I have a good job, I have lots of friends—but I don't see them now. I guess I'm OK looking. I went to college, but I could have done better.

THERAPIST: If you had to weigh out the evidence for and against the idea that you are a loser, would it be 50/50, 60/40, 40/60, or what? [WEIGHING EVIDENCE]

PATIENT: I'd say the evidence is 90% I am not a loser and 10% I am a loser.

THERAPIST: What do your friends think of you? What do they like about you?

PATIENT: They generally think I'm a pretty decent guy. I guess they'd say I'm a good listener, I don't judge people, I'm reliable, generous, and I have a sense of humor.

THERAPIST: Would they think you're a loser? [DOUBLE STANDARD]

PATIENT: No. They see me differently.

THERAPIST: Do they see you more accurately than you see yourself?

PATIENT: Perhaps.

THERAPIST: Let's go back to your evidence that you're a loser. Read over what you wrote in relation to how your friends see you. If you had to weigh the evidence that you are a loser, would it be 50/50, 60/40, 40/60, or what? [EXAMINE THE EVIDENCE]

PATIENT: I'd say that the evidence is about 5% that I'm a loser and 95% that I'm not.

THERAPIST: Does thinking about this issue in a larger context make you feel any differently?

PATIENT: I guess I feel less depressed and less hopeless.

THERAPIST: It seems that you have this idea that "Unless I have a girlfriend right now, then I'm a loser." [IDENTIFYING ASSUMPTION]

PATIENT: Yeah. That's the way it feels right now.

THERAPIST: Let's write down that thought and put a line down the center of the page again. Let's look at the advantages and disadvantages of this thought for you. [COST–BENEFIT ANALYSIS]

PATIENT: I guess the only advantage I can think of is that it might motivate me to find another girl-friend.

THERAPIST: How about the disadvantages?

PATIENT: I'm miserable, I get really tense in a relationship because I think I need it. I make some bad choices. It's not good for me.

THERAPIST: OK. If you didn't believe this notion, how would you be better off?

PATIENT: I'd be more independent. I wouldn't stay in a bad relationship.

THERAPIST: Weighing the advantages and disadvantages, are they 50/50, or something else? [COST–BENEFIT ANALYSIS]

PATIENT: I'd say about 20/80—far more disadvantages.

THERAPIST: When you are not involved with someone, what things do you like doing?

PATIENT: I like my work. I like coming up with new ideas about marketing. I like working out, movies, restaurants, seeing my friends, reading.

THERAPIST: If you were to do some of those things this week, what do you predict would happen?

PATIENT: I'll feel better. [PLEASURE PREDICTING]

THERAPIST: On a scale from 0% to 100%, where 100% represents the best you can ever imagine feeling, how would you feel if you saw your friends?

PATIENT: I'd have to guess about 60%.

THERAPIST: If you felt better doing those things, what does that say about the thought that you need a girlfriend to feel happy? [EXAMINING EVIDENCE AGAINST ASSUMPTION]

PATIENT: It means it's not true. But I used to get more pleasure from these things.

THERAPIST: Are you discounting the positives here? Would you feel better staying home and just thinking how bad you are feeling or would you feel better seeing friends?

PATIENT: Seeing friends would be better.

THERAPIST: Let's draw a figure of a pie. Let's say your entire life in the last 10 years would be the whole pie. How much of that pie represents your time with Rita? (*Draws pie chart.*) [USING PIE TECHNIQUE]

PATIENT: Only a very small piece.

THERAPIST: And in how much of that pie were you really, really depressed?

PATIENT: Only the last 3 weeks.

THERAPIST: What does that say about your *needing* a relationship with Rita?

PATIENT: I guess when I look at this pie, it really is clear. In fact, I wasn't that happy *with* her. I was happier before I met her!

THERAPIST: Let's do a role play. I'll be your negative thoughts and you challenge me. OK? [ROLE PLAYING AGAINST THOUGHT]

PATIENT: I'll try.

THERAPIST: [as negative] Rita is the only source of happiness for you.

PATIENT: That's not true. I had a lot of good times without her.

THERAPIST: She was perfect.

PATIENT: She was a pain at times! I think she had shallow values.

THERAPIST: You are totally flawed and have nothing to offer anyone.

PATIENT: That's false, too. I'm a decent guy. I have a lot of things to offer. I'm kind, generous, thoughtful, attractive, smart.

THERAPIST: OK. How do you feel now?

PATIENT: I'm feeling a lot better.

THERAPIST: What if your best friend were going through a breakup and felt the way you felt? What advice would you give him? [GIVING ADVICE TO A FRIEND]

PATIENT: I'd tell him to move on. She wasn't worth it.

THERAPIST: OK. Let's think of some things you could do to help yourself over the next week. How about keeping track of these negative thoughts and challenging them? You can use the Daily Record of Negative Thoughts. And it might be interesting for you to keep track of how you feel using the Activity Schedule. [ASSIGNING DAILY RECORD OF NEGATIVE THOUGHTS; ACTIVITY SCHEDULE]

NEXT SESSION

THERAPIST: (*Therapist reviews prior session, asks for feedback, and reviews homework.*) Let's look at your activity schedule. What were you doing when you felt the best during the past week?

PATIENT: I was seeing my friends, going to the health club, and working at the office.

THERAPIST: I notice that none of these things has anything to do with Rita.

PATIENT: Yeah, but I felt really bad when I was home at night alone. I kept thinking what a loser I am to be alone.

THERAPIST: So when you are thinking about Rita, you feel bad? And you also feel bad when you think that you are a loser because you are alone that evening? [LOOKING FOR VARIATIONS IN A SPECIFIC BELIEF] Did you write down some of these thoughts and try to challenge them?

PATIENT: I tried. (*Reading from his form*) "I'm a loser." My challenge was "I'm not really a loser. I'm just me."

THERAPIST: How effective was the challenge?

PATIENT: Not very effective.

THERAPIST: It sounded more like an affirmation—like, "I'm OK"—rather than really attacking the negative thought and trying to defeat it. Let's take the thought "I'm a loser." What thoughts go with that belief?

PATIENT: I think that maybe I don't really have anything to offer. There are a lot of these guys making a lot more money than I make.

THERAPIST: What does that realization, that comparison, make you think about yourself?

PATIENT: I really have nothing going for me.

THERAPIST: So that thought might put you at the zero point on the scale?

PATIENT: Sometimes I feel close to zero.

THERAPIST: OK, let's look at what that would mean—being a zero. [SETTING A ZERO POINT FOR EVALUATION] Let's see, someone who is at zero would be the ugliest, stupidest, most immoral, hostile, and boring person that we could imagine. Is that you?

PATIENT: No. I think I'm OK looking. I'm in decent shape. I went to college, but I didn't get the best grades. But I'm pretty decent, I guess. [EXAMINING THE EVIDENCE]

THERAPIST: Imagine if you were a zero on any of these things. Wouldn't that be completely different from the way you really are?

PATIENT: Yeah. I'm not a zero.

THERAPIST: When you think about the people who are doing so much better than you, whom do you have in mind?

PATIENT: I saw this guy on CNBC who was worth 200 million dollars. He has his own company.

THERAPIST: How many people have that kind of money?

PATIENT: Almost no one.

THERAPIST: What is the average income in the United States? [DEPOLARIZING COMPARISONS]

PATIENT: I'd guess about $40,000.

THERAPIST: So, if you compared yourself to the average, you're doing better than average?

PATIENT: Yeah. But I'm not as rich as some of these people.

THERAPIST: Who is?

PATIENT: Almost no one.

THERAPIST: When we compare ourselves to the extremes, we are bound to feel we have less. Wouldn't it be more realistic to compare yourself to people in the middle? Or even at the bottom? [APPLYING THE CONTINUUM]

PATIENT: I tend to always think about people who are doing better.

THERAPIST: Let's use a continuum. Let's draw a line from left to right and put 100% at the far right and 0% at the far left. This continuum represents degree of success. For someone your age, what would be the least amount of success and the most amount of success possible?

PATIENT: I'd say that 0% would be someone in a coma, and 100% would be someone who has a billion dollars.

THERAPIST: Where would we put someone who is average, above average, and below average?

PATIENT: Well average for my age might actually be around $25,000, above average would be around $40,000, and below average might be $20,000. I make about $55,000—so for someone my age, I'm significantly above average. [DIVERSIFYING COMPARISONS]

THERAPIST: How do you reconcile that rating with being a loser?

PATIENT: I'm not a loser. But I could do better.

THERAPIST: Isn't that true for everyone? Sometimes we are afraid that our worst fantasy will come true. What is your worst fantasy about success?

PATIENT: Oh, going back to my college reunion and talking to Larry, who is very successful, and I would be out of work, no money. I'd feel like a loser.

THERAPIST: OK, so this is your worst fantasy about not succeeding? [ELICITING FEARED FANTASY]

PATIENT: Yeah, I'd be humiliated.

THERAPIST: Let's do a role play where you confront this feared fantasy in the form of Larry. I'd like you to play the role of Larry, being really condescending and obnoxious. I'll play you being rational and assertive. [ROLE PLAYING THE FEARED FANTASY]

PATIENT: [as Larry, the obnoxious classmate] So, John, I see that you made it to the reunion. I guess you heard that I sold my company and made a billion dollars.

THERAPIST: [As John, challenging the obnoxious classmate] Congratulations. I am sure that you are happy.

PATIENT: But I see that you aren't that successful. I noticed you didn't bring anyone. My wife is a beauty contest winner.

THERAPIST: It seems you like to brag about things that you acquire. Why is that?

PATIENT: I'm just being realistic.

THERAPIST: Well, I've learned that other people's acquisitions don't detract from my quality of life. I have friends, I've had relationships, I'm experiencing my life, day to day, without needing to acquire a billion dollars to make myself feel worthwhile.

PATIENT: But if you don't have a girlfriend, you can't be happy.

THERAPIST: I find that you have a pretty shallow system of values. I have many happy and meaningful experiences with and without women. Don't you?

PATIENT: Yeah, but you should have a girlfriend.

THERAPIST: Why should I? I think the best way for me to do things is to be with people I find rewarding. You're not someone I find rewarding to be with. (*Stepping outside of the role play*) How does this sound to you?

PATIENT: I guess if I met someone like that at the reunion, I'd think he was a jerk.

THERAPIST: You'd be right. Perhaps you can remind yourself of what that sounds like when you criticize yourself.

PATIENT: Yeah, I'd think a guy like him was a jerk.

THERAPIST: One way of changing the way you think is to recall times when you felt a lot better. I'd like you to close your eyes. Relax. Let your arms hang to the side. Breathe slowly. Let's go back in your memory to a time when you felt really good about yourself. Try to get that feeling in you of "I feel really at peace with myself." [MOOD INDUCTION]

PATIENT: It's hard for me to do.

THERAPIST: I know. Just let your mind relax. Repeat in your mind, "I'm really at peace. I feel calm."

PATIENT: I have the image of my mother's face. I can see her hair. Her eyes. She's telling me she's proud of me.

THERAPIST: Let's hold that image for a while. Try to feel what she is feeling toward you.

PATIENT: She's feeling love. She cares about me. She accepts me. [COMPASSIONATE MIND]

THERAPIST: Let's hold that image of Mom's face, her eyes, her hair. What is she saying?

PATIENT: She says that everything will be OK, that there are a lot of women who would cherish me, who would love me.

THERAPIST: How do you feel in this image?

PATIENT: I feel calm, relaxed.

THERAPIST: How do you feel about yourself?

PATIENT: I accept myself more.

THERAPIST: Open your eyes now. What I'd like you to do is to write down the kinds of things that your compassionate, loving mother would say to you about the difficulties that you are having. We are going to open the compassionate and loving mind in you. Over the next week, every day I'd like you to write down some of the things your mother, or anyone who is compassionate and loving toward you, might say to you about any difficulties that you are having. [ASSIGNING DAILY RECORD OF COMPASSIONATE THOUGHTS]

PATIENT: OK.

NEXT SESSION

THERAPIST: We discussed how you have been listening to the critical part of your mind—the part that tells you that you are not good enough, the part that tells you that you are a loser and will be alone forever. We discussed how this part is different from the compassionate, caring, accepting, and loving part of your mind, the part that is represented by the image of your mother. How did you feel last week?

PATIENT: I felt a release. I felt the tension lifting from me, like I wasn't so bad, and there was some hope for me.

THERAPIST: Let's review some of the homework that you did. I suggested that you try to think about the kinds of loving and compassionate things your mother would say to you during these difficult times. Did you write something down?

PATIENT: (*Looking at homework paper*) Yes, I wrote down "You have always been kind, you have a lot of energy, a lot to offer, and Rita might not be the right person for you. It was OK to feel the things that you felt, and it is OK to feel the pain. It only shows how open and sensitive you are."

THERAPIST: How did you feel, writing down these compassionate statements your mother might say?

PATIENT: I felt better. I just wish that I could keep these good thoughts in mind.

THERAPIST: A lot of times we get caught up in what is happening right now. For example, because you and Rita just broke up, we are focusing on your feelings in response to that breakup right now. But let's imagine that we put you in a time machine and took you into the future about 1 year from now. What would we be talking about? [USING THE TIME MACHINE]

PATIENT: Probably how I am doing on my job or about the new women I am dating.

THERAPIST: Why would Rita seem less important?

PATIENT: Well, I'd realize that there are other things in life.

THERAPIST: Other things that turn out to be more important for you. I know that a breakup can feel bad at times, but it's sometimes helpful to think about it in perspective. Can you think of some things that could be worse than breaking up with Rita?

PATIENT: (*laughing*) Other than still being with her?

THERAPIST: Yeah. What are some possible things that happen to people that are worse than a breakup with Rita? [PUTTING THINGS IN PERSPECTIVE]

PATIENT: Having a terrible illness, losing a family member, losing my job, being depressed forever.

THERAPIST: OK., we could go on, I'm sure. But why would these other things be worse?

PATIENT: They would have long-term or permanent implications.

THERAPIST: How is that different from your breakup with Rita?

PATIENT: Well, that relationship was bound to be limited in its duration. We would have broken up sooner or later.

THERAPIST: Another way of looking at it—putting it in perspective—is to think of all the things that you can do, even though your relationship is over with Rita. What can you still do?

PATIENT: I can still see my friends, work, exercise, learn, meet new women . . . everything, except see Rita.

THERAPIST: It sounds like, if we put this in perspective, losing Rita might not feel as bad as it did, say, a week ago. And that perspective also might help you reduce your self-criticism. You seem to criticize yourself because you think that something terrible has happened that shows that you are a loser. Is it really going to be as terrible as it seems or feels? [DECATASTROPHIZING]

PATIENT: Probably not. It helps to know that I have a lot of options.

THERAPIST: One way of looking at this—to put it in perspective—is to ask how others might see your life right now. [BORROWING SOMEONE ELSE'S PERSPECTIVE]

PATIENT: They might think that things are not so bad. I have a good job, lots of friends, I'm relatively attractive—and when I'm not depressed, I have a sense of humor.

THERAPIST: Could something positive emerge from this breakup? [FINDING THE POSITIVE IN THE NEGATIVE]

PATIENT: Well, maybe the positive aspect is one of cutting my losses—a relationship that wasn't working is over.

THERAPIST: Are you also learning something in this experience? [POSITIVE REFRAME]

PATIENT: I might be learning that I don't need a relationship to be happy or to think that I am worthwhile.

THERAPIST: So, even though you might be feeling miserable for a while, there is some growth taking place. Could this growth, this new learning, help you in making better choices about women in the future?

PATIENT: Yeah. I need to think about what will work better for me.

THERAPIST: Another way of putting your experience in perspective might be to think about the problems that you need to solve in your life. Rather than criticize yourself, you could think about the kinds of things that are causing you problems and how you could solve them. [PROBLEM SOLVING]

PATIENT: Let's see. I feel lonely and sad and I can't seem to get myself motivated—those are my problems.

THERAPIST: OK. Let's take the first problem, feeling lonely. There are a couple of things that we could approach this one. Let's start with planning time with friends. [ACTIVITY SCHEDULING]

PATIENT: Since the breakup with Rita, I've been spending a lot of time by myself.

THERAPIST: Why is that?

PATIENT: I guess I feel like I'm a burden to my friends. I keep talking about the breakup.

THERAPIST: How does it feel when you focus on the breakup with your friends?

PATIENT: I feel better knowing that my friends are supportive, but I feel down after a while. It's like reliving the whole separation over and over.

THERAPIST: It's important to feel supported. But there's another way that your friends can be supportive to you: by talking with you about the positive things you are doing. [ACTING AS IF; ACTING AGAINST THE FEELING]

PATIENT: So, rather than obsessing about Rita, I could talk about other things that I'm doing? But don't I have to get all of these bad feelings out? Won't they just well up inside me?

THERAPIST: No. The more you dwell on these things, the more important they seem. Check it out. How do you feel after you've been talking about how bad you feel? [EXAMINING EVIDENCE]

PATIENT: Worse.

THERAPIST: Now this doesn't mean that you should *never* talk about your feelings. But what if you decided to limit your focus on this topic to 5 or 10 minutes? Then talk about what your friend is doing or what you are doing—things that are positive. How does that sound?

PATIENT: Yeah. OK. Let's see. My friend Norm is doing well in his job, and I could talk about that. I could talk about the scuba diving that I want to do. I could talk about the project at work that my boss gave me.

THERAPIST: How do you feel at this moment?

PATIENT: Better.

THERAPIST: Just shifting away from Rita for a while makes you feel better. [LOOKING FOR VARIATIONS IN A SPECIFIC BELIEF]

PATIENT: Right. I'm too focused on her.

THERAPIST: OK. So refocusing on the positives rather than dwelling on the negatives with your friends can be helpful. Let's see, we're trying to deal with loneliness. Let's make a list of a number of people whom you have talked to or done things with in the past year or so, and see if we can find some "use" for them.

PATIENT: There's Norm, Bill, Paul, Nancy, Tom, Fran, Carol, Betsy, Sam . . .

THERAPIST: OK. You can expand that list when you get home. What I'd like you to do is schedule some time with some of these people over the next week. This contact could include just touching base on the phone, having lunch or dinner, having coffee, making a plan for the future. One rule, though. [ACTIVITY SCHEDULING]

PATIENT: What's that?

THERAPIST: Limit the time talking about Rita to 5 minutes.

PATIENT: It's a deal. But I haven't talked to some of these people for a while. They'll think it's odd for me to call.

THERAPIST: What if you called and said, "Hey, I know we haven't talked for a while, but I just wanted to catch up on how things are with you." How do you think they would respond? [TESTING PREDICTIONS]

PATIENT: Probably glad to hear from me.

THERAPIST: Is it worth a try?

PATIENT: I'll do it.

THERAPIST: OK. So we have one solution to the loneliness—calling friends. We know that when you're feeling lonely, you are also feeling down and probably criticizing yourself, right?

PATIENT: Yeah.

THERAPIST: What kinds of things are you saying to yourself that make you feel so down? [EXPLAINING HOW THOUGHTS CREATE FEELINGS]

PATIENT: I'm thinking that I'm a loser because I'm alone. If I had anything going for me, I'd have a girlfriend.

THERAPIST: Sounds circular: I'm alone, therefore I'm a loser. I'm a loser, therefore, I'm alone. [REDUCTIO AD ABSURDUM]

PATIENT: That's how my mind works. Pretty sick, huh?

THERAPIST: No, it's how a lot of people think when they feel down. Let's look at your thoughts when you are alone. You criticize yourself when you are alone—imagine how it would be if you had several friends there with you, telling you what a loser you are. You'd feel down, right? Are there times you are alone when you feel OK? [EXPLAINING HOW THOUGHTS CREATE FEELINGS]

PATIENT: Yeah, if I'm distracted, watching a game on television, or working, or reading a book.

THERAPIST: So, being alone *per se*, isn't always so depressing. It's these negative thoughts. You mentioned a number of friends—Norm, Bill, Fran, and Betsy. Have they ever been without a partner? [DOUBLE STANDARD; EXAMINING EVIDENCE]

PATIENT: Yeah, all of them. In fact, right now Norm and Fran and Betsy are not involved with anyone special.

THERAPIST: Are they losers?

PATIENT: No! They're terrific people.

THERAPIST: So why are they alone?

PATIENT: Because they choose to be. They aren't with anyone special because that's not where it is for them right now. [APPLYING ALTERNATIVE INTERPRETATION]

THERAPIST: Could we say the same thing for you?

PATIENT: Possibly.

THERAPIST: Could we look at your being alone as a positive choice along the lines of "I'd rather be alone than be with someone who is not right for me"?

PATIENT: That's how I see them. Maybe it's true . . . maybe I'm better off being alone than being with Rita.

THERAPIST: Is being alone temporary or permanent? [USING THE TIME MACHINE]

PATIENT: Oh, I'm sure that I'll have a girlfriend eventually.

THERAPIST: But I'll bet that you can talk to someone today and see someone tomorrow? You have these friends, right?

PATIENT: Right. I could call Norm or Bill.

THERAPIST: So, being alone is something that you experience for a few hours. You can always call friends.

PATIENT: That's true.

THERAPIST: Let's see. When you criticize yourself for being alone, you're thinking that being alone is the same thing as being a loser. Then we looked at the fact that your friends are alone and they aren't losers. We also can look at being alone as temporary, and we can see it as a positive or healthy choice. How does this sound?

PATIENT: It's better than criticizing myself. You're right. I'm tougher on myself than I am on others.

THERAPIST: We need to change that self-directed harshness. Ask yourself, "If I had a friend who was feeling down because of a breakup, what advice would I give him or her?" [GIVING ADVICE TO A FRIEND]

PATIENT: I'd tell him or her to get on with his or her life. But I don't really feel like seeing people right now.

THERAPIST: Well, we can make a distinction between what you feel like doing and what you are willing to do. Because you're depressed right now, you don't feel like seeing friends, but are you willing to act *against* the way you feel? This is an important idea—to act as if you're not depressed. It's like acting against what you feel like doing. [ACTING AS IF]

PATIENT: You mean, see people even when I don't feel like it?

THERAPIST: Right. Have you ever done things you didn't feel like doing?

PATIENT: Yeah. Like going to work. Or exercising.

THERAPIST: What happens?

PATIENT: I sometimes end up feeling like doing it once I get into it.

THERAPIST: OK. Would you be willing to experiment? How much pleasure do you think you would get if you stayed home or didn't call a friend? [PLEASURE PREDICTING]

PATIENT: Probably zero.

THERAPIST: How much pleasure (from 0 to 10 where 10 is the most pleasure possible) would you get if you called a friend or saw a friend?

PATIENT: Maybe 3 out of 10.

THERAPIST: OK. Let's experiment. Keep track of your pleasure when you are sitting home alone ruminating, and compare it with the pleasure you feel when you call or see a friend. Let's see what happens when you act *as if* you were not depressed. [ACTIVITY SCHEDULING; ACTING AS IF]

PATIENT: Won't that be phony—trying to act as if I don't feel something?

THERAPIST: In a sense it is phony, but it's a positive form of phony. We often act against the way we feel, so that we can get things done and feel better. For example, you might feel like having a large piece of chocolate cake, but you decide it's not good for your diet. Or you might not feel like exercising, but you go anyway. How do you feel after you decide not to do what you feel like doing, instead doing what you think might be good for you? [COST–BENEFIT ANALYSIS]

PATIENT: Better. Like I got something done.

THERAPIST: It's a great power to be able to do what you don't feel like doing. This is the kind of self-discipline that gives you a sense that you are more in control of your life. We can use the pleasure predicting and activity scheduling to see how things work out. For example, how much pleasure do you predict you'll get if you call Norm? [PLEASURE PREDICTING]

PATIENT: Probably 6 out of 10.

THERAPIST: OK. How about the amount of pleasure you'll get if you go to the gym and work out?

PATIENT: Probably 0 to start, but probably about 5 after I get into it.

THERAPIST: Does it seem that sometimes things start with a low amount of pleasure but end up giving you more pleasure?

PATIENT: Yeah. Exercise is one of those things.

THERAPIST: OK. Now let's see what we can do with these self-critical thoughts. Over the last couple of weeks you've had thoughts like "I'm a loser . . . I have nothing to offer . . . I'm not successful." Let's see if we can develop some rational responses you could carry around with you and use to challenge these thoughts. (*taking out an index card*) We use these little cards. We call them "flash cards" because you can carry them around and challenge your negative thinking in a flash. Let's write "I'm a loser" on one side of this card. Now let's write out five challenges to this negative thought. Where would you begin? [ARGUING BACK AT THE THOUGHT; EXAMINING EVIDENCE]

PATIENT: Well, I'm intelligent, attractive, I have good values.

THERAPIST: OK. Let's write those on the flip side of the card. Anything else?

PATIENT: I have friends who think I'm a good guy. I have a decent job.

THERAPIST: OK. So these are the rational responses. Whenever you begin thinking that you are a loser, just take this card out and look at the rational responses. You can even add some new rational responses.

PATIENT: OK. But how about this thought—because it's true? There are people who are more successful than I am. What do you make of that thought?

THERAPIST: What is the implication of your veritable statement? [VERTICAL DESCENT; EXAMINING UNDERLYING ASSUMPTION]

PATIENT: I don't know. Maybe that I'm not that successful.

THERAPIST: How successful do you need to be?

PATIENT: Good question. I'd like to make more money.

THERAPIST: Probably most people would prefer to make more money. But does that mean that you are not successful at some things? Are you assuming that because other people are more successful, then you are *not* successful?

PATIENT: Yeah. Well it's a matter of degree. I do have some success in some areas of my life. Friends, health, I have a reasonably good job.

THERAPIST: How does your current status compare to 5 years ago? [CONSIDERING PROGRESS VS. PERFECTION]

PATIENT: I was still in college. I didn't know what I wanted to do. My friendships were not as meaningful.

THERAPIST: What if we were to look at the fact that you have been making progress?

PATIENT: I guess I have. I'm supporting myself. My friendships are better. I think I understand things more.

THERAPIST: We can contrast making progress versus trying to aim for perfection. [CONSIDERING PROGRESS VS. PERFECTION]. The thing about perfection is that you will never achieve it. But you can always make progress.

PATIENT: I feel that the breakup was a setback.

THERAPIST: Did you learn anything? [POSITIVE REFRAME]

PATIENT: Yeah. I learned that a relationship with the wrong person comes to an end, and I learned how to identify and challenge my negative thoughts.

THERAPIST: Is that progress?

PATIENT: I guess it is. But it was painful.

THERAPIST: Sometimes progress is painful. Let's go back to your concern that other people are doing better. What if we were to change the question around? What if we were to ask how *you* are doing better, or how *you* can learn, or how *you* can make progress? [CONSIDERING PROGRESS VS. PERFECTION; POSITIVE REFRAME]

PATIENT: That's a lot better for me.

THERAPIST: How is it better?

PATIENT: Because I can always think of ways of making progress for myself.

THERAPIST: Even when we have losses in our lives, we can learn something from them that we can use. This new learning can give a lot of meaning to our experiences.

PATIENT: I hope I can keep that in mind.

SUMMARY

These few sessions illustrate the diversity and flexibility of the cognitive therapist. The individual who focuses on self-criticism can be led, through the Socratic dialogue, to a new understanding of his or her experiences. The therapist can help self-critical patients identify the negative thoughts, the cognitive distortions, the motivation to modify their thinking, and the evidence and logic underlying the negative beliefs. Through guided discovery, the therapist assists patients in recognizing that their negative beliefs and sad feelings are partly dependent on their own behavior and thinking—that is, on their social isolation, passivity, and rumination. The therapist invites patients to consider alternatives to these negative patterns, while examining patients' rationale for isolation (e.g., "I'm a burden"). Specific interpersonal behaviors are suggested—for example, "Limit complaining about the loss," "Focus on what the other person is doing," or "Describe some positive things you are doing." The therapist engages patients in pleasure predicting and activity scheduling to modify the rumination and passivity that contribute to the self-critical mood.

Throughout the interaction, the therapist reminds patients of the double standard they are applying, by engaging them in role plays with fictional others. This exercise helps patients distance themselves from their negative beliefs and provides rational responses that can access on their own. Furthermore, patients are asked to imagine a compassionate voice (in our case illustration, exemplified by John's mother's kindness), to further bolster a soothing, accepting, forgiving, and nurturing counterpart to the negative and self-critical voice. Flash cards are utilized to further reinforce the rational responses. Patients' continual comparisons with others are countered with comparisons of the self to the self; progress and learning emphasized, rather than hierarchical evaluation. Finally, the loss itself—along with the pain experienced—are reframed in a positive light in terms of what has been learned and what can help in the future.

CHAPTER 12

—

Concluding Comments

Cognitive therapy is a multifaceted approach that is not reducible to techniques, case conceptualization, treatment modules, empirically validated approaches, schema work, or analysis of resistance. It is all of these things. However, I believe that techniques are really the fundamental place to begin. I need to reiterate my support of the use of experiential approaches, schema-focused work, and case conceptualization—but these should not be used in the absence of techniques that have made cognitive therapy so effective.

Often novice practitioners of cognitive therapy believe that they are doing good cognitive therapy when they have "conceptualized" or "explained" patients' problems. These therapists may believe that therapy involves constructing a life history and theory about patients that satisfies them (the therapists). In contrast, good case conceptualization entails utilizing both the overall case history and conceptualization of the various levels of cognitive and emotional processing, but also numerous active interventions for modifying the negative automatic thoughts, assumptions, conditional rules, and core schemas (see Needleman, 1999; Persons, 1993). The stress here is on *interventions*. Cognitive therapy may be known for its Socratic dialogue, but its purpose is to actively intervene and move the agenda of self-efficacy forward. It is not simply *understanding*—it is *change*.

The techniques we have examined were organized around specific levels of analysis. For example, eliciting and categorizing thoughts (the focus of Chapter 1) is a fundamental starting place. The therapist is well-served by developing a taxonomy of negative thoughts and assumptions that can inform the case conceptualization and direct the testing and challenging of these thoughts. As noted throughout this text, negative thoughts are not necessarily distortions; some are true. The essential component here is to identify biased slants on viewing experience (e.g., negative filters) and exaggerated and judgmental interpretations of experience. Demanding and unrealistic assumptions and rules are the fuel for the automatic thoughts. Individuals who believe that they should be perfect or they are failures may do fine until they experience a setback in their accomplishments. This setback will trigger a flood of negative thoughts (e.g., "I always fail" or "I'll amount to nothing") and activate the underlying schema (e.g., "I'm a loser").

Indeed, the fundamental vulnerability conferred by negative cognitive schemas should be a focus even when patients are feeling better. These negative schemas and assumptions lie dormant, until they are activated by events that are schema-relevant. Thus, even when patients are not anxious or depressed, it may be helpful to examine the earlier periods of depression or anxiety: What were the triggers? What automatic thoughts and assumptions were activated? What dysfunctional coping styles were utilized? It is better to be ready—to inoculate patients against recurrences of their core problems—than to congratulate oneself on having "cured" the patient.

Perhaps because I have seen many patients with recurrent problems (e.g., histories of several episodes of major depression) and patients with comorbid conditions (e.g., generalized anxiety disorder, social phobia, and major depression), I have begun to view a considerable percentage of our patients as having a chronic diathesis. This diathesis may best be understood, I believe, in terms of cognitive, such as negative attributional style (Alloy, Reilly-Harrington, Fresco, Whitehouse, & Zechmeister, 1999) or dysfunctional assumptions, rules, and schemas (Ingram et al., 1997). The identification of useful techniques that counter the foundational components of this diathesis can be particularly helpful for patients. As patients near the end of their more regular phase of treatment, it is helpful for the therapist to work on this cognitive diathesis (e.g., schemas or assumptions) and to review, with the patient, the techniques that were most helpful. For example, the patient whose depression has taken the form of self-criticism might be instructed to monitor self-critical thoughts, examine the costs and benefits of these thoughts, weigh the evidence for and against the thoughts, challenge the assumptions of perfectionism, apply a compassionate mind approach for self-loathing, and utilize the double-standard question. These techniques can be summarized on flash cards, to be read daily and to be used whenever a negative thought about the self arises.

Indeed, I believe that patients' application of these techniques facilitate a generalization of the therapy between sessions and after therapy is completed. Keeping a tab of which techniques worked—and which did not—can streamline treatment for follow-up sessions or for relapses that can be more quickly reversed if we know, for each patient, which techniques worked best.

The multitude of techniques described in this volume argues against the criticism of cognitive therapy as a shallow or "quick to learn" therapy. These techniques require practice and self-correction. I have often found that therapists who become the most effective are inclined to use these techniques on their most difficult patients—themselves. I recall, when I first began a private practice, how I was flooded with negative thoughts about whether I would ever have a successful practice. I was filled with negative fortune telling, discounting the positive, negative filters, and emotional reasoning. I was driven by perfectionistic and demanding standards that fed into my overly positive self-schema. When I began using these techniques on my own troubled mind, I realized how powerful they really are. I also realized the necessity of repeating the exercises—very much like trying to train someone who had not exercised in years.

I would suggest to the reader, having read this book, to apply each and every technique to yourself. Become a consumer of cognitive therapy. This will help you understand much better how the techniques "feel"; sometimes you will feel some relief and sometimes you will feel that something is missing. As you begin to realize that one technique is not working enough for you, try the other techniques. Often the initial techniques—identifying the thoughts and assumptions—prove to be less of a manner of modifying a thought and feeling and more of an inquiry that leads you to a deeper level of conceptualization. And this deeper level of conceptualization may then be amenable to the use of the techniques.

References

Adler, A. (1964). *Social interest: A challenge to mankind* (J. Linton & R. Vaughan, Trans.). New York: Capricorn Books. (Originally published 1924)

Alden, L. E., & Bieling, P. (1998). Interpersonal consequences of the pursuit of safety. *Behaviour Research and Therapy, 36*(1), 53–64.

Alloy, L. B., Reilly-Harrington, N., Fresco, D. M., Whitehouse, W. G., & Zechmeister, J. S. (1999). Cognitive styles and life events in subsyndromal unipolar and bipolar disorders: Stability and prospective prediction of depressive and hypomanic mood swings. *Journal of Cognitive Psychotherapy, 13,* 21–40.

Ayer, A. J. (1946). *Language, truth, and logic* (2nd ed.). London: Gollancz.

Beck, A. T. (1970). Cognitive therapy: Nature and relation to behavior therapy. *Behavior Therapy, 1*(2), 184–200.

Beck, A. T. (1976). *Cognitive therapy and the emotional disorders.* New York: International Universities Press.

Beck, A. T., Butler, A. C., Brown, G. K., Dahlsgaard, K. K., Newman, C. F., & Beck, J. S. (2001). Dysfunctional beliefs discriminate personality disorders. *Behaviour Research and Therapy, 39,* 1213–1225.

Beck, A. T., Emery, G., & Greenberg, R. L. (1985). *Anxiety disorders and phobias: A cognitive perspective.* New York: Basic Books.

Beck, A. T., Freeman, A., & Associates. (1990). *Cognitive therapy of personality disorders.* New York: Guilford Press.

Beck, A. T., Rush, A. J., Shaw, B. F., & Emery, G. (1979). *Cognitive therapy of depression.* New York: Guilford Press.

Beck, A. T., Wright, F. D., Newman, C. F., & Liese, B. S. (1993). *Cognitive therapy of substance abuse.* New York: Guilford Press.

Beck, J. S. (1995). *Cognitive therapy: Basics and beyond.* New York: Guilford Press.

Bieling, P. J., Beck, A. T., & Brown, G. K. (2000). The Sociotropy–Autonomy Scale: Structure and implications. *Cognitive Therapy and Research, 24*(6), 763–780.

Blatt, S. J. (1974). Levels of object representation in anaclitic and introjective depression. *Psychoanalytic Study of the Child, 29*(10), 7–157.

Blatt, S. J., & Zuroff, D. C. (1992). Interpersonal relatedness and self-definition: Two prototypes for depression. *Clinical Psychology Review, 12*(5), 527–562.

Borkovec, T. D., Alcaine, O. M., & Behar, E. (in press). Avoidance theory of worry and generalized anxiety disorder. In R. G. Heimberg, C. L. Turk, & D. S. Mennin (Eds.), *Generalized anxiety disorder: Advances in research and practice.* New York: Guilford Press.

Borkovec, T. D., & Hu, S. (1990). The effect of worry on cardiovascular response to phobic imagery. *Behaviour Research and Therapy, 28,* 69–73.

Borkovec, T. D., & Inz, J. (1990). The nature of worry in generalized anxiety disorder: A predominance of thought activity. *Behaviour Research and Therapy, 28,* 153–158.

Burns, D. D. (1989). *The feeling good handbook: Using the new mood therapy in everyday life.* New York: William Morrow.

Burns, D. D. (1999). *The feeling good handbook.* New York: Quill.

Cason, D. R., Resick, P. A., & Weaver, T. L. (2002). Schematic integration of traumatic events. *Clinical Psychology Review, 22*(1), 131–153.

Caspar, F., Pessier, J., Stuart, J., Safran, J. D., Samstag, L. W., & Guirguis, M. (2000). One step further in assessing how interpretations influence the process of psychotherapy. *Psychotherapy Research, 10*(3), 309–320.

Clark, D. A., Steer, R. A., Beck, A. T., & Ross, L. (1995). Psychometric characteristics of revised sociotrophy and autonomy scales in college students. *Behaviour Research and Therapy, 33*(3), 325–334.

Copi, I. M., & Cohen, C. (1994). *Introduction to logic* (9th ed.). Upper Saddle River, NJ: Prentice Hall.

Dryden, W., & DiGiuseppe, R. (1990). *A primer on rational–emotive therapy.* Champaign, IL: Research Press.

Dugas, M. J., Buhr, K., & Ladouceur, R. S. (in press). The role of intolerance of uncertainty in the etiology and maintenance of generalized anxiety disorder. In R. G. Heimberg, C. L. Turk, & D. S. Mennin (Eds.), *Generalized anxiety disorder: Advances in research and practice.* New York: Guilford Press.

Dugas, M. J., & Ladouceur, R. (1998). Analysis and treatment of generalized anxiety disorder. In V. E. Caballo (Ed.), *International handbook of cognitive-behavioural treatments of psychological disorders* (pp. 197–225). Oxford, UK: Pergamon Press.

Dweck, C. S., Davidson, W., Nelson, S., & Enna, B. (1978). Sex differences in learned helplessness: II. The contingencies of evaluative feedback in the classroom, and III. An experimental analysis. *Developmental Psychology, 14,* 268–276.

Ellis, A. (1994). *Reason and emotion in psychotherapy* (2nd ed.). Secaucus, NJ: Carol.

Finucane, M., Alhakami, A., Slovic, P., & Johnson, S. (2000). The affect heuristic in judgments of risks and benefits. *Journal of Behavioral Decision Making, 13,* 1–13.

Freeman, A., Pretzer, J., Fleming, B., & Simon, K. (1990). *Clinical applications of cognitive therapy.* New York: Plenum Press.

Freeston, M. H., Rheaume, J., Letarte, H., & Dugas, M. J. (1994). Why do people worry? *Personality and Individual Differences, 17,* 791–802.

Greenberg, L. S. (2001). *Toward an integrated affective, behavioral, cognitive psychotherapy for the new millennium.* Paper presented at the meeting of the Society for the Exploration of Psychotherapy Integration.

Greenberg, L. S. (2002a). Integrating an emotion-focused approach to treatment into psychotherapy integration. *Journal of Psychotherapy Integration, 12*(2), 154–189.

Greenberg, L. S. (2002b). *Emotion-focused therapy: Coaching clients to work through their feelings.* Washington, DC: American Psychological Association.

Greenberg, L. S., & Paivio, S. (1997). *Working with emotions in psychotherapy.* New York: Guilford Press.

Greenberg, L. S., & Safran, J. D. (1987). *Emotion in psychotherapy: Affect, cognition, and the process of change.* New York: Guilford Press.

Greenberg, L. S., Watson, J. C., & Goldman, R. (1998). Process-experiential therapy of depression. In L. S. Greenberg & J. C. Watson (Eds.), *Handbook of experiential psychotherapy* (pp. 227–248). New York: Guilford Press.

Greenberger, D., & Padesky, C. A. (1995). *Mind over mood.* New York: Guilford Press.

Grey, N., Holmes, E., & Brewin, C. R. (2001). Peritraumatic emotional "hot spots" in memory. *Behavioural and Cognitive Psychotherapy, 29,* 367–372.

Guidano, V. F., & Liotti, G. (1983). *Cognitive processes and the emotional disorders.* New York: Guilford Press.

Hackmann, A., Clark, D. M., & McManus, F. (2000). Recurrent images and early memories in social phobia. *Behaviour Research and Therapy, 38,* 601–610.

Halpern, D. (2003). *Thought and knowledge: An introduction to critical thinking.* Mahwah, NJ: Erlbaum.

Hanson, N. R. (1958). *Patterns of discovery: An inquiry into the conceptual foundations of science.* Cambridge, UK: Cambridge University Press.

Harter, S. (1999). *The construction of the self: A developmental perspective.* New York: Guilford Press.

Harvey, A. G. (2001a). "I can't sleep, my mind is racing!" An investigation of strategies of thought control in insomnia. *Behavioural and Cognitive Psychotherapy, 29*(1), 3–11.

Harvey, A. G. (2001b). Insomnia: Symptom or diagnosis? *Clinical Psychology Review, 21*(7), 1037–1059.

Hastie, R. (1980). *Person memory: The cognitive basis of social perception.* Hillsdale, NJ: Erlbaum.

Hersen, M. (2002). *Clinical behavior therapy: Adults and children.* New York: Wiley.

Husserl, E. (1960). *Cartesian meditations: an introduction to phenomenology.* The Hague: Nijhoff.

Ingram, R. E., Miranda, J., & Segal, Z. V. (1998). *Cognitive vulnerability to depression.* New York: Guilford Press.

Kabat-Zinn, J., & University of Massachusetts Medical Center/Worcester Stress Reduction Clinic. (1991). *Full catastrophe living: Using the wisdom of your body and mind to face stress, pain, and illness.* New York: Dell.

Kahneman, D. (1995). Varieties of counterfactual thinking. In N. J. Roese & J. J. Olson (Eds.), *What might have been: The social psychology of counterfactual thinking* (pp. 375–396). Mahwah, NJ: Erlbaum.

Kahneman, D., & Tversky, A. (1979). Prospect theory: An analysis of decision under risk. *Econometrica, 47,* 263–291.

Kassinove, H., & Tafrate, R. C. (2002). *Anger management: The complete treatment guidebook for practitioners.* Atascadero, CA: Impact.

Kelly, G. A. (1955). *The psychology of personal constructs* (1st ed.). New York: Norton.

Kessler, R. C., Walters, E. E., & Wittchen, H.-U. (in press). Epidemiology of generalized anxiety disorder. In R. G. Heimberg, C. L. Turk, & D. S. Mennin (Eds.), *Generalized anxiety disorder: Advances in research and practice.* New York: Guilford Press.

Kuhn, T. S. (1970). *The structure of scientific revolutions* (2nd ed.). Chicago: University of Chicago Press.

Leahy, R. L. (1996). *Cognitive therapy: Basic principles and applications.* Northvale, NJ: Aronson.

Leahy, R. L. (1997). *Practicing cognitive therapy: A guide to interventions.* Northvale, NJ: Aronson.

Leahy, R. L. (1999). Decision making and mania. *Journal of Cognitive Psychotherapy: An International Quarterly, 13,* 83–105.

Leahy, R. L. (2001a). Depressive decision making: Validation of the portfolio theory model. *Journal of Cognitive Psychotherapy: An International Quarterly, 15,* 341–362.

Leahy, R. L. (2001b). *Overcoming resistance in cognitive therapy.* New York: Guilford Press.

Leahy, R. L. (2002). A model of emotional schemas. *Cognitive and Behavioral Practice, 9*(3), 177–191.

Leahy, R. L. (in press). Cognitive therapy of generalized anxiety disorder. In R. G. Heimberg, C. L. Turk, & D. S. Mennin (Eds.), *Generalized anxiety disorder: Advances in research and practice.* New York: Guilford Press.

Leahy, R. L., & Beck, A. T. (1988). Cognitive therapy of depression and mania. In R. Cancro & A. Georgotas (Eds.), *Depression and mania* (pp. 517–537). New York: Elsevier.

Leahy, R. L., & Holland, S. J. (2000). *Treatment plans and interventions for depression and anxiety disorders.* New York: Guilford Press.

Mahoney, M. J. (1991). *Human change processes: The scientific foundations of psychotherapy.* New York: Basic Books.

McKay, M., & Fanning, P. (2000). *Self-esteem: A proven program of cognitive techniques for assessing, improving, and maintaining your self-esteem.* Oakland, CA: New Harbinger.

Mennin, D. S., Turk, C. L., Heimberg, R. G., & Carmin, C. N. (in press). Focusing on the regulation of emotion: A new direction for conceptualizing and treating generalized anxiety disorder. In M. A. Reinecke & D. A. Clark (Eds.), *Cognitive therapy over the lifespan: Theory, research and practice.* Cambridge, UK: Cambridge University Press.

Miranda, J., & Persons, J. B. (1988). Dysfunctional attitudes are mood-state dependent. *Journal of Abnormal Psychology, 97*(1), 76–79.

Miranda, J., Persons, J. B., & Byers, C. N. (1990). Endorsement of dysfunctional beliefs depends on current mood state. *Journal of Abnormal Psychology, 99*(3), 237–241.

Needleman, L. D. (1999). *Cognitive case conceptualization: A guidebook for practitioners.* Mahwah, NJ: Erlbaum.

Nolen-Hoeksema, S. (2000). The role of rumination in depressive disorders and mixed anxiety/depressive symptoms. *Journal of Abnormal Psychology, 109,* 504–511.

Papageorgiou, C., & Wells, A. (2000). Treatment of recurrent major depression with attention training. *Cognitive and Behavioral Practice, 7*(4), 407–413.

Pennebaker, J. W. (1993). Putting stress into words: Health, linguistic, and therapeutic implications. *Behaviour Research and Therapy, 31,* 539–548.

Pennebaker, J. W., & Beall, S. K. (1986). Confronting a traumatic event: Toward an understanding of inhibition and disease. *Journal of Abnormal Psychology, 95,* 274–281.

Persons, J. B. (1993). Case conceptualization in cognitive-behavior therapy. In K. T. Kuehlwein & H. Rosen (Eds.), *Cognitive therapies in action: Evolving innovative practice* (pp. 33–53). San Francisco, CA: Jossey-Bass.

Persons, J. B., & Miranda, J. (1992). Cognitive theories of vulnerability to depression: Reconciling negative evidence. *Cognitive Therapy and Research, 16*(4), 485–502.

Popper, K. R. (1959). *The logic of scientific discovery.* New York: Basic Books.

Purdon, C. (1999). Thought suppression and psychopathology. *Behaviour Research and Therapy, 37,* 1029–1054.

Purdon, C., & Clark, D. A. (1993). Obsessive intrusive thoughts in nonclinical subjects: I. Content and relation with depressive, anxious and obsessional symptoms. *Behaviour Research and Therapy, 31*(8), 713–720.

Rachman, S. (1993). Obsessions, responsibility and guilt. *Behaviour Research and Therapy, 31,* 149–154.

Reinecke, M. A., Dattilio, F. M., & Freeman, A. (Eds.). (1996). *Cognitive therapy with children and adolescents: A casebook for clinical practice.* New York: Guilford Press.

Resick, P. A. (2001). *Stress and trauma.* Philadelphia, PA: Psychology Press.

Segal, Z. V., & Ingram, R. E. (1994). Mood priming and construct activation in tests of cognitive vulnerability to unipolar depression. *Clinical Psychology Review, 14*(7), 663–695.

Segal, Z. V., Williams, M. J. G., & Teasdale, J. D. (2002). *Mindfulness-based cognitive therapy for depression: A new approach to preventing relapse.* New York: Guilford Press.

Selman, R. L. (1980). *The growth of interpersonal understanding.* New York: Academic Press.

Simon, H. A. (1983). *Reason in human affairs.* Stanford, CA: Stanford University Press.

Smucker, M. R., & Dancu, C. V. (1999). *Cognitive-behavioral treatment for adult survivors of childhood trauma: Imagery rescripting and reprocessing.* Northvale, NJ: Aronson.

Snyder, M., & White, P. (1982). Moods and memories: Elation, depression, and the remembering of the events of one's life. *Journal of Personality, 50*(2), 149–167.

Tompkins, M. A. (1996). Cognitive-behavioral case formulation: The case of Jim. *Journal of Psychotherapy Integration, 6*(2), 97–105.

Tversky, A., & Kahneman, D. (1974). Judgment under uncertainty: Heuristics and biases. *Science, 185*(4157), 1124–1131.

Velten, E., Jr. (1968). A laboratory task for induction of mood states. *Behaviour Research and Therapy, 6*(4), 473–482.

Wells, A. (1997a). *Cognitive therapy of anxiety disorders: A practice manual and conceptual guide.* Chichester, UK: Wiley.

Wells, A. (1997b). Belief about worry and intrusions . . . *Journal of Anxiety Disorders, 11*(3), 279–296.

Wells, A. (1999). A metacognitive model and therapy for generalized anxiety disorder. *Clinical Psychology and Psychotherapy, 6,* 86–95.

Wells, A. (2000). *Emotional disorders and metacognition: Innovative cognitive therapy.* New York: Wiley.

Wells, A. (in press). Metacognitive beliefs in the maintenance of worry and generalized anxiety disorder. In R. G. Heimberg, C. L. Turk, & D. S. Mennin (Eds.), *Generalized anxiety disorder: Advances in research and practice.* New York: Guilford Press.

Wells, A., & Papageorgiou, C. (1995). Worry and the incubation of intrusive images following stress. *Behaviour Research and Therapy, 33*(5), 579–583.

York, D., Borkovec, T., Vasey, M., & Stern, R. (1987). Effects of worry and somatic anxiety induction on thoughts, emotion and physiological activity. *Behaviour Research and Therapy, 25*(6), 523–526.

Young, J. E. (1990). *Cognitive therapy for personality disorders: A schema-focused approach.* Sarasota, FL: Professional Resource Exchange.

Young, J. E., & Flanagan, C. (1998). Schema-focused therapy for narcissistic patients. In E. F. Ronningstam (Ed.), *Disorders of narcissism: Diagnostic, clinical, and empirical implications* (pp. 239–262). Washington, DC: American Psychiatric Press.

Index

Bold text indicates a technique, *italic* indicates a form/handout, *f* indicates a figure, and *t* indicates a table.